GESTATIONAL TROPHOBLASTIC DISEASE

GESTATIONAL TROPHOBLASTIC DISEASE

Edited by

B. W. Hancock

Professor of Clinical Oncology, YCRC Department of Clinical Oncology, The University of Sheffield, Weston Park Hospital, Sheffield, UK

E. S. Newlands

Professor of Cancer Medicine, Department of Medical Oncology, Charing Cross Hospital, London, UK

R. S. Berkowitz

William H. Baker Professor of Gynecology, Harvard Medical School; Director of Gynecology and Gynecologic Oncology, Brigham and Women's Hospital and Dana Farber Cancer Institute, Boston, USA

CHAPMAN & HALL MEDICAL

London · Weinheim · New York · Tokyo · Melbourne · Madras

Published by Chapman & Hall, 2–6 Boundary Row, London SE1 8HN, UK

Chapman & Hall, 2–6 Boundary Row, London SE1 8HN, UK

Chapman & Hall GmbH, Pappelallee 3, 69469 Weinheim, Germany

Chapman & Hall USA, 115 Fifth Avenue, New York NY 10003, USA

Chapman & Hall Japan, ITP-Japan, Kyowa Building, 3F, 2-2-1

Hirakawacho, Chiyoda-ku, Tokyo 102, Japan

Chapman & Hall Australia, 102 Dodds Street, South Melbourne, Victoria 3205, Australia

Chapman & Hall India, R. Seshadri, 32 Second Main Road, CIT East, Madras 600 035, India

---

First edition 1997

Typeset in 10/12 Palatino by Keyset Composition, Colchester

Printed in Great Britain at the University Press, Cambridge

ISBN 0 412 631008

A catalogue record for this book is available from the British Library

Library of Congress Catalog Card Number: 96-86255

∞ Printed on acid-free text paper, manufactured in accordance with ANSI/NISO Z39.48-1992 (Permanence of Paper).

CONTENTS

CONTRIBUTORS

KENNETH D. BAGSHAWE
Emeritus Professor of Medical Oncology,
Department of Surgery, 4 North,
Charing Cross Hospital,
Fulham Palace Road,
London W6 8RF,
UK

ROSS S. BERKOWITZ
William H. Baker Professor of Gynecology,
Harvard Medical School,
Director of Gynecology and Gynecologic Oncology, Brigham and Women's Hospital, and Dana Farber Cancer Institute,
75 Francis Street,
Boston,
Massachusetts 02115,
USA

LAURENCE A. COLE
Associate Professor in Reproduction and Cancer Biology, hCG Research Laboratory,
Department of Obstetrics and Gynecology,
Yale University School of Medicine,
New Haven,
Connecticut 06510,
USA

A. C. EVANS JR
Fellow, Department of Obstetrics and Gynecology,
Division of Gynecologic Oncology,
Box 3079,
Duke University Medical Center,
Durham,
North Carolina 27710,
USA

ROSEMARY A. FISHER
Senior Research Fellow and Honorary Lecturer,
Department of Medical Oncology,
Charing Cross Hospital,
Fulham Palace Road,
London W6 8RF,
UK

DONALD P. GOLDSTEIN
Director, New England Trophoblastic Disease Center,
Brigham and Women's Hospital,
333 Longwood Avenue – Suite 520,
Boston,
Massachusetts 02115,
USA

CHARLES B. HAMMOND
E. C. Hamblen Professor and Chairman,
Department of Obstetrics and Gynecology,
Duke University Medical Center,
Durham,
North Carolina 27710,
USA

BARRY W. HANCOCK
Professor and Director, YCRC Department of Clinical Oncology,
The University of Sheffield,
Weston Park Hospital,
Sheffield S10 2SJ,
UK

HOWARD D. HOMESLEY
Head, Section on Gynecologic Oncology,
Comprehensive Cancer Center of Wake Forest University,
Medical Center Boulevard,
Winston-Salem,
North Carolina 27157-1065,
USA

SEUNG JO KIM
Director of Korea Research Institute for Trophoblastic Disease,
Kangham St Mary's Hospital,
Catholic University Medical College,
Seoul,
Korea

JOHN R. LURAIN
John and Ruth Brewer Professor of Gynecologic Oncology,
Prentice Women's Hospital,
333 East Superior Street,
Chicago,
Illinois 60611,
USA

HO-KEI MA
Professor and Head,
Department of Obstetrics and Gynecology,
6/F Professorial Block,
Queen Mary Hospital,
Pokfulam Road,
Hong Kong

DAVID R. MILLAR
Honorary Consultant Gynaecologist,
Jessop Hospital for Women and North of England Trophoblastic Tumour Service,
Leavygreave Road,
Sheffield S3 7RE,
UK

EDWARD S. NEWLANDS
Professor of Cancer Medicine,
Department of Medical Oncology,
Charing Cross Hospital,
London W6 8RF,
UK

HEXTAN Y. S. NGAN
Senior Lecturer,
Department of Obstetrics and Gynecology,
6/F Professorial Block,
Queen Mary Hospital,
Pokfulam Road,
Hong Kong

FERNANDO J. PARADINAS
Senior Lecturer and Honorary Consultant Histopathologist,
Histopathology Department,
Charing Cross and Westminster Hospital Medical School,
Fulham Palace Road,
London W6 8RF,
UK

GORDON J. S. RUSTIN
Director of Medical Oncology,
Mount Vernon Centre for Cancer Treatment,
Mount Vernon Hospital,
Northwood,
Middlesex HA6 2RN,
UK

JOHN T. SOPER
Professor, Department of Obstetrics and Gynecology,
Division of Gynecologic Oncology,
Box 3079,
Duke University Medical Center,
Durham,
North Carolina 27710,
USA

LARI B. WENZEL
Director of Psychosocial Oncology Research,
AMC Cancer Research Center,
1600 Pierce Street, Denver
Colorado 80214,
USA

LING-CHUI WONG
Reader, Department of Obstetrics and Gynecology,
6/F Professorial Block,
Queen Mary Hospital,
Pokfulam Road,
Hong Kong

FOREWORD

Effective treatment of trophoblastic tumors, choriocarcinoma, became possible with the introduction of cycle-specific chemotherapy agents some 35 years ago. This textbook is a remarkable collection of essays from first- and second-generation trophoblast centers, by the originators of this therapeutic revolution and by some of the second and third generation of physicians whom they trained. It is a significant multi-author endeavor to cover this fascinating field that combines genetic aberration and therapeutic pitfalls which require both clinical skill and experience to achieve successful outcome.

The pathologic features and the discussion of the clinical manifestation of trophoblastic disease were steeped in controversy at the end of the nineteenth century. As we near the end of the twentieth century, the knowledge concerning the genetic basis, the pathophysiology, the clinical categorization as well as the means of treating trophoblastic disease are much more firmly established and are all well described in this text. It is, therefore, remarkable that the diagnostic criteria and the methods of staging and assessment used in different centers as well as the way therapy is approached are still so widely divergent, and that in spite of the wealth of information opinion and practice are still so disparate. Hopefully, however, these writings will stimulate rigorous discussion that will permit consensus.

The shining spark of truth cometh forth only after the clash of differing opinions.

Paris Talks, 1909, Abdul Baha

Ernest I. Kohorn MA, MChir (Cantab), FRCS, FRCOG
New Haven, Connecticut
January 1996

INTRODUCTION

Kenneth D. Bagshawe

It is just 100 years since Marchand[1] identified choriocarcinoma as a tumor arising from placental villous trophoblast. Earlier descriptions of similar tumors had failed to identify their tissue of origin. Gestational trophoblastic disease (GTD) is the terminological umbrella now used to span the spectrum of cellular proliferations ranging from the various forms of hydatidiform mole through invasive mole and choriocarcinoma to placental site tumors[2]. Each form of GTD presents its own particular set of problems ranging from social to therapeutic.

These proliferations are unique in several respects. In the first place, there is no known homolog of hydatidiform mole in any other species although this could possibly be masked by maternal placentophagy. The rare identification of choriocarcinoma-like tumors remains restricted to a rhesus monkey[3] and an armadillo[4]. In the human, histologically characterized choriocarcinoma behaves in a broadly similar fashion whether it is genetically identical with the host as in a germ cell origin, or whether it arises from a normal conception or an androgenetic hydatidiform mole.

Gestational trophoblastic tumors have long been regarded as naturally occurring allografts in the maternal host as befits their fetal origin. At the same time the low incidence of fetal involvement by choriocarcinoma following term delivery remains unexplained. Whether they are allografts or not depends on the precise definition of allograft. Mammalian evolution has depended on the failure of the maternal immune system to reject the fetus and on the unique role of trophoblast. Thus, gestational trophoblastic tumors have a normal set or a complete set of paternal genes and it was assumed for some years that they and normal trophoblast expressed paternally derived antigens of the human leukocyte antigen (HLA) system. Evidence mounted during the 1960s and 1970s that this was not so. Recent work by[5] has confirmed this and shown that HLA G expression by trophoblast is a unique mechanism for abrogating immune rejection. It may be a reasonable assumption that trophoblastic tumors inherit this mechanism so that immune mechanisms are unlikely to account for their sensitivity to cytotoxic chemotherapy.

It is now more than 35 years since the sensitivity of invasive mole and choriocarcinoma to cytotoxic drugs was first recognized[6]. They remain the most sensitive and most curable of all human cancers. Apart from speculation about the contribution of the immune response to this sensitivity there has been little expression of

Gestational Trophoblastic Disease.
Edited by B.W. Hancock, E.S. Newlands and R.S. Berkowitz.
ISBN 0 412 63100 8

interest as to why choriocarcinoma should, in most cases, be so responsive.

It is an issue that is not without relevance to the understanding of cytotoxic action in human cancer in general. It is probably facile to attribute the responsiveness simply to a low propensity to drug resistance and indeed drug resistance can develop in choriocarcinoma and placental site tumor, particularly where inappropriate treatment is given. On the other hand, multi-drug resistant invasive mole has not, to my knowledge, been described.

It was suggested[7] that a progressive reduction in a tumor cell population could only be achieved with conventional cytotoxic chemotherapy under certain conditions. Tumor growth results from the fact that cell losses are less than cell gains but the margin between losses and gains, varies substantially between different cancers. The analysis was based on an antimetabolite such as methotrexate and assumed that cytotoxic action was intermittent and the duration of each administration or set of administrations was determined by the sensitivity of one or more normal cell renewal compartments. In general, drug exposure time is shorter in duration than the rest phase between successive drug exposures. Further, it was proposed that the rate of cell kill was related to and limited by the size of the growth fraction of the tumor cell population, i.e. the fraction of cells in cycle. If these assumptions were justified then it was argued that the rate of spontaneous cell loss from natural causes is critical to progressive reduction in the tumor cell population. That is to say the cytotoxic drug-induced cell kill plus the spontaneous loss rate in the tumor cell population can in the course of a complete treatment cycle exceed the rate of tumor cell accumulation in the rest phase.

It will be noted that the vulnerability of normal renewal cell populations derives from the fact that over a period of time spontaneous losses equal cell additions. In contrast to tumors, normal renewal cell tissues are organized for rapid recovery from toxic insults.

The thesis is therefore that choriocarcinoma is curable because the magnitude of spontaneous losses approaches that of cell gains. Losses and gains are not readily quantifiable although this may now be a lesser problem than when the proposal was first made. Supporting evidence for a high rate of cell loss in choriocarcinoma is evident in the relatively small number of viable cells present in comparison with the total tumor mass. The intravascular cells and perivascular location of choriocarcinoma cells suggest they may be unusually vulnerable to anoxia and hence growth occurs only in close proximity to the capillaries at the periphery of tumor masses. A second and perhaps critical mechanism is the differentiation of a proportion of the stem cell population of cytotrophoblast into syncytium which is an 'end' cell. Mitoses are rarely, if ever, to be found in syncytium and these cells appear to be short-lived, so this constitutes a substantial exit route from the clonogenic population.

A personal unpublished observation is that the amount of syncytium seen in autopsy material from drug-resistant choriocarcinoma is less than that seen in pre-chemotherapy material. This could be the subject of formal study. It is also relevant that placental site trophoblastic tumor which is more frequently drug-resistant than gestational choriocarcinoma shows markedly less syncytium formation.

The implication of the suggestion that the natural cell loss rate from a tumor is critical to its response to conventional cytotoxic therapy is that complete responsiveness is inherent in the biology of some tumors but not, unfortunately, in the majority of common cancers. If this were to be proven it would challenge the widely held view that the failure of cytotoxics to be curative of common cancers is the result of natural or acquired drug resistance at the biochemical level. Whilst this undoubtedly occurs, the correlation between drug resistance at the clinical and biochemical levels does not appear to be supported by a substantial body of evidence.

I have dwelt on this subject at some length because some of the motivation in the early years of chemotherapy for trophoblastic tumors was the hope that it would point the way towards the curability of more common tumors. However, curability with conventional cytotoxic therapy may be dependent on the biology of the tumor.

There was also the hope, even the expectation, that tumor markers comparable to human chorionic gonadotropin (hCG) would be found for many other cancers. Whilst there has been a proliferation of tumor-associated antigens none of them, except perhaps α-fetoprotein in some germ cell tumors, provide information comparable to that provided by hCG for trophoblastic tumors.

The screening programs for persistent trophoblastic disease following evacuation of hydatidiform mole have been instrumental in the near elimination of fatalities from the sequelae to mole and have done so at low cost. The fact that there are wide differences in intervention policy resulting in a three- to four-fold difference in the frequency of intervention is less important than the fact that the different policies are successful. If the more frequent intervention in the USA results, as has been suggested, from a fear of litigation over late intervention, perhaps unnecessary intervention will become equally persuasive in time.

The evolution of knowledge about hCG has been sustained now for almost 70 years and it continues to evolve, as does the methodology for its detection. Nothing illustrates this better than a comparison of the rarely available biological pregnancy tests with toads, mice and rabbits in the 1950s to the present time when 'over-the-counter' pregnancy tests are universally available. Nevertheless, the methodology of assays is of critical importance and many, indeed most, of the commercial sandwich assays are inferior for monitoring purposes[8] to long-established radioimmunoassays employing polyclonal antisera.

Apart from its role in monitoring the course of trophoblastic tumors hCG has proved to be a useful target antigen for immunoscintigraphy. Whilst the technique is not yet widely available and has to compete with the array of computed tomography, ultrasound and magnetic resonance imaging, early studies using ^{131}I-labeled anti-hCG antibodies were amongst the first to show potential both for locating small residual tumor masses and for therapeutic targeting[8].

Antibodies directed at tumor-associated antigens remain the only class of molecule to be taken up selectively in a wide range of cancers. Since conventional chemotherapy has not achieved the selectivity required to eliminate the generality of cancers, the case for exploiting antibodies was evident from the early immunoscintigraphic studies. Interesting results have recently been reported with radiolabeled antibodies in lymphoma and with drug–antibody conjugates in xenograft models. But the potential appears greatest for antibody–enzyme conjugates which are able to generate cytotoxic substances at tumor sites[9] from subsequently administered prodrugs, thereby allowing much greater cytotoxic concentrations to be achieved in tumors than in normal tissues.

If such potential is fulfilled then the link between the mid-twentieth-century studies on trophoblastic tumors and the control of other cancers will have been forged.

REFERENCES

1. Marchand, F. (1895) Über die sogenannten 'decidualen' Geschwulste im Anschluss an normale Geburt. Abort, Blasenmole,

und extrauterin Schwangerschaft. *Monatsschr. Geburtshilfe Gynäkol.*, **1**, 419–38.

2. WHO Scientific Group Report (1983) Gestational trophoblastic diseases. *WHO Tech. Rep. Ser. 692*, Geneva.
3. Lindsey, J.R., Wharton, L.R., Woodruff, J.D. and Baker, H.J. (1969) Intrauterine choriocarcinoma in a rhesus monkey. *Pathol. Vet.*, **6**, 378–84.
4. Marin-Padella, M. and Benirshke, K. (1963) Thalidomide induced alterations in the blastocyst and placenta of an armadillo, *Dasypus novemcintas mexicanus*, including a choriocarcinoma. *Am. J. Pathol.*, **43**, 999–1016.
5. Chumbley, G., King, A., Holmes, N. and Loke, Y.W. (1993) *In situ* hybridisation and Northern Blot demonstration of HLA-G mRNA in human trophoblast populations by locus-specific oligonucleotide. *Hum. Immunol.*, **37**, 17–22.
6. Li, M.C., Hertz, R. and Spencer, D.B. (1956) Effect of methotrexate upon choriocarcinoma and chorioadenoma. *Proc. Soc. Exp. Biol. Med.*, **93**, 361–6.
7. Bagshawe, K.D. (1968) Tumor growth and anti-mitotic action: the role of spontaneous cell losses. *Br. J. Cancer*, **22**, 698–713.
8. Begent, R.H.J., Searle, F., Stanway, G. *et al.* (1980) Radioimmunolocalisation of tumours by external scintigraphy after administration of ^{131}I antibody to human chorionic gonadotrophin. *J. R. Soc. Med.*, **73**, 824–30.
9. Bagshawe, K.D. (1989) Towards generating cytotoxic agents at cancer sites. *Br. J. Cancer*, **60**, 275–89.

Genetics 2

Rosemary A. Fisher

2.1 GENETIC ORIGINS

Gestational trophoblastic diseases (GTD) include complete (CHM) and partial hydatidiform mole (PHM), invasive mole and the malignant trophoblastic tumors choriocarcinoma and placental site trophoblastic tumors (PSTT). While many genetic studies have been carried out in relation to CHM and PHM, genetic studies of the trophoblastic tumors have been limited to a large extent by the availability of fresh material. The introduction of molecular techniques, in particular those which can be used in conjunction with fixed material, has facilitated both diagnosis and further studies of the pathogenesis of this unusual group of diseases.

2.1.1 HYDATIDIFORM MOLES

Karyotypes of hydatidiform mole

Early genetic studies of hydatidiform mole (HM) showed that they were not only pathologically abnormal but that they were also genetically unusual. The first observation was that most molar pregnancies were female. Barr bodies – darkly staining bodies found in the interphase nuclei of female cells[1] – were shown to be present in the majority of HM[2]. This was confirmed by cytogenetic studies which showed that most HM had the female karyotype, 46, XX[3–6].

Cytogenetic studies also revealed a small proportion of HM with triploid karyotypes[7, 8]. Correlation of the morphology of HM with studies of their karyotype led Vassilakos and his colleagues[9,10] to suggest that the two pathological entities CHM and PHM were genetically distinct. They found all CHM to have a diploid 46,XX karyotype, while PHM were mainly triploid or trisomic for a single chromosome. In their study PHM were classified as conceptuses with a fetus, cord or amniotic membranes and a placenta comprising both normal and cystic villi. Hyperplasia, present in some cases, was not marked. When hyperplasia was included as a prerequisite for the pathological diagnosis of PHM, Szulman and Surti[11,12] showed that PHM were almost always triploid, an observation subsequently confirmed by other groups[13–15]. Thus, PHM was shown to be a separate entity and not, as had previously been suggested by Hertig and Edmonds[16], a transitional stage between normal placenta and CHM.

Parental origin of CHM

While the distinction between CHM and PHM was being elucidated, other groups

Gestational Trophoblastic Disease.
Edited by B.W. Hancock, E.S. Newlands and R.S. Berkowitz.
ISBN 0 412 63100 8

went on to show that it was in fact the CHM with the apparently normal diploid karyotype which was the genetically more unusual tissue. Cytogenetic polymorphisms – inherited staining patterns on chromosomes – can be used as markers to enable the parental origin of molar tissue to be identified. Using these techniques two groups demonstrated that CHM were in fact androgenetic in origin,[17,18] all 46 chromosomes in the HM being paternally derived. This surprising observation was soon confirmed by other groups[13,19–22].

Several different mechanisms could account for the presence of two paternal chromosome complements in a conceptus (Figure 2.1). During gametogenesis DNA replication is normally followed by the first meiotic division in which the two chromosomes of each pair separate, one going to each pole of the cell as the cytoplasm divides. A second division in which the centromeres of the chromosomes divide results in the sister chromatids of each chromosome moving to opposite poles of the cell. In this way male meiosis results in the formation of four gametes each with a haploid chromosome complement. During the first meiotic division recombination, i.e. exchange of genetic material, between homologous pairs of chromosomes gives rise to genetic variation in potential offspring and as a consequence recombination of polymorphic regions of the chromosome. Investigation of these polymorphic regions has enabled the origin of both CHM and PHM to be determined.

Early studies of cytogenetic polymorphisms in CHM found that homologous chromosome pairs were homozygous for all informative markers examined[17,18]. Since cytogenetic polymorphisms are centromeric these observations are compatible with fertilization by a diploid sperm arising from failure at the second meiotic division (Figure 2.1a) or fertilization of an egg by a single sperm which subsequently duplicates (Figure 2.1b). Examination of polymorphic enzyme markers which are distal to the centromere, in combination with cytogenetic studies[13,21,22], made it possible to distinguish between these two mechanisms. Homozygosity for both centromeric markers and enzyme polymorphisms in 46,XX molar tissue suggested that CHM arose by duplication of a haploid sperm. Since 46,YY CHM have not been reported, duplication of a sperm with a Y chromosome is presumed to be non-viable.

Duplication of a haploid sperm could not account for the small proportion of CHM with a 46,XY karyotype[3,6,23]. In 1981 Ohama *et al.*[24] described four androgenetic 46,XY CHM in which half the informative polymorphisms studied were homozygous but half heterozygous, suggesting that 46,XY CHM arose by dispermy (Figure 2.1c). Several other examples of 46,XY CHM have since been reported[25–27]. Theoretically, fertilization of an egg by two sperm should also give rise to 46,XX dispermic CHM and these have now been described[28,29]. The incidence of dispermic CHM varies in different series, in part due to the number of informative polymorphisms which may need to be examined in order to identify heterozygosity in a 46,XX CHM[30]. Where highly polymorphic markers, such as restriction fragment length polymorphisms of DNA, have been used to examine the origin of CHM (Figure 2.2a,b) the incidence of dispermic CHM has been shown to be in the region of 20–25%[30,33,34].

Despite the androgenetic nature of the nuclear genome, analysis of DNA polymorphisms has shown that the mitochondrial DNA of CHM, as in a normal conceptus, is maternally derived[35–37]. These findings suggest that CHM arise from the fusion of one or two sperm with a mature but enucleate egg. The fate of the maternal chromosomes in CHM is unclear. During the first meiotic division of oogenesis the chromosomes separate, one set remaining in the nucleus

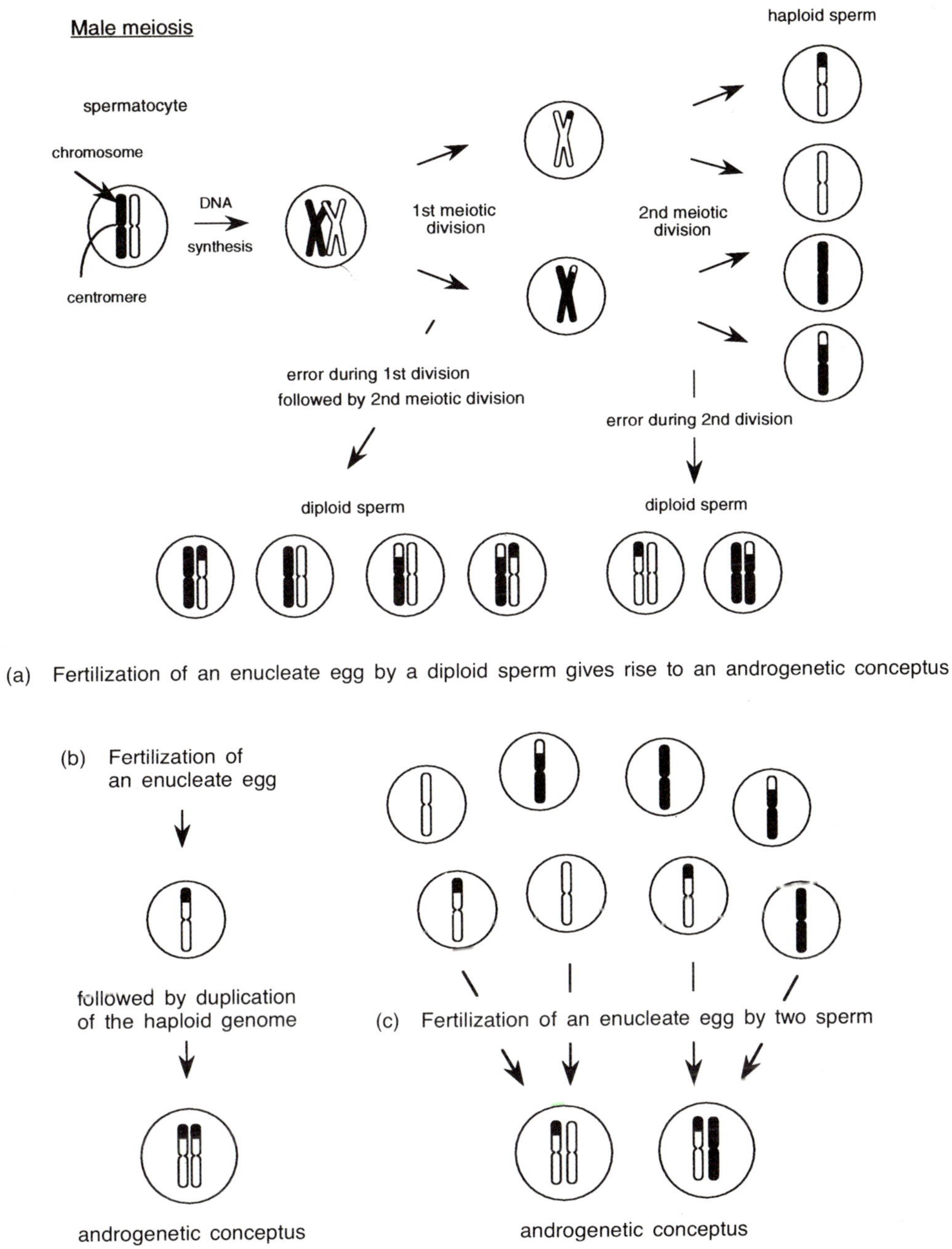

Figure 2.1 Possible mechanisms of origin giving rise to two paternal chromosome complements in CHM. For simplification a single pair of chromosomes and a single recombination event has been illustrated. Fertilization of an anucleate egg by (a) a sperm which has failed to undergo normal meiotic division, (b) a haploid sperm which subsequently duplicates or (c) two sperm, results in a diploid androgenetic conceptus.

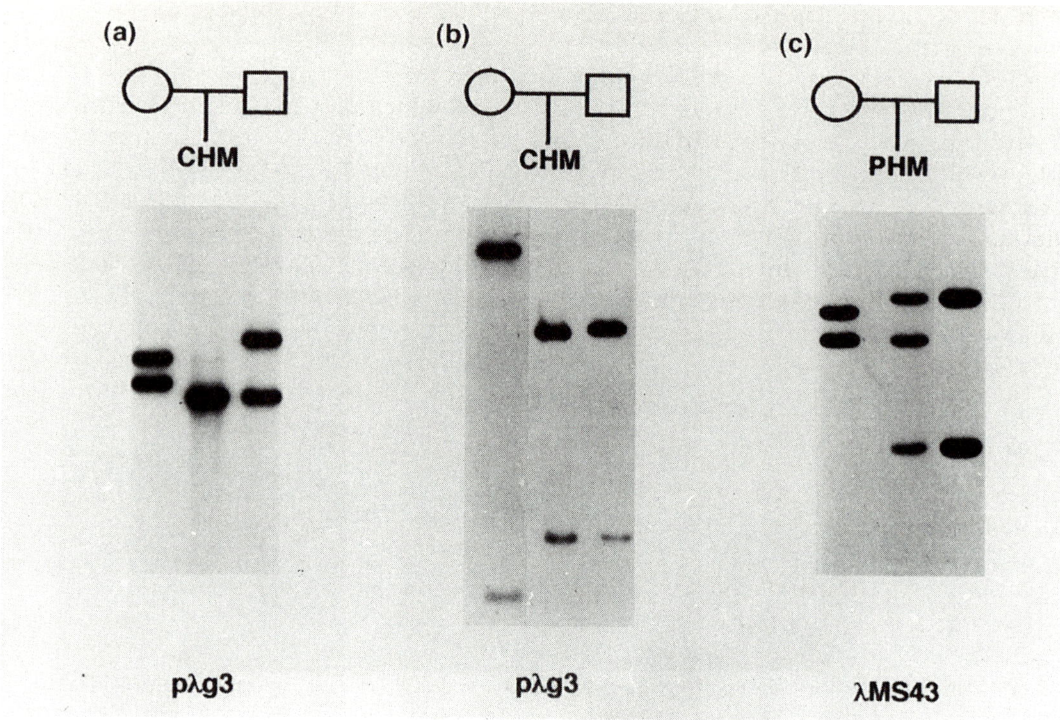

Figure 2.2 Restriction fragment length polymorphisms detected following digestion with the restriction enzyme Hinf1 and hybridization with the locus specific minisatellite probes pλg3[31] or λMS43[32] in (a) an androgenetic CHM, homozygous for the smaller paternal allele, (b) an androgenetic CHM, heterozygous for paternal alleles and therefore dispermic in origin, and (c) a PHM having one maternal and two paternal contributions to the genome.

while the other is extruded as a polar body. Following fertilization the second meiotic division occurs. The sister chromatids separate, one set remaining to form the pronucleus of the mature oocyte while the other is extruded as a second polar body. One explanation for loss of the maternal chromosomes might be extrusion of both maternal sets of chromosomes or chromatids into one of the polar bodies during meiosis. Alternatively, maternal chromosomes may be present but degenerate. Fluorescence microscopy of living human oocytes has shown that some oocytes, which at the light microscope level appear to have no chromosomes, when viewed using electron microscopy do in fact have a number of pyknotic chromosomes located throughout the cytoplasm[38]. Thus maternal chromosomes may be absent or degenerate.

Parental origin of PHM

PHM are distinct from CHM in that they are triploid and have a maternal contribution to the genome[13,14,39] (Figure 2.2c). Several mechanisms may account for a triploid conceptus, the most likely being failure at the first or second meiotic division during gametogenesis to produce either a diploid sperm or egg, or fertilization of an egg by two sperm. These mechanisms have all been shown to occur in triploid material from spontaneous abortions[40–43].

Studies of cytogenetic and enzyme polymorphisms in molar tissue obtained clinically[14], or from a series of spontaneous abortions[39] confirmed that PHM were triploid and in almost all cases diandric, the additional chromosome set being paternally derived (Figure 2.2c). In diandric PHM, examination of genetic polymorphisms has shown an origin by dispermy to be proven or possible in all cases[14,34,39].

Cytogenetically unusual HM

Occasional HM have been described which are neither androgenetic diploids nor diandric triploids. Amongst CHM, rare tetraploid and triploid cases which are androgenetic in origin have been identified[44]. Tetraploid PHM have also been reported[34,44–46]. Like triploid PHM, these HM generally have an excess of paternal genomes, their most likely origin being fertilization of an egg by three sperm or two sperm, one of which is diploid, although two cases of tetraploid PHM with apparently equal contributions from each parent have also been described[34,47]. Diploid PHM are reported but many may represent misdiagnosis of diploid hydropic abortion or CHM[48] or twin pregnancy consisting of CHM and normal fetus[49].

The morphology of the few aneuploid HM which have been described [14,15,50,51] generally reflects their basic karyotype; hypodiploid HM are morphologically CHM while hypotriploid or hypertriploid HM are PHM. In one study selective culture of stromal or trophoblast cells from CHM showed an aneuploid population of cells to be present in the trophoblast cultures from most CHM[52]. This has recently been confirmed by *in situ* hybridization to pathological sections of CHM with chromosome-specific probes. While villous trophoblast and stromal cells were found to be diploid, a high proportion of polyploid cells were found in the extravillous trophoblast[53].

An interesting subgroup of HM may be rare cases of diploid HM with a normal or biparental genotype with a genetic contribution from both parents[15,33,54–58]. Where the origin of these cases has been determined by cytogenetic analysis of cultured cells it is possible that the normal cells represent preferential growth of a second population of cells from an unrecognized twin[44]. This is unlikely to be the case where molecular genetic analysis has been performed. Further studies of specific chromosomes in these cases may increase our understanding of the pathogenesis of molar pregnancies.

2.1.2 GESTATIONAL TROPHOBLASTIC TUMORS

The genetics of gestational trophoblastic tumors (GTT) has been less well studied than those of HM. Monitoring of disease by measurement of serum human chorionic gonadotropin (hCG) levels and the development of successful chemotherapeutic regimens has meant that surgical intervention, and hence fresh tumor tissue for investigation, is rare.

Invasive mole

Cytogenetic studies of invasive HM have shown the majority to be diploid, with a high proportion of cells in the tetraploid range[5], A detailed study of four invasive moles by Wake *et al.*[28] found them to be diploid – three 46,XX and one 46,XY – reflecting their origin from CHM. In one case the antecedent HM was also examined and shown to be identical to the invasive mole for all markers examined. Interestingly, all four invasive moles appeared to be derived from the rarer dispermic type of HM. Two further cases of invasive mole have been described as aneuploid, with a modal number of 46[59].

Choriocarcinoma

Choriocarcinoma may follow any type of pregnancy, approximately equal numbers following normal pregnancy, non-molar abortion or HM[60]. The nature of the antecedent pregnancy will determine the genetics of the tumor, those following term pregnancies or non-molar abortions having both maternal and paternal chromosomes, while those deriving from CHM will be androgenetic in origin. Cytogenetic analysis of cell lines and a small number of choriocarcinoma have shown a more aberrant karyotype than invasive mole. Choriocarcinoma shows a wide variation in karyotype, most being aneuploid, with modes in the hyperdiploid and hypotetraploid range whether they follow term births, HM or spontaneous abortion[5,61–66]. Although karyotypes of choriocarcinomas show a wide range of abnormalities, including chromosomal gains, losses and rearrangements, unlike many other tumor types which exhibit specific rearrangements, no specific chromosomal abnormalities have yet been associated with trophoblastic tumors.

Placental site trophoblastic tumor

Very few data are currently available on the genetics of PSTT. Although these tumors are less often associated with an antecedent molar pregnancy, it has been confirmed using DNA analysis that, like choriocarcinoma, they may arise from both HM and normal term pregnancy[67]. Cytogenetic analysis of a single PSTT by Lathrop *et al.*[68] showed it to be diploid.

2.2 GENETIC DIAGNOSIS

2.2.1 DIAGNOSTIC PROBLEMS

Hydatidiform moles

It is estimated that the risk of choriocarcinoma following HM is in the order of 1000 times more likely than after a normal conception[69]. Studies in which HM have been characterized as CHM or PHM have shown that it is the CHM which are likely to require treatment for persistent trophoblastic disease (PTD)[9,10,34,70]. In the UK approximately one in 12 patients with CHM requires treatment for PTD[70] which in the absence of a pathological diagnosis, may be invasive mole, choriocarcinoma or PSTT. Estimates of the percentage of patients with PHM which do not resolve, following evacuation of the molar pregnancy, range from 0.5%[71] to 5%[72], although even the lower of these figures is likely to be an overestimate due to the large number of PHM which go undiagnosed[48,60,73]. Differences in the risk of developing PTD following CHM, PHM or hydropic abortion make it important to distinguish between these conceptions.

Although diagnosis is usually possible on the basis of morphology, poor sampling or necrosis where an HM has been retained for a long period can make a pathological diagnosis difficult[48] and genetic confirmation of diagnosis useful. The introduction of ultrasound scanning has led to earlier diagnosis and termination of suspected molar pregnancy. At an earlier gestational age the distinction between CHM and PHM is less marked[48] and genetic diagnosis is again useful for confirmation.

Twin pregnancies with CHM and normal conceptus may also pose diagnostic problems. PHM are characterized by a range of villi from normal to cystic and show evidence of the presence of a fetus or fetal development, generally in the form of fetal red blood cells in the villi. Twin pregnancies consisting of normal twin and CHM may also show similar characteristics. A review of the literature[74] has shown that a patient with CHM in a twin pregnancy has a significantly greater risk of PTD than with a singleton CHM and that the disease tends to be more aggressive. It is therefore particularly important to make the distinction between twin pregnancy with CHM and PHM both for appropriate management of the pregnancy and subsequent follow-up. Several cases have been reported where genetic studies have been used to identify CHM in twin pregnancies[75–83] or in multiple conceptions [84–87].

A third situation where a genetic diagnosis is useful is in the very rare type of CHM where fetal red blood cells (FRBCs), a feature of PHM, are present in some molar villi[88]. We have recently examined a series of seven HM which were shown to be diploid on flow cytometry, to have the conspicuous trophoblastic hyperplasia typical of CHM but to have some FRBCs in a small number of villi. Genetic diagnosis showed six of the seven cases to be androgenetic and therefore CHM[58]. In one of these cases it was also possible to carry out molecular genetic analysis of DNA prepared from a small area of amnion in the sample. This was shown to derive from a genetically normal twin having both a maternal and paternal genome. That the presence of FRBCs in the molar villi might derive from a twin pregnancy in other cases in the series is currently being investigated. It is possible that two similar cases – a 'diploid PHM'[11] and a case of CHM with some FRBCs[15] might also form part of this unusual group.

A distinction between monospermic and dispermic CHM can only be made on the basis of genetic polymorphisms, there being no morphological difference between these two conditions[89]. At present the clinical significance of this distinction is not clear. Data from a recent series suggest there is no difference in the incidence of PTD following monospermic or dispermic CHM[34]. This is supported by the observation that Y chromosome-positive CHM do not have a greater chance of metastases than Y chromosome-negative CHM[90].

Gestational trophoblastic tumors

GTT are a unique group of tumors in that they are allografts arising, not from the patient's own tissue, but from a genetically distinct conceptus. They are also unique in their response to cytotoxic drugs. GTT are characterized morphologically by the presence of cytotrophoblast and syncytiotrophoblast cells and biochemically by the production of hCG. Problems in diagnosis of GTT may arise because trophoblastic differentiation and hCG production sometimes occur in non-gestational tumors[91]. Patients with non-gestational tumors showing trophoblastic differentiation may respond to current chemotherapy but long-term survival is uncommon. It is therefore important to distinguish between a gestational or non-gestational tumor with trophoblastic characteristics.

Using genetic techniques it is now possible to determine the gestational or non-gestational origin of trophoblastic tumors. A tumor which is gestational in origin will reflect the genome of the pregnancy in which it arose and will therefore have paternal and maternal genes if it derives from a normal pregnancy or spontaneous abortion, or paternal genes if it originates in a CHM. In any case the presence of paternal genes will distinguish it from a non-gestational carcinoma with trophoblastic metaplasia which will have a genome that reflects that of the host.

The nature of the pregnancy, molar or non-molar, in which a tumor arises cannot be determined morphologically but is important clinically, tumors which arise following an HM having a more favorable prognosis. The time interval between a pregnancy and the diagnosis of a tumor is also a factor in determining the appropriate chemotherapeutic regime[92]. Therefore ascertainment of the nature of the causative pregnancy and the time interval between that pregnancy and the diagnosis of the tumor will enable better patient management. Clinically, the immediately antecedent pregnancy is perceived as the causative pregnancy. However, in a patient with multiple

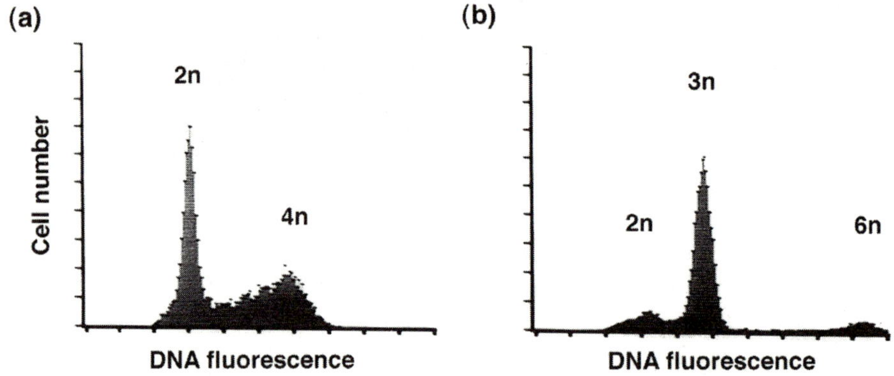

Figure 2.3 Flow cytometry of cells from (a) CHM and (b) PHM tissue. In the case of CHM a major diploid (2n) peak is observed, with a smaller tetraploid (4n) peak which represents dividing CHM cells. In PHM a small diploid peak is present which corresponds to contaminating host cells, while the major triploid peak (3n) and smaller 6n peak represent resting and dividing cells of the PHM respectively.

pregnancies it is not possible to be sure clinically that the last recognized pregnancy is the one in which the tumor arose. Results from studies of antibodies to major histocompatability antigens in the serum of patients with choriocarcinoma[93] have suggested that the antecedent pregnancy is not always the causative pregnancy in cases of GTT, an observation which has now been confirmed by molecular genetic studies[94–96].

2.2.2 DIAGNOSTIC TECHNIQUES

Determination of cell ploidy

Ploidy of both HM and GTT has been determined by karyotype analysis. However, these techniques generally require cell culture and good-quality metaphase spreads for analysis. An assessment of ploidy can be made by other techniques. In particular, flow cytometry, a technique based on the level of fluorescence emitted from labeled nuclei, has been useful in distinguishing diploid CHM from triploid PHM[97–100] (Figure 2.3) and in identifying the more unusual tetraploids HM[47]. Flow cytometry has the advantage that it can be applied to cells recovered from formalin-fixed paraffin-embedded blocks[101]. Determination of cell ploidy can also be made by fluorochrome staining of interphase nuclei[102] or *in situ* hybridization with chromosome-specific probes[53]. Triploid cells are distinguished from diploid by the presence of three spots rather than two for each probe used.

Flow cytometry and *in situ* hybridization have revealed more heterogeneity in CHM cells than previously found in most cytogenetic studies. Single cases of an apparently haploid CHM[34] and apparently haploid PHM[103] have been identified by flow cytometry. Some studies of cell ploidy have also identified aneuploid[104] or polyploid[53,100,103] populations of cells in CHM. It was suggested by Martin *et al.*[104] that ploidy correlated with clinical course although this has not been confirmed by other groups[100, 103]. Proliferative activity was found to be higher in CHM than non-molar placenta[98,100,105]. However, this was not found to be a predictor of prognosis[98,100,104,105].

Using flow cytometry, both choriocarcinoma[71,105–107] and PSTTs[107–109] have generally been shown to be diploid despite the varied karyotypes identified in choriocarcinomas by cytogenetic analysis. In some cases this may reflect the high proportion of infiltrating host cells present in pathological blocks of tumor tissue which will be diploid.

Studies of cell ploidy can confirm pathological diagnosis in some cases by distinguishing CHM from PHM or PHM from hydropic abortions. However, these techniques cannot distinguish between molar and non-molar triploids. Distinction between these two types of conception requires examination of polymorphic markers and demonstration of two paternal contributions to the genome for confirmation. Analysis of polymorphic markers is also required to determine the origin of GTTs.

Molecular genetic studies

Major advances in the diagnosis and classification of HM and in the diagnosis of trophoblastic tumors came with the introduction of molecular genetic techniques which use DNA polymorphisms as a basis for determining the parental origin of molar or tumor tissue. These polymorphisms, in particular the hypervariable minisatellite polymorphisms[31,32,110] are very much more informative than the cytogenetic or enzyme polymorphisms previously used[30,34].

In studies of molar pregnancies restriction fragment length polymorphisms[56], DNA fingerprinting[33,111,112] and the locus-specific minisatellite probes[30,33,34,80,113] (Figure 2.2) have all been used to confirm the androgenetic origin of CHM, to distinguish monospermic from dispermic CHM, to confirm the diandric origin of PHM or distinguish CHM with twin from PHM.

More rapid diagnosis has been made possible by the use of the polymerase chain reaction (PCR) to amplify

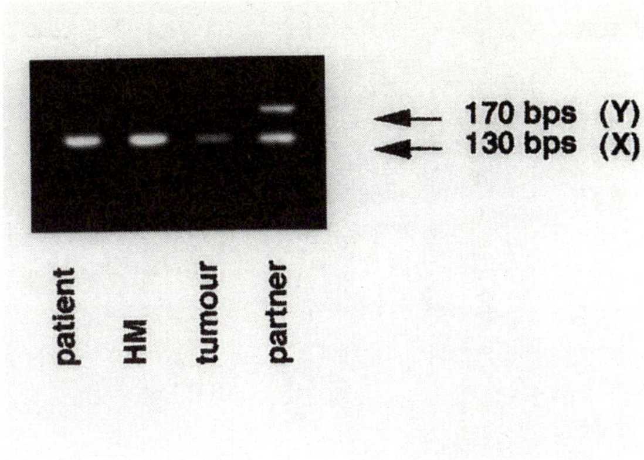

Figure 2.4 PCR amplification of DNA with primers for sex chromosome-specific sequences[115]. DNA from the patient shows only the 130 bps X chromosome-specific band, while DNA from her partner has both the X chromosome-specific and 170 bps Y chromosome-specific fragment. DNA samples prepared from a paraffin-embedded pathological block of HM and tissue from a subsequent choriocarcinoma are both Y chromosome-negative and therefore female.

sex chromosome-specific sequences[90],114] (Figure 2.4), variable-number tandem repeats (VNTRs)[82,114,116,117] and microsatellite, or short tandem repeat, polymorphisms[118] in DNA from molar tissue. This has reduced the requirement for large amounts of tissue, while gel electrophoresis, followed by ethidium bromide staining of PCR products, enables DNA analysis to be carried out without the use of radio-labeled probes[119]. Perhaps the greatest advantage of these techniques, particularly for the pathologist, is that the microsatellite sequences are short enough to be amplified even in degraded DNA prepared from pathological blocks[118,119] (Figure 2.5). Preparation of DNA from pathological blocks has the advantage that adjacent sections can be cut, one stained to identify trophoblast tissue and a second used for dissection of tumor cells for

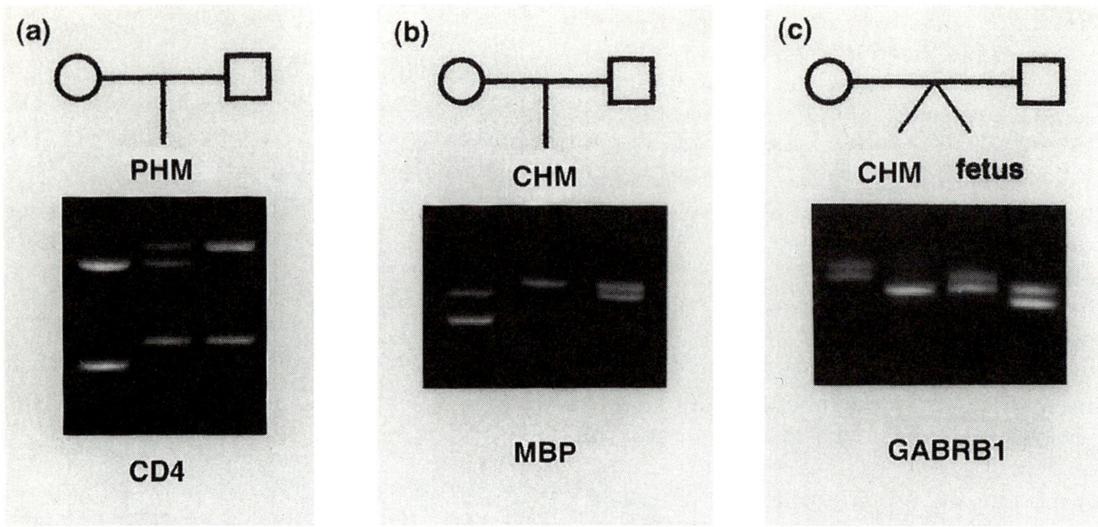

Figure 2.5 Microsatellite polymorphisms detected following PCR amplification with primers for the pentanucleotide repeat CD4[120], or the tetranucleotide repeats MBP[121] or GABRB1[122] in (a) a PHM having one maternal and two paternal contributions to the genome, (b) an androgenetic CHM, homozygous for the larger paternal allele and (c) a twin pregnancy comprising an androgenetic CHM and coexisting twin with biparental genome.

DNA preparation, thus minimizing any contamination from host cells.

The most recent modification of these techniques has been the incorporation of a fluorescently labeled primer into the PCR reaction followed by automated sizing of the products using an automated DNA sequencer and Genescan software[119]. This type of technology allows large numbers of polymorphisms to be examined from different regions of the genome simultaneously and provides a rapid means of determining genetic origin of both molar and tumor tissue (Figure 2.6).

Restriction fragment length polymorphisms of DNA[67,94,96,125–127], PCR amplification of VNTR polymorphisms in DNA[95], sex chromosome-specific sequences[96,119] and microsatellite polymorphisms[119,128] (Figure 2.6) have all been used to examine trophoblastic tumours. These reports together with two cytogenetic studies[61,129] have provided information on the origin of 19 cases of trophoblastic tumor. Four tumors were found to be non-gestational, seven to have a genetic origin consistent with a preceding term pregnancy or spontaneous abortion and four with an origin from an antecedent molar pregnancy.

However, in at least four cases the causative pregnancy was not the clinically antecedent pregnancy. In two the immediately antecedent pregnancy was a term pregnancy, while the tumor tissue was clearly androgenetic in origin[94,95]. In both cases the patients had a history of molar pregnancy, 4 and 10 years prior to diagnosis of the tumor respectively and in one case this was proven to be the causative pregnancy[119]. In a further case reported by Arima *et al.*[96] two term female pregnancies were followed by a PSTT which was shown by sex chromosome-specific sequences to

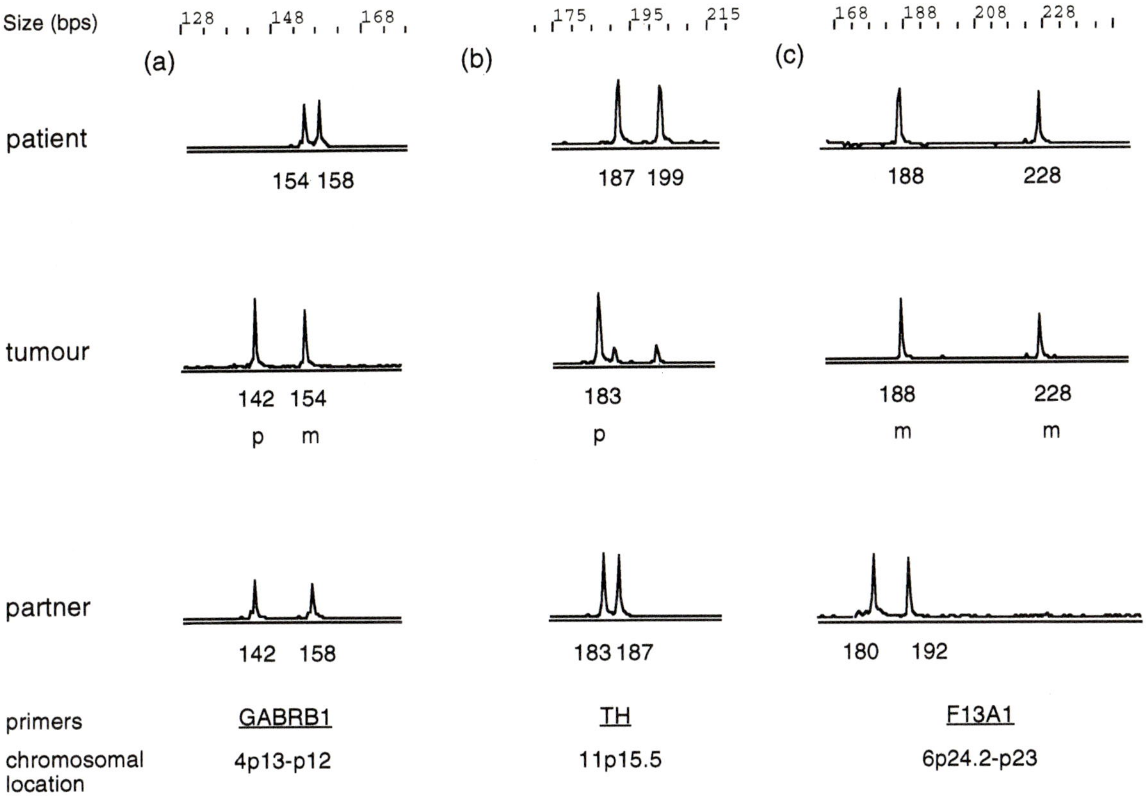

Figure 2.6 Microsatellite polymorphisms detected following PCR amplification with fluorescently labeled primers for the tetranucleotide repeats GABRB1, TH[123] or F13A1[124] in (a) a post-term PSTT with a maternal (m) and paternal (p) contribution to the genome, (b) a post-mole GTT which is androgenetic in origin and (c) a non-gestational tumor which has two alleles identical to those in the patient, and no paternally derived alleles. The two smaller peaks in case (b) represent amplification of contaminating host DNA from maternal cells which infiltrate the tumor.

have arisen in an unrecognized male pregnancy. Perhaps the most intriguing case is that in which a pregnancy with CHM was followed 12 months later by a choriocarcinoma which was shown genetically to have arisen in a normal conception, having both a maternal and paternal contribution to the genome[96].

Molecular genetic studies have also been useful in distinguishing between recurrent HM, i.e. a new conceptus, and PTD from a previous HM[130]. We have also carried out microsatellite genotyping in two cases where molar tissue was identified in the uterus five and seven months after evacuation of a CHM. Comparison of polymorphisms in DNA extracted from pathological blocks of molar tissue with those in maternal tissue showed molar tissue from the second evacuation to be genetically distinct from the previous CHM, and therefore recurrent CHM, in both cases.

These results demonstrate the importance of genetic studies in the management of GTT. The ability to identify microsatellite polymorphisms in fixed material now provides a rapid, accurate technique which can be used to determine the origin of trophoblastic tumors. The ability to isolate trophoblast cells from the peripheral blood of pregnant women and to perform PCR analysis of these cells[131] suggests that it may be possible in future to carry out non-invasive diagnosis of trophoblastic tumors using a combination of these techniques.

2.3 GENETIC FACTORS IN PATHOGENESIS

2.3.1 HYDATIDIFORM MOLES

Reports of HM in more than one member of a family[132–134] in homozygous twins[135] and patients with recurrent HM[134,136–138] suggest that, in some cases at least, genetic factors may be present, resulting in a tendency to produce defective eggs. Karyotyping of patients with molar pregnancies and their partners has not generally shown them to have any significant increase in constitutional abnormalities at the cytogenetic level[139].

2.3.2 GESTATIONAL TROPHOBLASTIC TUMORS

The single most important factor associated with the development of GTT is a history of pregnancy with CHM. Although a relatively high proportion of CHM progress to GTT compared with other types of pregnancy, the majority of CHM still resolve spontaneously. One of the important questions in the management of patients with HM is predicting which HM will progress to GTT. Since histopathological grade has not been shown to have prognostic significance[140] the search continues for genetic factors which might identify those CHM at risk.

Origin of CHM

The most obvious genetic distinction within CHM is their monospermic or dispermic origin. Although it was originally suggested that the dispermic CHM had the more malignant potential[28,54,141,142], recent studies in which molecular genetic techniques have been used to examine the origin of HM[34, 90] have not found the origin of CHM to have clinical significance.

ABO blood group

It has been shown that CHM in patients with a blood group unlike that of their partner are more likely to progress to a GTT[143–145]. Since the genotype of an androgenetic CHM reflects that of the partner, it follows that patients with HM of unlike blood group may be at greater risk of PTD. The recent development of techniques for ABO genotyping of DNA[146–148] has made it possible to determine the ABO group of molar tissue. A small study in which the ABO type of patients was compared with that of their HM found that CHM with blood groups unlike the patient showed no greater risk of developing to a trophoblastic tumor[149]. Interestingly, a significantly greater proportion of CHM with an O phenotype progressed to a GTT than those with other phenotypes, suggesting that blood group O in CHM may be a risk factor for the development of GTT.

Oncogenes

Many tumor types are associated with activation of oncogenes or loss of tumor suppressor genes. Studies of oncogene expression in CHM have shown an increased expression of c-fms in CHM[150] although neither c-fms or c-myc expression was shown to correlate with clinical course. Mutations in the p53 tumor suppressor gene have been observed in choriocarcinoma cell lines[151] although no mutations have been found in the small number of CHM examined[152]. Further studies of oncogenes and tumor suppressor genes are required to elucidate their role in the pathogenesis of trophoblastic tumors.

2.3.3 GENOMIC IMPRINTING

Hydatidiform moles

More recent studies of the pathogenesis of HM have focused on the role of genomic imprinting in HM and GTT. Several lines of evidence suggest that abnormal development in CHM is due to the presence of two paternal genomes. Despite the androgenetic origin of the nuclear genome, the mitochondrial DNA of CHM, as in a normal conceptus, is maternally derived. This together with the observation that ovarian teratomas, genetically analogous to CHM but having a maternally derived diploid karyotype[153] and very different pathology to HM, suggests that abnormal development in CHM is due to the paternal nuclear genome.

Further evidence for the role of the paternal genome in molar development comes from studies of the parental origin of PHM which have been shown, like CHM, to have two paternal sets of chromosomes. Digynic triploids with two maternal contributions to the nuclear genome are generally associated with non-molar placenta[39] and thus in most PHM, as in CHM, the characteristic abnormal pathology is associated with the presence of two paternal genomes.

HM thus appear to be an example of genomic imprinting, a phenomenon first described in lower Diptera[154] but now known to occur in humans, whereby genes function differently depending on their parental origin. Where only paternal chromosomes are present a CHM develops, trophoblastic hyperplasia is marked and no fetus is present. In PHM the presence of a maternal genome is associated with more moderate trophoblastic hyperplasia and fetal development.

Further evidence for the association between the paternal genome and trophoblastic development comes from mouse models[155,156]. Experiments involving nuclear transfer in mice have shown that normal development during mouse embryogenesis requires both maternal and paternal contributions to the genome. In these models relatively good trophoblast differentiation occurs in androgenetic embryos with two male pronuclei compared with gynogenetic embryos having two female pronuclei[156] demonstrating an association between the paternal genome and extraembryonic development analogous to that seen in HM.

In view of the close association between the paternal genome and molar development, rare cases of CHM which are diploid but have both a maternal and paternal contribution to the genome[15,33,55,58] may in fact be paternally disomic for part of the genome important in molar development[34]. These cases may be of particular interest in understanding the pathogenesis of HM.

Several genes which are imprinted, i.e. where only the maternal or paternal copy is expressed, have now been identified in humans[157]. The androgenetic CHM provides an interesting tissue in which to examine the expression of these imprinted genes. Two closely linked genes, insulin-like growth factor 2 (IGF-2) which is normally transcribed from the paternal allele, and H19, a putative tumor suppressor gene[158] normally expressed only from the maternal allele, have both been examined in CHM. IGF-2 shows the expected pattern of expression, being present in CHM tissue[159] but not ovarian teratomas[160]. Surprisingly, H19, which is normally transcribed from the maternal allele, is expressed in CHM[160–163] suggesting a failure to repress the paternal allele. Whether there are differences in H19 expression between HM which resolve spontaneously and those which progress to PTD remains to be answered.

Gestational trophoblastic tumors

Since early studies of CHM showed them to be homozygous it was suggested that development of GTD might be related to homozygosity for deleterious recessive genes[17]. Dispermic CHM which are homozygous for only some loci would therefore be expected to show less frequent progression to GTD. That there is no evidence that monospermic CHM are more likely to progress to GTD suggests that it is the paternal nature of the genome rather than homozygosity for specific genes which is the important factor in tumorigenesis.

There is now both indirect and direct evidence that genomic imprinting is important in the development of some types of tumor. Preferential involvement of specific parental alleles is associated with loss of tumor suppressor genes in several childhood tumors[164,165], the loss generally being the maternal allele. Association of excess paternal genes with tumorigenesis is implicated in the Beckwith–Wiedemann syndrome, which may result from unipaternal disomy or paternal duplication of part of chromosome 11 and in which affected individuals show predisposition to embryonal tumors[166]. More direct evidence comes from studies of tumors such as Wilms' tumor, where loss of the normal imprinting pattern (LOI) has been observed for IGF-2 and H19[167,168].

Recent studies have shown both H19 and IGF-2 to be expressed in choriocarcinoma[163, 169] which are derived from CHM, although in cases where both HM and choriocarcinoma were examined the level of H19 appeared to be less in the tumour than the preceding CHM[163]. Studies of H19 and IGF-2 in choriocarcinoma cell lines, some of which derive from tumors that followed term pregnancies, showed biallelic expression of one or both genes[169] suggesting that LOI may be an important factor in the development of GTT. Further studies are required to define the role of imprinting in the development of trophoblastic tumors.

2.4 SUMMARY

The majority of HM can be divided on the basis of genetics into PHM, monospermic and dispermic CHM. The genetic diagnosis of PHM and CHM correlates well with their pathological diagnosis and there are many circumstances where a genetic diagnosis provides confirmation of pathological findings or resolves diagnosis in pathologically unusual cases. Genetic diagnosis has proved important in the management of patients with trophoblastic tumors, in particular the differential diagnosis between the gestational or non-gestational origin of trophoblastic tumors. The development of techniques based on PCR amplification of microsatellite DNA polymorphisms now enables rapid, accurate diagnosis of both fresh and fixed tissue from GTD. HM represents an extreme example of genomic imprinting. Studies of imprinting in GTD should increase our understanding of its role in both molar and normal development.

ACKNOWLEDGEMENTS

The author would like to thank the late Professor S.D. Lawler for her helpful criticism of the manuscript.

REFERENCES

1. Barr, M.L. and Bertram, E.G. (1949) A morphological distinction between neurones of the male and female and the behaviour of the nucleolar satellite during accelerated nucleoprotein synthesis. *Nature*, **163**, 676–7.
2. Park, W.W. (1957) The occurrence of sex chromatin in chorionepitheliomas and hydatidiform moles. *Journal of Pathology and Bacteriology*, **74**, 197–206.
3. Sasaki, M., Fukuschima, T. and Makino, S.

(1962) Some aspects of the chromosome constitution of hydatidiform moles and normal chorionic villi. *Gann*, **53**, 101–6.

4. Makino, S., Sasaki, M.S. and Fukuschima, T. (1963) Preliminary notes on the chromosomes of human chorionic lesions. *Proceedings of the Japanese Academy*, **39**, 54–8.
5. Makino, S., Sasaki, M.S. and Fukuschima, T. (1965) Cytological studies of tumours. XLI. Chromosomal instability in human chorionic lesions. *Okajimas Folia Anatomica Japonica*, **40**, 439–65.
6. Bourgoin, P., Baylet, R., Ballon, C. and Grattepanche, H. (1965) Exploration d'une hypothèse sur l'étiopathogénie des môles hydatidiformes: étude chromosomique. *Revue Française de Gynécologie et d'Obstétrique*, **60**, 673–84.
7. Makino, S., Sasaki, M.S. and Fukuschima, T. (1964) Triploid chromosome constitution in human chorionic lesions. *Lancet*, **ii**, 1273–5.
8. Boue, J.G., Boue, A. and Lazer, P. (1967) Les aberrations chromosomiques dans les avortements. *Annales de Génétique (Paris)*, **10**, 179–87.
9. Vassilakos, P. and Kajii, T. (1976) Hydatidiform mole: two entities. *Lancet*, **i**, 259.
10. Vassilakos, P., Riotton, G. and Kajii, T. (1977) Hydatidiform mole: two entities. A morphological and cytogenetic study with some clinical considerations. *American Journal of Obstetrics and Gynecology*, **127**, 167–70.
11. Szulman, A.E. and Surti, U. (1978) The syndromes of hydatidiform mole. I. Cytogenetic and morphologic correlations. *American Journal of Obstetrics and Gynecology*, **131**, 665–71.
12. Szulman, A.E. and Surti, U. (1978) The syndromes of hydatidiform mole. II. Morphologic evolution of the complete and partial mole. *American Journal of Obstetrics and Gynecology*, **132**, 20–7.
13. Lawler, S.D., Pickthall, V.J., Fisher, R.A. *et al.* (1979) Genetic studies of complete and partial hydatidiform moles. *Lancet*, **ii**, 58.
14. Lawler, S.D., Fisher, R.A., Pickthall, V.J. *et al.* (1982) Genetic studies on hydatidiform moles. I. The origin of partial moles. *Cancer Genetics and Cytogenetics*, **5**, 309–20.
15. Jacobs, P.A., Hunt, P.A., Matsuura, J.S. and Wilson, C.C. (1982) Complete and partial hydatidiform mole in Hawaii: cytogenetics, morphology and epidemiology. *British Journal of Obstetrics and Gynaecology*, **89**, 258–66.
16. Hertig, A.T. and Edmonds, H.W. (1940) Genesis of hydatidiform mole. *Archives of Pathology*, **30**, 260–91.
17. Kajii, T. and Ohama, K. (1977) Androgenetic origin of hydatidiform mole. *Nature*, **268**, 633–4.
18. Wake, N., Takagi, N. and Sasaki, M. (1978) Adrogenesis as a cause of hydatidiform mole. *Journal of the National Cancer Institute*, **60**, 51–7.
19. Jacobs, P.A., Hassold, T.J., Matsuyama, A.M. and Newlands, I.M. (1978) Chromosome constitution of gestational trophoblastic disease. *Lancet*, **ii**, 49.
20. Wake, N., Shiina, Y. and Ichinoe, K. (1978) A further cytogenetic study of hydatidiform mole, with reference to its androgenetic origin. *Proceedings of the Japanese Academy, Series B*, **54**, 533–7.
21. Jacobs, P.A., Wilson, C.M., Sprenkle, J.A. *et al.* (1980) Mechanism of origin of complete hydatidiform mole. *Nature*, **286**, 714–16.
22. Lawler, S.D., Povey, S., Fisher, R.A. and Pickthall, V.J. (1982) Genetic studies of hydatidiform moles. II. The origin of complete moles. *Annals of Human Genetics*, **46**, 209–22.
23. Surti, U., Szulman, A.E. and O'Brien, S. (1979) Complete (classic) hydatidiform mole with 46,XY karyotype of paternal origin. *Human Genetics*, **51**, 153–5.
24. Ohama, K., Kajii, T., Okamoto, E. *et al.* (1981) Dispermic origin of XY hydatidiform moles. *Nature*, **29**, 551–2.
25. Pattillo, R.A., Sasaki, S., Katayama, K.P. *et al.* (1981) Genesis of 46,XY hydatidiform mole. *American Journal of Obstetrics and Gynecology*, **141**, 104–5.
26. Surti, U., Szulman, A.E. and O'Brien, S. (1982) Dispermic origin and clinical outcome of three complete hydatidiform moles with 46,XY karyotype. *American Journal of Obstetrics and Gynecology*, **144**, 84–7.
27. Fisher, R.A., Sheppard, D.M. and Lawler, S.D. (1984) Two patients with complete hydatidiform mole with 46,XY karyotype. *British Journal of Obstetrics and Gynaecology*, **91**, 690–3.

28. Wake, N., Seki, T., Fujita, H. *et al.* (1984) Malignant potential of homozygous and heterozygous complete moles. *Cancer Research*, **44**, 1226–30.
29. Fisher, R.A. and Lawler, S.D. (1984) Heterozygous complete hydatidiform moles: do they have a worse prognosis than homozygous complete moles? *Lancet*, **ii**, 51.
30. Fisher, R.A., Povey, S., Jeffreys, A. J. *et al.* (1989) Frequency of heterozygous complete hydatidiform moles, estimated by locus-specific minisatellite and Y chromosome-specific probes. *Human Genetics*, **82**, 259–63.
31. Wong, Z., Wilson, V., Jeffreys, A.J. and Thein, S.L. (1986) Cloning a selected fragment from a human DNA 'fingerprint': isolation of an extremely polymorphic minisatellite. *Nucleic Acids Research*, **14**, 4605–16.
32. Wong, Z., Wilson, V., Patel, I. *et al.* (1987) Characterisation of a panel of highly variable minisatellites cloned from human DNA. *Annals of Human Genetics*, **51**, 269–88.
33. Kovaks, B.W., Shahbahrami, B., Tast, D. E. and Curtin, J.P. (1991) Molecular genetic analysis of complete hydatidiform moles. *Cancer Genetics and Cytogenetics*, **54**, 143–52.
34. Lawler, S.D., Fisher, R.A. and Dent, J. (1991) A prospective study of hydatidiform mole. *American Journal of Obstetrics and Gynecology*, **164**, 1270–7.
35. Wallace, D.C., Surti, U., Adams, C.W. and Szulman, A.E. (1982) Complete moles have paternal chromosomes but maternal mitochondrial DNA. *Human Genetics*, **61**, 145–7.
36. Edwards, Y.H., Jeremiah, S.J., McMillan, S.L. *et al.* (1984) Complete hydatidiform moles combine maternal mitochondria with a paternal nuclear genome. *Annals of Human Genetics*, **48**, 119–27.
37. Azuma, C., Saji, F., Tokugawa, Y. *et al.* (1991) Application of gene amplification by polymerase chain reaction to genetic analysis of molar mitochondrial DNA: the detection of anuclear empty ovum as the cause of complete mole. *Gynecologic Oncology*, **40**, 29–33.
38. van Blerkom, J. and Henry, G. (1988) Cytogenetic analysis of living oocytes: cellular basis and developmental consequences of perturbations in chromosomal organization and complement. *Human Reproduction*, **3**, 777–90.
39. Jacobs, P.A., Szulman, A.E., Funkhouser, J. *et al.* (1982) Human triploidy: relationship between parental origin of the additional haploid complement and development of partial hydatidiform mole. *Annals of Human Genetics*, **46**, 223–31.
40. Lauritsen, J.G. (1976) Aetiology of spontaneous abortion. *Acta Obstetricia et Gynecologica Scandinavica, Supplement*, **52**, 1–29.
41. Kajii, T. and Niikawa, N. (1977) Origin of triploidy and tetraploidy in man: 11 cases with chromosome markers. *Cytogenetics and Cell Genetics*, **18**, 109–25.
42. Jacobs, P.A., Angell, R.R., Buchanan, I.M. *et al.* (1978) The origin of human triploids. *Annals of Human Genetics*, **42**, 49–57.
43. Uchida, I.A. and Freeman, V.C.P. (1985) Triploidy and chromosomes. *American Journal of Obstetrics and Gynecology*, **151**, 65–9.
44. Vejerslev, L.O., Fisher, R.A., Surti, U. and Wake, N. (1987) Hydatidiform mole: cytogenetically unusual cases and their implications for the present classification. *American Journal of Obstetrics and Gynecology*, **157**, 180–4.
45. Sheppard, D.M., Fisher, R.A., Lawler, S.D. and Povey, S. (1982) Tetraploid conceptus with three paternal contributions. *Human Genetics*, **62**, 371–4.
46. Surti, U., Szulman, A.E., Wagner, K. *et al* (1986) Tetraploid partial hydatidiform moles: two cases with a triple paternal contribution and a 92,XXXY karyotype. *Human Genetics*, **72**, 15–21.
47. Lage, J.M., Weinberg, D.S., Yavner, D.L. and Bieber, F.R. (1989) The biology of tetraploid hydatidiform moles: histopathology, cytogenetics and flow cytometry. *Human Pathology*, **20**, 419–25.
48. Paradinas, F.J. (1994) The histological diagnosis of hydatidiform moles. *Current Diagnostic Pathology*, **1**, 24–31.
49. Szulman, A.E. and Surti, U. (1985) Strict clinicopathological criteria in the diagnosis of partial hydatidiform mole: a plea renewed. *American Journal of Obstetrics and Gynecology*, **152**, 1107–8.

50. Berkowitz, R.S., Sandstrom, M., Goldstein, D.P. and Driscoll, S.G. (1982) 45,X complete hydatidiform mole. *Gynecologic Oncology*, **14**, 279–83.
51. Vejerslev, L.O., Dissing, J., Hansen, H.E. and Poulsen, H. (1987) Hydatidiform mole: genetic origin in polyploid conceptuses. *Human Genetics*, **76**, 11–19.
52. Habibian, R. and Surti, U. (1987) Cytogenetics of trophoblasts from complete hydatidiform moles. *Cancer Genetics and Cytogenetics*, **29**, 271–87.
53. van de Kaa, C.A., Hanselaar, A.G.J.M., Hopman, A.H.N. *et al.* (1993) DNA cytometric and interphase cytogenetic analyses of paraffin-embedded hydatidiform moles and hydropic abortions. *Journal of Pathology*, **170**, 229–38.
54. Davis, J.R., Surwit, E.A., Garay, J.P. and Fortier, K.J. (1984) Sex assignment in gestational trophoblastic neoplasia. *American Journal of Obstetrics and Gynecology*, **148**, 722–5.
55. Vejerslev, L.O., Dissing, J. and Hansen, H.E. (1987) Hydatidiform mole: genetic markers in diploid abortuses with macroscopic villous enlargement. *Cancer Genetics and Cytogenetics*, **26**, 143–55.
56. Ko, T.–M., Hsieh, C.-Y., Ho, H.-N. *et al.* (1991) Restriction fragment length polymorphism analysis to study the genetic origin of hydatidiform mole. *American Journal of Obstetrics and Gynecology*, **164**, 901–6.
57. Vejerslev, L.O., Sunde, L., Hansen, B.F. *et al.* (1991) Hydatidiform mole and fetus with normal karyotype: support of a separate entity. *Obstetrics and Gynecology*, **77**, 868–74.
58. Fisher, R.A., Paradinas, F.J., Soteriou, B.A. *et al* (1996). Diploid hydatidiform moles with fetal red blood cells in molar villi: 2-Genetics. *Journal of Pathology*, in press.
59. Yang, Y.H., Kwak, H.M., Park, T.K. *et al.* (1986) Comparative cytogenetic and clinicopathologic studies on gestational trophoblastic neoplasia, especially hydatidiform mole. *Yonsei Medical Journal*, **27**, 250–60.
60. WHO Scientific Group (1983) Gestational Trophoblastic Disease. World Health Organization Technical Report Series 692.
61. Wake, N., Tanaka, K.I., Chapman, V. *et al.* (1981) Chromosomes and cellular origin of choriocarcinoma. *Cancer Research*, **41**, 3137–43.
62. Sasaki, S., Katayama, P.K., Roesler, M. *et al.* (1982) Cytogenetic analysis of choriocarcinoma cell lines. *Acta Obstetrica Gynaecologica Japonica*, **34**, 2253–6.
63. Sekiya, S., Shirotake, S., Kaiho, T. *et al.* (1983) A newly established human gestational choriocarcinoma cell line and its characterization. *Gynecologic Oncology*, **15**, 413–21.
64. Okabe, T., Sasaki, N., Matsuzaki, M. *et al.* (1983) Establishment and characterization of a new human functional cell line from a choriocarcinoma. *Cancer Research*, **43**, 4920–6.
65. Sheppard, D.M., Fisher, R.A. and Lawler, S.D. (1985) Karyotypic analysis and chromosome polymorphisms in four choriocarcinoma cell lines. *Cancer Genetics and Cytogenetics*, **16**, 251–9.
66. Lawler, S.D. and Fisher, R.A. (1986) Genetic aspects of gestational trophoblastic tumours, in *Trophoblastic Diseases* (ed. K. Ichinoe), Igaku-Shoin, Tokyo, New York, pp. 23–33.
67. Fisher, R.A., Paradinas, F.J., Newlands, E.S. and Boxer, G.M. (1992) Genetic evidence that placental site trophoblastic tumours can originate from a hydatidiform mole or a normal conceptus. *British Journal of Cancer*, **65**, 355–8.
68. Lathrop, J.C., Lauchlan, S., Nayak, R. and Ambler, M. (1988) Clinical characteristics of placental site trophoblastic tumor (PSST). *Gynecologic Oncology*, **31**, 32–42.
69. Bagshawe, K.D. and Lawler, S.D. (1982) Choriocarcinoma, in *Cancer Epidemiology and Prevention*, (eds D. Schottenfeld and J.F. Fraumeni), Saunders, Philadelphia, pp. 909–24.
70. Bagshawe, K.D., Dent, J. and Webb, J. (1986) Hydatidiform mole in England and Wales 1973–83. *Lancet*, **ii**, 673–7.
71. Bagshawe, K.D., Lawler, S.D., Paradinas, F.J. *et al.* (1990) Gestational trophoblastic tumours following initial diagnosis of partial hydatidiform mole. *Lancet*, **335**, 1074–6.
72. Rice, L.W., Berkowitz, R.S., Lage, J.M. *et al.* (1990) Persistent gestational trophoblastic tumor after partial hydatidiform mole. *Gynecological Oncology*, **36**, 358–6.

73. Jeffers, M.D., O'Dwyer, P., Curran, B. *et al.* (1993) Partial hydatidiform mole: a common but underdiagnosed condition. A 3-year retrospective clinicopathological and DNA flow cytometric analysis. *International Journal of Gynecological Pathology*, **12**, 315–23.
74. Steller, M.A., Genest, D.R., Bernstein, M.R. *et al.* (1994) Natural history of twin pregnancy with complete hydatidiform mole and coexisting fetus. *Obstetrics and Gynecology*, **83**, 35–42.
75. Honda, J., Ihara, S., Sato, A. *et al.* (1980) Hydatidiform mole concurrent with normal pregnancy (twins) following clomiphene therapy. *Acta Obstetrica Gynaecologica Japonica*, **32**, 2041–3.
76. Fisher, R.A., Sheppard, D.M. and Lawler, S.D. (1982) Twin pregnancy with complete hydatidiform mole (46,XX) and fetus (46,XY): genetic origin proved by analysis of chromosome polymorphisms. *British Medical Journal*, **284**, 1218–20.
77. Ohama, K., Ueda, K., Okamoto, E. and Fujiwara, A. (1985) Two cases of dizygotic twins with androgenetic mole and normal conceptus. *Hiroshima Journal of Medical Sciences*, **34**, 371–5.
78. Vejerslev, L.O., Dueholm, M. and Nielsen, F.H. (1986) Hydatidiform mole: cytogenetic marker analysis in twin gestation. Report of two cases. *American Journal of Obstetrics and Gynecology*, **155**, 614–17.
79. Jauniaux, E., de Lannoy, E., Moscoso, G. and Campbell, S. (1990) Diagnostic prénatal des pathologies molaires associées à un foetus. Revue de la littérature récente à propos d'un cas. *Journal de Gynécologie Obstétrique et Biologie de la Réproduction (Paris)* **19**, 941–6.
80. Hsu, C.C., McConnell, J., Ko, T.M. and Braude, P.R. (1993) Twin pregnancy consisting of a complete hydatidiform mole and a fetus: genetic origin determined by DNA typing. *American Journal of Obstetrics and Gynecology*, **100**, 867–9.
81. Miller, D., Jackson, R., Ehlen, T. and McMurtrie, E. (1993) Complete hydatidiform mole coexistent with a twin live fetus: clinical course of four cases with complete cytogenetic analysis. *Gynecologic Oncology*, **50**, 119–23.
82. Osada, H., Iitsuka, Y., Matsui, H. and Sekiya, S. (1995) A complete hydatidiform mole coexisting with a normal fetus was confirmed by variable number tandem repeat (VNTR) polymorphism analysis using polymerase chain reaction. *Gynecologic Oncology*, **56**, 90–3.
83. van de Kaa, C.A., Robben, J.C.M., Hopman, A.H.N. *et al.* (1995) Complete hydatidiform mole in twin pregnancy: differentiation from partial mole with interphase cytogenetic and DNA cytometric analysis on paraffin embedded tissue. *Histopathology*, **26**, 123–9.
84. Ohmichi, M., Tasaka, K., Suehara, N. *et al.* (1986) Hydatidiform mole in a triplet pregnancy following gonadotrophin therapy. *Acta Obstetricia et Gynecologica Scandinavica*, **65**, 523–4.
85. Azuma, C., Saji, F., Takemura, M. *et al.* (1992) Triplet pregnancy involving complete hydatidiform mole and two fetuses: genetic analysis by deoxyribonucleic acid fingerprint. *American Journal of Obstetrics and Gynecology*, **166**, 664–7.
86. van de Geijn, E.J., Yedema, C.A., Hemrika, D.J. *et al.* (1992) Hydatidiform mole with coexisting twin pregnancy after gamete intrafallopian transfer. *Human Reproduction*, **7**, 568–72.
87. Hoshi, K., Morimura, Y., Azuma, C. *et al.* (1994) A case of quadruplet pregnancy containing complete mole and three fetuses. *American Journal of Obstetrics and Gynecology*, **170**, 1372–3.
88. Paradinas, F.J. and Fisher, R.A. (1995) Pathology and molecular genetics of trophoblastic disease. *Current Obstetrics and Gynaecology*, **5**, 6–12.
89. Kajii, T., Kurashige, H., Ohama, K. and Uchino, F. (1984) XY and XX complete moles: clinical and morphologic correlations. *American Journal of Obstetrics and Gynecology*, **150**, 57–64.
90. Mutter, G.L., Pomponio, R.J., Berkowitz, R.S. and Genest, D.R. (1993) Sex chromosome composition of complete hydatidiform moles: relationship to metastasis. *American Journal of Obstetrics and Gynecology*, **168**, 1547–51.
91. Braunstein, G.D., Vaitukaitis, J.L., Carbone, P.P. and Ross, G.T. (1973) Ectopic produc-

tion of human chorionic gonadotrophin by neoplasms. *Annals of Internal Medicine*, **78**, 39–45.

92. Bagshawe, K.D. (1976) Risk and prognostic factors in trophoblastic neoplasia. *Cancer*, **38**, 1373–85.
93. Lawler, S.D., Klouda, P.T. and Bagshawe, K.D. (1976) The relationship between HLA antibodies and the causal pregnancy in choriocarcinoma. *British Journal of Obstetrics and Gynaecology*, **83**, 651–5.
94. Fisher, R.A., Newlands, E.S., Jeffreys, A.J. *et al.* (1992) Gestational and non-gestational trophoblastic tumours distinguished by DNA analysis. *Cancer*, **69**, 839–45.
95. Suzuki, T., Goto, S., Nawa, A. *et al.* (1993) Identification of the pregnancy responsible for gestational trophoblastic disease by DNA analysis. *Obstetrics and Gynecology*, **82**, 629–34.
96. Arima, T., Imamura, T., Amada, S. *et al.* (1994) Genetic origin of malignant trophoblastic neoplasms. *Cancer Genetics and Cytogenetics*, **73**, 95–102.
97. Fisher, R.A., Lawler, S.D., Ormerod, M.G. *et al.* (1987) Flow cytometry used to distinguish between complete and partial hydatidiform moles. *Placenta*, **8**, 249–56.
98. Hemming, J.D., Quirke, P., Womack, C. *et al.* (1987) Diagnosis of molar pregnancy and persistent trophoblastic disease by flow cytometry. *Journal of Clinical Pathology*, **40**, 615–20.
99. Lage, J.M., Driscoll, S.G., Yavner, D.L. *et al.* (1988) Hydatidiform moles: application of flow cytometry in diagnosis. *American Journal of Clinical Pathology*, **89**, 596–600.
100. Fukunaga, M., Ushigome, S., and Sugishita, M. (1993) Methods in pathology: application of flow cytometry in diagnosis of hydatidiform moles. *Modern Pathology*, **6**, 353–9.
101. Hedley, D.W., Friedlander, M.L., Taylor, L.W. *et al.* (1983) Method for analysis of cellular DNA content of paraffin-embedded pathological material using flow cytometry. *Journal of Histochemistry and Cytochemistry*, **3**, 1333–5.
102. Tommerup, N. and Vejerslev, L.O. (1985) Identification of triploidy by DA/DAPI staining of trophoblastic interphase nuclei. *Placenta*, **6**, 363–7.
103. Lage, J.M., Mark, S.D., Roberts, D.J. *et al.* (1992) A flow cytometric study of 137 fresh hydropic placentas: correlation between types of hydatidiform moles and nuclear DNA ploidy. *Obstetrics and Gynecology*, **79**, 403–10.
104. Martin, D.A., Sutton, G.P., Ulbright, T.M. *et al.* (1989) DNA content as a prognostic index in gestational trophoblastic neoplasia. *Gynecologic Oncology*, **34**, 383–8.
105. Hemming, J.D., Quirke, P., Womack, C. *et al.* (1988) Flow cytometry in persistent trophoblastic disease. *Placenta*, **9**, 615–21.
106. Gardner, H.A.R. and Lage, J.M. (1992) Choriocarcinoma following a partial hydatidiform mole: a case report. *Human Pathology*, **23**, 468–71.
107. Fukunaga, M. and Ushigome, S. (1993) Malignant trophoblastic tumors: immunohistochemical and flow cytometric comparison of choriocarcinoma and placental site trophoblastic tumors. *Human Pathology*, **24**, 1098–106.
108. Eckstein, R.P., Russell, P., Friedlander, M.L. *et al.* (1985) Metastasizing placental site trophoblastic tumor: a case study. *Human Pathology*, **16**, 632–6.
109. Kotylo, P.K., Michael, H., Davis, T.E. *et al.* (1992) Flow cytometric DNA analysis of placental-site trophoblastic tumors. *International Journal of Gynecological Pathology*, **11**, 245–52.
110. Armour, J.A.L., Povey, S., Jeremiah, S. and Jeffreys, A.J. (1990) Systematic cloning of human minisatellites from ordered arrays of charomid libraries. *Genomics*, **8**, 501–12.
111. Saji, F., Tokugawa, Y., Kimura, T. *et al.* (1989) A new approach using DNA fingerprinting for the determination of androgenesis as a cause of hydatidiform mole. *Placenta*, **10**, 399–405.
112. Takahashi, H., Kanazawa, K., Ikarashi, T. *et al.* (1990) Discrepancy in the diagnoses of hydatidiform mole by macroscopic findings and the deoxyribonucleic acid fingerprint method. *American Journal of Obstetrics and Gynecology*, **163**, 112–13.
113. Cho, S. and Kim, S.J. (1993) Genetic study of hydatidiform moles by restriction fragment length polymorphisms (RFLPs)

analysis. *Journal of Korean Medical Science*, **8**, 446–52.
114. Fisher, R.A. and Newlands, E.S. (1993) Rapid diagnosis and classification of hydatidiform moles using the polymerase chain reaction. *American Journal of Obstetrics and Gynecology*, **168**, 563–9.
115. Witt, M. and Erickson, R.P. (1989) A rapid method for detection of Y-chromosome DNA from dried blood specimens by the polymerase chain reaction. *Human Genetics*, **82**, 271–4.
116. Fukuyama, R., Takata, M., Kudoh, J. *et al.* (1991) DNA diagnosis of hydatidiform mole using the polymerase chain reaction. *Human Genetics*, **87**, 216–18.
117. Fujita, N., Tamura, S., Shimizu, N. and Nozawa, S. (1994) Genetic analysis of hydatidiform mole and non-molar abortion using the polymerase chain reaction method. *Acta Obstetricia et Gynecologica Scandinavica*, **73**, 719–25.
118. Lane, S.A., Taylor, G.R. Ozols, B. and Quirke, P. (1993) Diagnosis of complete molar pregnancy by microsatellites in archival material. *Journal of Clinical Pathology*, **46**, 346–8.
119. Fisher, R.A., Soteriou, B., Meredith, L. *et al.* (1995) Previous hydatidiform mole identified as the causative pregnancy of choriocarcinoma following birth of normal twins. *International Journal of Gynecological Cancer*, **5**, 64–70.
120. Edwards, M.C., Clemens, P.R., Tristan, M. *et al.* (1991) Pentanucleotide repeat length polymorphism at the human CD4 locus. *Nucleic Acids Research*, **19**, 4791.
121. Polymeropoulos, M.H., Xiao, H. and Merril, C.R. (1992) Tetranucleotide repeat polymorphism at the human myelin basic protein gene (MBP). *Human Molecular Genetics*, **1**, 658.
122. Dean, M., Lucas-Derse, S., Bolos, A. *et al.* (1991) Genetic mapping of the $\beta 1$ GABA Receptor gene to human chromosome 4, using a tetranucleotide repeat polymorphism. *American Journal of Obstetrics and Gynecology*, **49**, 621–6.
123. Polymeropoulos, M.H., Xiao, H., Rath, D.S. and Merril, C.R. (1991) Tetranucleotide repeat polymorphism at the human tyrosine hydroxylase gene (TH). *Nucleic Acids Research*, **19**, 3753.
124. Polymeropoulos, M.H., Rath, D.S., Xiao, H. and Merril, C.R. (1991) Tetranucleotide repeat polymorphism at the human coagulation factor XIII A subunit gene (F13A1). *Nucleic Acids Research*, **19**, 4306.
125. Fisher, R.A., Lawler, S.D., Povey, S. and Bagshawe, K.D. (1988) Genetically homozygous choriocarcinoma following pregnancy with hydatidiform mole. *British Journal of Cancer*, **58**, 788–92.
126. Azuma, C., Saji, F., Nobunaga, T. *et al.* (1990) Studies of the pathogenesis of choriocarcinoma by analysis of restriction fragment length polymorphisms. *Cancer Research*, **50**, 488–91.
127. Osada, H., Kawata, M., Yamada, M. *et al.* (1991) Genetic identification of pregnancies responsible for choriocarcinomas after multiple pregnancies by restriction fragment length polymorphism analysis. *American Journal of Obstetrics and Gynecology*, **165**, 682–8.
128. Bower, M., Brock, C., Fisher, R.A. *et al.* (1995) Gestational choriocarcinoma. *Annals of Oncology*, **6**, 503–8.
129. Chaganti, R.S.K., Kodura, P.R.K., Chakraborty, R. and Jones, W.B. (1990) Genetic origin of a trophoblastic choriocarcinoma. *Cancer Research*, **50**, 6330–3.
130. Roberts, D.J. and Mutter, G.L. (1994) Advances in the molecular biology of gestational trophoblastic disease. *Journal of Reproductive Medicine*, **39**, 201–8.
131. Mueller, U.W., Hawes, C.S., Wright, A.E. *et al.* (1990) Isolation of fetal trophoblast cells from peripheral blood of pregnant women. *Lancet*, **336**, 197–200.
132. Ambani, L.M., Vaidya, R.A., Rao, C.S. *et al.* (1980) Familial occurrence of trophoblastic disease: report of recurrent molar pregnancies in sisters in three families. *Clinical Genetics*, **18**, 27–9.
133. Parazzini, F., La Vecchia, C., Franceschi, S. and Mangali, G. (1984) Familial trophoblastic disease: case report. *American Journal of Obstetrics and Gynecology*, **149**, 382–3.
134. Kircheisen, R. and Schroeder-Kurth, T. (1991). Familiäres Blasenmolen-Syndrom und genetische Aspekte dieser gestörten

Trophoblastentwicklung. *Geburtshilfe Frauenheilk.*, **51**, 569–71.

135. La Vecchia, C., Franceschi, S., Fasoli, M. and Mangioni, C. (1982). Gestational trophoblastic neoplasias in homozygous twins. *Obstetrics and Gynecology*, **60**, 250–2.
136. Wu, F.Y.W. (1972) Recurrent hydatidiform mole, a case report of nine consecutive molar pregnancies. *Obstetrics and Gynecology*, **41**, 200–4.
137. Patek, E. and Johnson, P. (1978) Recurrent hydatidiform mole, report of a case with five recurrences. *Acta Obstetricia et Gynecologica Scandinavica*, **57**, 381–3.
138. Federschneider, J.M., Goldstein, D.P., Berkowitz, R.S. *et al.* (1980) Natural history of recurrent molar pregnancy. *Obstetrics and Gynecology*, **55**, 457–9.
139. Vejerslev, L.O., Fisher, R.A., Surti, U. and Wake, N. (1987) Hydatidiform mole: parental chromosome aberrations in partial and complete moles. *Journal of Medical Genetics*, **24**, 613–15.
140. Genest, D.R., Laborde, O., Berkowitz, R.S. *et al.* (1991) A clinicopathologic study of 153 cases of complete hydatidiform mole (1980–1990): histologic grade lacks prognostic significance. *Obstetrics and Gynecology*, **78**, 402–9.
141. Kajii, T. (1980) Androgenetic origin of hydatidiform moles: its bearing on carcinogenesis. *Gann Monographs in Cancer Research*, **25**, 189–94.
142. Wake, N., Fujino, T., Hoshi, S. *et al.* (1987) The propensity to malignancy of dispermic heterozygous moles. *Placenta*, **8**, 319–26.
143. Bagshawe, K.D., Rawlins, G., Pike, M.C. and Lawler, S.D. (1971) ABO blood-groups in trophoblastic neoplasia. *Lancet*, **i**, 553–7.
144. Bagshawe, K.D. (1982) Some facets of trophoblastic neoplasia in man. *Journal of Reproduction and Fertility, Supplement*, **31**, 175–9.
145. Lawler, S.D. and Fisher, R.A. (1987) Immunogenicity of hydatidiform moles. *Placenta*, **8**, 195–9.
146. Yamamoto, F.-I., Clausen, H., White, T. *et al.* (1990) Molecular basis of the histo-blood group ABO system. *Nature*, **345**, 229–33.
147. Ugozzoli, L. and Wallace, R.B. (1992) Application of an allele-specific polymerase chain reaction to the direct determination of ABO blood group genotypes. *Genomics*, **12**, 670–4.
148. Johnson, P.H. and Hopkinson, D.A. (1992) Detection of ABO blood group polymorphism by denaturing gradient gel electrophoresis. *Human Molecular Genetics*, **1**, 341–4.
149. Fisher, R.A., Johnson, P.H., Povey, S. *et al.* (1993) ABO Genotyping of complete hydatidiform moles. *Disease Markers*, **11**, 179–85.
150. Cheung, A.N.Y., Srivastava, G., Pittaluga, S. *et al.* (1993) Expression of c-myc and c-fms oncogenes in trophoblastic cells in hydatidiform mole and normal human placenta. *Journal of Clinical Pathology*, **46**, 204–7.
151. Yaginuma, Y., Yamashita, T., Takuma, N. *et al.* (1995) Analysis of the p53 gene in human choriocarcinoma cell lines. *British Journal of Cancer*, **71**, 9–12.
152. Cheung, A.N., Srivastava, G., Chung, L.P. *et al.* (1994) Expression of the p53 gene in trophoblastic cells in hydatidiform moles and normal human placentas. *Journal of Reproductive Medicine*, **39**, 223–7.
153. Parrington, J.M., West, L.F. and Povey, S. (1984) The origin of ovarian teratomas. *Journal of Medical Genetics*, **21**, 4–12.
154. Crouse, H.V. (1960) The controlling element in sex chromosome behaviour in Sciara. *Genetics*, **45**, 1429–43.
155. Surani, M.A.H., Barton, S.C. and Norris, M.L. (1984) Development of reconstituted mouse eggs suggests imprinting of the genome during gametogenesis. *Nature*, **308**, 548–50.
156. Barton, S.C., Surani, M.A.H. and Norris, M.L. (1984) Role of maternal and paternal genomes in mouse development. *Nature*, **311**, 374–6.
157. Surani, M.A. (1994) Genomic imprinting: control of gene expression by epigenetic inheritance. *Current Opinion in Cell Biology*, **6**, 390–5.
158. Hao, Y., Crenshaw, T., Moulton, T. *et al.* (1993) Tumour-suppressor activity of H19 RNA. *Nature*, **365**, 764–7.
159. Rachmilewitz, J., Goshen, R., Ariel, I. *et al.*

(1992) Parental imprinting of the human H19 gene. *FEBS Letters*, **309**, 25–8.

160. Mutter, G.L., Stewart, C.L., Chaponot, M.L. and Pomponio, R.J. (1993) Oppositely imprinted genes H19 and insulin-like growth factor 2 are coexpressed in human androgenetic trophoblast. *American Journal of Human Genetics*, **53**, 1096–102.
161. Ohlsson, R., Nystrom, A., Pfeifer-Ohlsson, S. *et al.* (1993) IGF2 is parentally imprinted during human embryogenesis and in the Beckwith–Wiedemann syndrome. *Nature Genetics*, **4**, 94–7.
162. Ariel, I., Lustig, O., Oyer, C.E. *et al.* (1994) Relaxation of imprinting in trophoblastic disease. *Gynecologic Oncology*, **53**, 211–19.
163. Walsh, C., Miller, S.J., Flam, F. *et al.* (1995) Paternally-derived H19 is differentially expressed in malignant and non-malignant trophoblast. *Cancer Research*, **55**, 1111–16.
164. Schroeder, W.T., Chao, L.Y., Dao, D.D. *et al.* (1987) Nonrandom loss of maternal chromosome 11 alleles in Wilms' tumour. *American Journal of Human Genetics*, **40**, 413–20.
165. Toguchida, J., Ishizaki, K., Sasaki, M.S. *et al.* (1989) Preferential mutation of paternally derived RB gene as the initial event in sporadic osteosarcoma. *Nature*, **338**, 156–8.
166. Henry, I., Bonaiti-Pellie, C., Chehensse, V. *et al.* (1991) Uniparental paternal disomy in a genetic cancer-predisposing syndrome. *Nature*, **351**, 665–7.
167. Rainier, S., Johnson, L.A., Dobry, C.J. *et al.* (1993) Relaxation of imprinted genes in human cancer. *Nature*, **362**, 747–9.
168. Ogawa, O., Eccles, M.R., Szeto, J. *et al.* (1993) Relaxation of insulin-like growth factor II gene imprinting implicated in Wilms' tumour. *Nature*, **362**, 749–51.
169. Hashimoto, K., Azuma, C., Koyama, M. *et al.* (1995) Loss of imprinting in choriocarcinoma. *Nature Genetics*, **9**, 109–10.

GLOSSARY

allele alternative forms of a gene located at the same site on a chromosome

androgenetic a conceptus in which all the chromosomes are derived from the male parent

aneuploid a chromosome complement that is not an exact multiple of the haploid number

centromere the primary constriction of a chromosome

chromatid one of two strands formed when a chromosome replicates

diploid the normal chromosome complement of the somatic cells of an individual; in humans, 46

haploid the number of chromosomes in a normal gamete

heterozygous having two different alleles

homolog one member of a pair of chromosomes

homozygous having two similar alleles

interphase the resting phase of the cell cycle

karyotype description of the chromosomal complement

meiosis nuclear division in gametogenesis during which the diploid chromosome number is reduced to haploid

metaphase the stage in nuclear division at which the chromosomes can be visualized as two chromatids joined at the centromere

tetraploid a chromosome complement that is four times the haploid number; in humans, 92

triploid a chromosome complement that is three times the haploid number; in humans, 69

trisomic having a single extra chromosome

EPIDEMIOLOGY 3

Seung J. Kim

Recently, the epidemiological investigation of the incidence and etiological factors in gestational trophoblastic disease (GTD) has received increased attention. It has been recognized that earlier attempts to estimate the incidence of hydatidiform mole (HM) and choriocarcinoma (CC) in various regions were limited by methodological difficulties of obtaining accurate rates. This chapter will review the literature on the epidemiology, with focus on the etiological risk factors of GTD.

3.1 DEFINITION OF GESTATIONAL TROPHOBLASTIC DISEASE

GTDs are either tumors or conditions which are allografts arising from a conceptus, which invade the tissues of the mother. The WHO Scientific Group[1] noted that there is considerable confusion in the literature regarding the terminology of GTD. This group therefore made the following recommendations for histopathological and clinical terminology in an attempt to standardize the reporting data. As histopathological entities, HM, invasive mole (IM) and CC arise from the trophoblastic epithelium. Unlike other types of the disease, placental site trophoblastic tumor (PSTT) is a tumor which arises from the trophoblast of the placental bed; it encompasses lesions of low- and high-grade malignancy and is characterized by the propagation of intermediate trophoblasts.

During the last decade, HM has been separated into two clinical and genetic entities: the complete hydatidiform mole (CHM) is androgenetically derived, while the partial hydatidiform mole (PHM) is a triploid conceptus[2].

Clinically the GTDs embrace HM, IM, PSTT and CC and therefore include both benign and malignant conditions.

The term 'gestational trophoblastic tumor' (GTT) defines a disease state in which there is clinical evidence of IM or CC and behaving in a malignant manner.

3.2 PROBLEMS AND LIMITATIONS IN THE INTERPRETATION OF PUBLISHED DATA

There are many differences in worldwide epidemiological reports of the incidence of GTD in various countries according to statistical differences and geographic variations. How can we interpret these differences?

For example, the epidemiology of GTD is not easily interpreted in many reports; there are considerable problems with using a pathology-based classification, since histological specimens are often unavailable and

Gestational Trophoblastic Disease.
Edited by B.W. Hancock, E.S. Newlands and R.S. Berkowitz.
ISBN 0 412 63100 8

the majority of cases are now managed using only clinical criteria. Therefore, there are serious obstacles in the interpretation of such worldwide reports. Grimes[3] pointed out that three obstacles, in terms of definition, detection and identification of disease, limit the value of much published data.

3.2.1 PROBLEMS IN DEFINITION AND TERMINOLOGY

Before the WHO Scientific Group meeting[1] there was no internationally agreed terminology of GTD. Many published data lacked a clear, precise and reproducible case definition of the disease[3]. Most studies of incidence antedate the discovery by Szulman and Surti[2] that HM encompasses two different disease entities, PHM and CHM, of different etiology. Also, previous classifications of HM and IM became obsolete; there is the additional problem that 'hydropic degeneration' has been confused with HM, and the terms 'destructive' and 'transitional' mole with IM.

Because of the extraordinary success of chemotherapy in the management of IM and CC, a histological diagnosis has limited clinical relevance. Thus there is a fundamental problem to understanding epidemiology involving histological classification because the therapies for PSTT, GTT and CC are similar.

Recently, however, developing diagnostic tools, e.g. color ultrasonography and magnetic resonance imaging (MRI), have established a more accurate anatomical diagnosis. Also, modern techniques to determine the precise cytogenetics of HM have not yet been applied at a service level; they will lead to reclassification of a proportion of cases in the future.

3.2.2 ERRORS IN CASE DETECTION

Another problem is errors in case reporting of GTD. It is now clear that many of the different incidences between different populations are caused by the over-reporting of GTD in hospital-based studies, particularly in developing countries which have more 'abnormal' pregnancies receiving hospital care. Under-reporting of GTD may also occur, especially in communities where medical attention is suboptimal. Even in developed countries with formal responsibility to report cases of HM, there is a documented under-reporting of 25%[4].

3.2.3 DIFFERENT DENOMINATORS FOR THE POPULATION AT RISK

The preferred denominator for any incidence of GTD is all women who have conceived in a given period. Since GTD follows all kinds of pregnancies, as a denominator, 'pregnancies' would include all live births, stillbirths, known abortions and ectopic pregnancies. For accurate estimation of population at risk, 'deliveries' is less reliable as a denominator, and 'live birth' is an approximation of the population at risk, because it excludes a number of pregnancies at risk. Because reports from various countries have calculated the incidences using differing denominators, simple comparison is likely to be erroneous. The incidence rates of GTD can be overestimated or underestimated according to whether they are hospital-based or population-based data.

Recently, however, there has been a great improvement in the case-finding methods used around the world and recent reports generally present the best information on both numerator and denominator.

3.3 GEOGRAPHICAL VARIATIONS IN THE INCIDENCE OF GTD

3.3.1 HYDATIDIFORM MOLE

It has been recognized for a long time that the incidence of HM varies between different countries, with the highest rates in parts of

Asia (Table 3.1). Although large regional differences in the incidence of HM have been reported, this variation may be attributable in large part to the methodological problems cited previously[3,5,6]. The highest rates are reported from Indonesia, the Philippines, Taiwan and Korea, based on older hospital-based studies. Following more recent and better controlled studies from various Asian countries, it is evident that the older hospital-based studies give inaccurate pictures of the rates of GTD.

In China, a nationwide study conducted by the National Co-ordination Research Group of Chorioma[7] and Song and Wu[8] found an incidence of 0.78 and 0.81 per 1000 pregnancies respectively, a rate within the range of that reported from Western countries. Also, in China, high rates have been reported in southern and coastal regions. The diversity of incidence of HM in China is very interesting; the incidence of molar pregnancy was significantly higher among women in southeast China than those in other parts of the country[7]. In Japan, better controlled studies from 20 different prefectures report that the incidence of HM ranges from 2.83 to 3.05 per 1000 live births in the data from a registration system for 16 829 cases of GTD from 1974 to 1982[9].

In Africa, the rates of GTD have ranged from 1.03 per 1000 deliveries in Uganda to 5.88 per 1000 deliveries in Nigeria. These reports are derived from older hospital-based studies.

Latin American reports also vary considerably, from 0.23 per 1000 pregnancies in Paraguay[10] to 4.62 per 1000 pregnancies in Mexico[11].

Regarding the USA and European countries, Hayashi *et al.*[12] reported 1.08 per 1000 pregnancies in American women and Bagshawe and Dent[13] reported a rate of 1.54 per 1000 live births in their study of England and Wales. Australian studies estimate similar rates to those from the USA and European countries. Within the USA, Hayashi *et al.*[12] found differences in rates of HM per 1000 pregnancies ranging from a low of 0.70 in New England to a high of 1.89 in the Rocky Mountain census regions. Overall, worldwide, rates in these population-based studies range from 0.2 to 2.9 cases per 1000 pregnancies, births or live births. On the other hand, rates from hospital-based studies range from 0.87 to 11.6 per 1000 deliveries (Table 3.1). These geographical differences in current incidence rates should be interpreted in the context of the previously mentioned obstacles; however, the fact that the disease incidence is relatively high in Asia, especially Southeast Asia, cannot be neglected. In addition, information from the study of temporal trends and the results of genetic studies should be accumulated.

3.3.2 CHORIOCARCINOMA

Estimations of the incidence of CC have been limited by some of the same problems as with HM. Similar rates have been reported in population-based studies from countries in Latin America (0.2 cases) and Europe (0.2–1.5 cases), but Japan reports 0.83 cases per 10 000 pregnancies and births (Table 3.2). On the other hand, rates from hospital-based studies ranged from 0.2 to 20.2 per 10 000 pregnancies and deliveries (Table 3.2).

Problems with definition and assessment of GTD and the use of different denominators and study intervals preclude a clear understanding of worldwide incidences.

3.4 TIME TRENDS IN INCIDENCE OF GTD

Information on temporal trends in the incidence of GTD is limited and very conflicting.

3.4.1 HYDATIDIFORM MOLE

In two US hospitals, between 1940 and 1964 the incidence of HM declined during World War II, then rose later to surpass the pre-war

Table 3.1 Selected incidences of hydatidiform mole reported by previous authors

		Rate per 1 000		
Country	*Authors*	*Pregnancies*	*Deliveries*	*Live births*
Population-based studies				
Latin America				
Paraguay	Rolon and de Lopez [10]	0.2	–	–
North America				
Canada	Yuen and Cannon [66]	0.83	–	–
Greenland	Nielsen and Hansen [16]	–	1.2	–
USA	Hayashi *et al* [12]	1.1	–	–
USA	Matsuura *et al.* [26]	0.8	(White Hawaiian)	
		1.75	(Filipino Orientals)	
North Asia				
Japan (20 prefectures)	Takeuchi [9,67]	1.96		3.0
China	NCRG [7]	0.8		
South Asia				
Singapore	Teoh *et al.* [20]	–	1.2	–
Europe				
Italy	Mazzann *et al.* [68]	0.7		–
Sweden	Flam and Rutgvist [4]	0.9	–	–
Netherlands	Franke *et al.* [69]			0.68
England and Wales	Bagshawe and Dent [13]			1.5
Oceania				
Australia	Olesnicky and Quinn [38]	0.57		0.7
United Arab Emirates	Graham and Fajardo [70]		2.0	
Hospital-based studies				
Africa				
Nigeria	Ogunbode [71]	–	4.8	–
Uganda	Leighton [72]	–	1.03	–
Latin America				
Mexico	Marquez-Monter *et al.* [11]	4.6	–	–
North America				
USA	Yen and MacMahon [14]	0.63	–	–
(Alaska)	Martin [53]	–	3.9	–
(Hawaii)	Jacobs *et al.* [73]	–	–	4.6
North Asia				
Japan	Nakano *et al.* [24]	1.9	2.6	–
Taiwan	Wei and Ouyang [74]	–	8.0	–
Korea	Kim [75]	–	7.9	–
China	Song *et al.* [23]		6.7	
South Asia				
Indonesia	Poen and Djojopranoto [76]	9.9	11.5	–
Malaysia	Ong *et al.* [77]	–	1.5	–
Philippines	Acosta-Sison [48]	5.0	–	–
Iran	Javey and Sajadi [78]	3.2	–	3.7
Israel	Matalon and Modan [15]	–	–	0.8
Europe				
Italy	Di Fabio and De Aloysio [79]	–	0.8	–
Oceania				
Australia (Sydney)	Steigrad [80]	0.9	1.0	–

Table 3.2 Selected incidences of choriocarcinoma reported by previous authors

Country	Authors	Rate per 1 000		
		Pregnancies	Deliveries	Live births
Population-based studies				
Latin America				
Paraguay	Rolon and de Lopez [10]	0.2	–	–
Jamaica	Sengupta *et al.* [81]	–	–	1.4
Puerto Rico	Aranda and Martinez (1968)	–	0.3	–
North America				
Canada	Brisson and Fabia [82]			0.4
South Asia				
Singapore	Teoh *et al.* [20]	–	2.3	–
North Asia				
Japan (20 prefectures)	Takeuchi [9]			0.83
Europe				
Sweden	Ringertz [83]	0.2	–	–
Hospital-based studies				
Africa				
Nigeria	Ayangade [84]	–	9.9	–
Latin America				
Mexico	Marquez-Monter [11]	3.5	–	–
Mexico	MacGregor *et al.* [85]	0.2	0.3	0.3
North America				
USA	Brewer and Gerbie [86]	0.5	0.6	–
USA	Yen and MacMahon [14]	0.3	–	–
East Asia				
Hong Kong	Chan [87]	–	7.5	–
Japan	Nakano *et al.* [24]	1.2	1.7	–
Taiwan	Wei and Ouyang [74]	–	20.2	–
Korea	Kim [75]	–	1.9	–
South Asia				
India	Pai [88]	19.1	–	–
Indonesia	Poen and Djojopranoto [76]	15.3	17.7	–
Philippines	Acosta-Sison [89]	8.7	–	–
Thailand	Srivannaboon *et al.* [90]	6.3	6.5	–
Israel	Matalon *et al.* [91]	–	–	0.5
Oceania				
Australia (Sydney)	Steigrad [80]	0.7	0.8	–

rate[14]. Among Jewish women in Israel from 1950 to 1965, the incidence steadily increased[15]. Among indigenous Greenlandic women from 1950 to 1974, the incidence increased significantly after 1965[16].

In the summary of the Japanese study of registration system data for GTD (16 829 HM) from 1974 to 1982, the incidence of HM per 100 000 women decreased yearly from 10.2 in 1974 to 7.9 in 1982, but interestingly the number per 1000 births was almost unchanged (range: 2.83–3.05), the average from 1974 to 1982 was 2.92 per 1000 births.

3.4.2 CHORIOCARCINOMA

Data on temporal trends in CC are even more limited. In Israel, the incidence of CC decreased significantly between 1950 and 1965; by 1960 to 1965, the rate was less than one-third of that for 1950 to 1954[15]. In the study of registration systems for CC in Japan the incidence of CC per 100 000 women decreased yearly from 0.31 in 1974 to 0.19 in 1982, or by about two-thirds over this period. It is also of note that the incidence per 10 000 births decreased slightly, from 0.86 in 1974 to 0.74 in 1982, with an average of 0.83[16a]. As described above, although the incidence of GTD in Asia is actually higher than in other regions, it cannot easily be ascribed to racial factors; maternal age, environmental and dietary factors and lifestyle should also be considered.

3.5 RISK FACTORS FOR GTD

A variety of risk factors have been considered to play a possible role in the causation of GTD but the etiology is still uncertain. However, many factors like viral infection[17, 18], poor nutrition, defective germ cell[19] prior pregnancies, maternal age, genetic factors, and environmental factors have been noted as possible etiological risk factors for GTD.

3.5.1 AGE FACTORS

Maternal age has consistently been identified as an important risk factor. Age-specific incidence reports usually reveal a 'J curve', with teenagers having a higher incidence, and women over 40 having a dramatically higher incidence[5,10,12,14–16,20,21].

The risk is slightly higher for pregnancies in those aged 15–20 years and much higher (about 20-fold) for a pregnancy in girls under 15 years. There is a progressive (above 10-fold) increase[13,15] in risk over the age of 40 years, so that for women over 50 years the risk that a pregnancy will result in HM is some 200 times greater than for those 20–35 years of age[22]. This increased incidence in the youngest and oldest age suggests that ova which are premature or postmature are at higher risk of developing HM. This appears to be a consistent finding in all regions and races[12,16,23–25].

Paternal age, however, has been found to be a significant risk factor in some studies but this is not a consistent finding[26,27], and in a Japanese study paternal age difference does not appear to be important[28].

3.5.2 REPRODUCTIVE AND OBSTETRIC HISTORY

Much of the literature confuses the two variables gravidity and parity. Very few studies have accounted for any of the variables of maternal age, age at first pregnancy, previous induced abortions, miscarriages, interpregnancy spacing and history of infertility. No studies have examined all of them.

Previous HM appears to be a strong and well-established risk factor for recurrent mole[15,26,27,29–32]. The relative risk of developing another HM ranges from 20 to 40 times that for the general population in reported studies[14,15,33].

It is reported that second moles occurred in 0.6–2.6%[31,32,34,35] of pregnancies occurring subsequent to a first HM.

Women who have given birth to twins may also be at increased risk of having an HM. In one study[36] the incidence of HM among such women was significantly higher than that for the general population.

In Rhode Island and Italy[29] parity was not associated with HM, after adjustment for maternal age. An Italian study[37] found an elevated risk of HM in nulliparous women with a history of miscarriage, and in another Italian study [29] difficulties in conception were significantly more common preceding the HM, but in Baltimore a history of infertility and menstrual problems was not related[27]. A recent report from Australia indicated an increased rate of

HM after artificial insemination by donor (AID) compared with normally conceived pregnancies[38]. It appears that a woman's ability to deliver a normal child reduces her risk of developing GTD. This may reflect the absence of adverse genetic or environmental factors which can cause abnormal fertilization resulting in GTD.

3.5.3 ETHNICITY

Data concerning possible ethnic factors in the incidence of GTD are provided from several studies carried out in polyracial societies. In the USA from 1970 to 1977, black women had half the rate of HM of non-black women[12] Matsura *et al*.[26] found that the rate of HM was 8.0 per 1000 pregnancies in Caucasians, 17.5 in Filipinos, 16.5 in Japanese and 7.7 in Hawaiians, and there were also differences in the rates among Oriental women born in Hawaii and those born in the Orient.

In the Singapore study from 1953 to 1965, the incidence of HM was one per 811 viable Chinese pregnancies and more frequently in the Indian and Eurasian population. However, there was no Caucasian patient in the entire 11-year period of their study. HM was found to be twice as common among Eurasians in Singapore as among Chinese and Malays[20]. There were considerable differences between provinces in China[8].

3.5.4 GENETIC FACTORS

The importance of genetic factors in the etiology of HM is exemplified by several observations. Some aspects of the wide variations in incidence seen between the different populations reported above may be due to genetic differences. The high incidence of HM and other trophoblastic tumors in certain areas, such as Indonesia, Taiwan, the Philippines and the East, was considered to be due to inbreeding[39]. Further, the risk of recurrence of HM in a subsequent pregnancy is 0.6–3%[15,35,40], which is similar to some polygenic conditions. The occurrence of recurrent HM in female siblings in a case report of three families[41] indicates that the proposed defect in the ovum could be due to a mutant gene. The ABO blood groups of patients and their husbands have not been found to be different from the normal population studied[42]. In one investigation[43] of women with HM in Japan, the frequency of Rh negative type was significantly lower than that of the general population. Cytogenetic studies in two series[19,44] gave a frequency of balanced translocations in women with CHM of 4.6% compared with a frequency of 0.6% for normal populations. It is possible that in women carrying a balanced translocation the chance of meiosis being disturbed is increased, so that empty or inactivated eggs may be more likely in these patients.

Karyotyping of the molar tissues has revealed most cases of PHM to have triploidy and trisomies[2,45], whereas CHM showed exclusively or predominantly a 46 XX female karyotype by Q polymorphism[19,46]. Some CHMs are the result of doubling of a haploid sperm, in which case they are genetically homozygous. Less commonly, CHM may be genetically heterozygous, resulting from the fertilization of an anucleate ovum (empty egg) by two sperms. This basic classification explains the majority of all CHMs. It is now possible to classify HMs accurately into PHM and CHM, and to subclassify CHM genetically into monospermic or dispermic variants by using the polymerase chain reaction with primers for a variable number of tandem repeat sequences and the Y chromosome-specific sequences[47].

3.5.5 FAMILIAL OCCURRENCE AND CLUSTERING

There are several reports of the influence of consanguinity, or family history, on the incidence of mole[5]. One study reported three families in India each having two or more sisters with HM in one or more pregnancies[41]. La Vecchia *et al.*[29] reported that among patients with molar pregnancy in Italy there was a history of HM in four of 100 relatives of the woman (three CHM, one CC) and in one of 100 relatives of the father (CHM) compared with no family history among 200 age-matched controls. There have been numerous reports of recurrent moles in single individuals, but very few reports of familial occurrence of molar pregnancies.

3.5.6 DIET AND NUTRITION

The information is inconclusive and is inextricably linked to socioeconomic status, and to geography. Although a dietary etiology for HM has been widely discussed, evidence supporting this hypothesis is weak. Early reports from the Philippines[48], Mexico[49] and Taiwan[50] speculated that nutritional deficiencies may play a role in the higher incidence of HM in regions where malnutrition was common. One laboratory study of 25 women with HM attempted to evaluate this hypothesis and it was observed that the serum albumin and total protein were significantly decreased compared with controls[51]. Two reports, however, from Hawaii[52] and on native Alaskans whose diet is high in animal protein[53] failed to find an association between HM and diet. Most recently, Berkowitz *et al.*[31] reported that dietary carotene above the median level of consumption in the control group appeared to reduce the risk of CHM (relative risk 0.6; $p = 0.02$). In the study of Parazzini *et al.*[54] there was also an inverse relation between HM and certain foods such as carotene. A significant trend for decreasing risk with increasing consumption of carotene and animal fat was noted. In contrast, recent studies have found no association with food intake of vitamin A or any other food (for example, the case–control study from China[30]).

3.5.7 ENVIRONMENTAL FACTORS

As yet no definite specific etiological factors have related GTD with environment. However, increasing attention has recently focused for the first time on several possible environmental agents as risk factors for HM.

Cigarette smoking

Cigarette smoking has been linked in some studies with increased risk of HM. Parazzini *et al.*[37] found a relative risk ratio (for CHM) of 2.6 in women who smoked less than 15 cigarettes and 2.2 for women who smoked more than 15 cigarettes a day. Berkowitz *et al.*[31] found no significant association. Surprisingly, cigarette smoking has been examined in only a few recent studies. La Vecchia *et al.*[29] found that duration of smoking was positively associated with increased risk. Compared with women who never smoked the increased risk of HM was 1.3 for women smoking ≤5 years, 2.3 for 5–9 years and 4.2 for ≥10 years. However, there was no association in other studies on the risk for smoking before or during the pregnancy[14,27,30,31].

Oral contraception and intrauterine contraceptive devices

There is conflicting evidence on the relationship between oral contraceptives and/or intrauterine contraceptive devices (IUCDs) before pregnancy and risk of HM. Past use of oral contraceptives was associated with an increased risk of HM in the study from China; the relative risk for four or more years of use was 2.6, and there was a significant trend of increasing risk according to years of use[30]. Palmer[55] found a six-fold increased risk of choriocarcinoma in women who had taken oral contraceptives for more than five years. However, no such association was found for invasive mole and CHM in the same study (whether this is due to the therapy, or an association with the underlying difficulty in conceiving as found by La Vecchia[29], or is just a chance finding is unclear). Previous use of an IUCD was significantly associated with HM in the Italian study[29] but less strongly related in that by Berkowitz *et al.*[31] and unrelated in the Baltimore study[27]. Two of 129 daughters of mothers who used diethylstilbestrol (DES) in pregnancy developed HM. The incidence (15.5 per 1000 pregnancies) is very high but is based on only two exposed cases and merits further study. Another study found no relation to DES exposure[27]. Such factors can be considered with maternal age and related only coincidentally.

Other environmental factors

Constakle and Hatch[56] have recently reviewed several studies from Southeast Asia which address the question of whether exposure to herbicides (including agent orange) is associated with an increased risk of HM. Two studies from South Vietnam provided rates of HM (and CC) seen in patients at the Gynaeco-Obstetrical Hospital of Ho Chi Minh City. The rate of HM and CC changed from 8.61 per 1000 pregnancies in 1952 to 8.7 in 1971, after which it rose to 45.4 in 1979, declining only slightly in the following two years. If herbicides were to influence directly the development of HM one would expect the epidemic and spraying to be more closely linked in time. Another hypothesis is that herbicides enter the food chain and take several years to affect reproductive processes. However, maternal age, parity and other important variables were not controlled. In Chinese women, on the other hand, usage of herbal medicine during the first trimester brought an increased risk of developing CHM. A report from Japan on an ecological investigation of exposure to ionizing radiation from 1974 to 1976 and the incidence of GTD raises the hypothesis that ionizing radiation may have a causal role[57]. Such studies have problems in method of study and interpretation of the results, but they seem to indicate that environmental factors are involved. Such risk factors acting at the perifertilization state could cause abnormal gametogenesis, to induce CHM or PHM.

3.6 RELATIVE RISK (ODDS RATIO) FOR CHM AND PHM

Many reports suggest that complete mole and partial mole share several epidemiological features. A number of sociodemographic factors identified as possible risk factors of GTD indicate similar risks for PHM and CHM where these conditions have been studied separately[54a]. In comparison with women who had had normal obstetric histories for both, the risk was elevated in nulliparous or low-parity women and in those reporting a personal history of infertility problems, spontaneous miscarriages, previous GTD or a family history of GTD.

Odds ratios were elevated for both histopathological subgroups in smokers; high educational level and maternal AB or A blood groups were associated respectively with an increased risk of PHM and CHM. No relationship emerged between the risk of either complete mole or partial mode and induced abortion, age at first pregnancy or alcohol consumption (Table 3.3). It is conceivable that more educated and probably more health-aware women tend to have a partial mole diagnosed more frequently after spontaneous abortion or to be referred for follow-up in specialist centers. Several identified risk factors, i.e. maternal age, ethnicity and genetic factors, for GTD were confirmed in many studies, providing more precise estimates of risks. Although absolute numbers are too limited for formal statistical evaluation or inference on the differences between the two histological entities, analysis suggests some similarities in the epidemiol-

Table 3.3 Corresponding relative risks of various factors reported to correlate with molar pregnancy occurrence

	Odds ratio	
Factors	*Complete mole*	*Partial mole*
Maternal age		
<20 year	1.5	
≥40 year	5.2	
Reproductive history		
Parity at conception		
0	0.9	0.7
≥3	0.8	0.5
Spontaneous miscarriages		
≥2	1.5–3.1	1.9
Infertility problems		
Yes	2.4–3.7	3.2
Contraception		
Oral pill user	1.1–2.6	
IUCD user	1.7–3.7	
Age of first pregnancy		
≥25	0.6	1.3
Molar pregnancy history		
Yes	16.0	
Family history		
Spontaneous abortion		
Yes	1.5	
Sociodemographic and lifestyle		
Education (year)		
≥12	0.9–2.1	2.1
Marital status		
Never married	2.1	2.1
Smoking		
Ex-smokers	1.1	0.7
Current smokers		
≥15 cigarettes per day	2.2	1.8
Alcohol consumption		
<2 drinks	2.1	1.4
ABO		
Maternal blood		
AB	2.1	1.2
A	1.7	0.9
Patient A/husband O	1.9	
Nutrition		
Vitamin A in diet above control median	0.6	

Source: Grimes [3], Matsuura *et al.* [26], Olesnicky and Quinn [38], Messerli *et al.* [27], La Vecchia *et al.* [29], Berkowitz *et al.* [31], Bracken [5], Brinton *et al.* [30].

ogy of complete and partial mole[37]. However, while maternal age is well recognized as a risk factor for CHM, it was not a risk factor for PHM[37].

3.7 RISK FACTORS FOR GTT (CC)

The majority of CCs derive from antecedent HM. However, CC can of course be associated with term delivery, stillbirth or spontaneous abortion. Choriocarcinoma has been reported to occur 1000 times more frequently after CHM than after normal pregnancy. The risk of CC transformation is much higher after CHM than after PHM. The clinically important factors are how such pregnancies occur and how malignant transformation after normal pregnancy can occur, but the etiological factors are still unknown.

3.7.1 AGE

The median age for women with CC is generally somewhat higher than that for normal pregnancy. Some reports[20] described slightly higher rates of CC for teenagers than for women aged 20–40 years, while others noted lower rates. As with HM, older women account for a minority of cases of CC due to their low fertility. The potential effect of the age of the father is unknown.

3.7.2 ETHNICITY

Little information is available on ethnic variability. In the Singapore study[20] the incidence was highest in Malaysians compared with other ethnic groups, but the data were rather inadequate, so that no definite conclusions could be drawn.

3.7.3 REPRODUCTIVE AND OBSTETRIC HISTORY

The data concerning the effect of gravidity, independent of age, are inadequate and no firm conclusions can be drawn. Bad obstetric histories with increased fetal wastage have been reported as increasing the risk of GTT[58,59]. It was found that the risk of GTT was 21, 31 and 34 times higher for women with one, two and three or more fetal losses, respectively, than those whose known pregnancies all ended in live births[58].

The higher proportion of CC following HM could be attributable either to the high incidence of HM in some countries or to a higher percentage of HM patients in those countries developing CC. The percentage of cases of CC preceded by HM ranges from 39%[58] to 83%[60] in reports published since 1960. Since HM is an uncommon pregnancy outcome, the high percentage of cases of choriocarcinoma which follow HM indicates that HM is a powerful risk factor for CC. One review reported that the risk of a woman with HM developing CC ranged from 2% to 25% in different studies[25] although it is doubtful if it even exceeds 5%[61].

3.7.4 OTHER FACTORS

Palmer[55] found a six-fold increased risk of CC in women who had taken oral contraceptives for more than five years, but no such association with HM in the same study. Based on the result of their case–control study, Buckley *et al.*[62] suggested that below-normal estrogen levels may predispose to CC. They proposed two different mechanisms that may explain the results: hormonal changes that may effect oocyte development, and low oestrogen levels that may be the result of an ovarian abnormality.

3.7.5 GENETIC FACTORS

As HM has been separated into two clinical and genetic entities (CHM and PHM), the incidence of developing GTT following the two separate pathological entities is also different. The incidence of GTT following a CHM is 2–20%[15], while GTT following

PHM is probably of the order of 0.5%. The variable genetic constitution of HM does make it possible to identify HM and distinguish between a PHM, a monospermic CHM and a dispermic CHM by using genetic analysis techniques such as cytogenetic polymorphism, enzyme polymorphism and restriction fragment length polymorphisms of DNA, and more recently polymerase chain reaction. The relative risk of a dispermic or a monospermic CHM progressing to a GTT has yet to be established, although it has been suggested that the dispermic CHM may have a higher malignancy potential[63].

3.7.6 MATERNAL AND PATERNAL BLOOD GROUP

Maternal blood groups of the mother and her consort have been studied but the data are inconclusive.

ABO group

Blood group A women with incompatible blood group consorts appear to have a higher risk of CC. Data from the USA[64] and the UK[42] for patients with CC showed a slight excess in group A above group O. The UK data suggested that the risk of a woman getting CC is also influenced by the blood group of her husband, and the effect was most marked in cases where CC was preceded by term delivery[42].

In a UK series of 115 patients with CC following term pregnancy or non-molar abortions at Charing Cross Hospital, for whom mating types were available, the ratio of incompatible/compatible matings was 2.19, indicating a predisposition to CC in the incompatible matings[22]. It is important that more large studies on blood group data should be done worldwide.

HLA types

Data are available on patients and husbands in a series treated for GTT. The overall frequencies of the HLA-A and HLA-B locus antigens in 225 Caucasian patients did not differ significantly from those of the normal control population[65]. However, the degree of incompatibility between husband and wife, as measured by the number of antigenic incompatibilities (0, 1 or 2), indicates that there is a trend for patients who are more compatible with their husbands for the B locus antigens to fall into the higher-risk treatment categories. Consanguinity as a risk factor will require evaluation in large-scale studies with modern cytogenetic techniques.

3.8 SUMMARY

Gestational trophoblastic disease is still an important reproductive health problem worldwide. The problem is that much information on GTD has come from less developed countries, where proper diagnostic tools and up-to-date treatment cannot be employed. Specifically, the incidence of HM and CC appears to be about twice as high in Japan and other Asian countries than in Western countries. Maternal age, previous HM, race and geographic region have been identified as clear risk factors for GTD. Etiological factors of GTD have long been studied but no definite causes have yet been found. However, it can be speculated that, during gametogenesis and fertilization, the risk factors may act synergistically. Genetic subclassification may be helpful in this context. Geographic variations of incidence exist but are inextricably linked with above-mentioned risk factors. Important prerequisites for accurate evaluation are common denominators, standard classification and definition of index cases, and same-study methodology. Further investigations on possible etiological factors based on case–control studies in different geographic settings are essential.

REFERENCES

1. WHO Scientific Group (1983) Gestational Trophoblastic Disease. *WHO Tech. Rep. Ser.*, **692**, 37.
2. Szulman, A.E. and Surti, U. (1978) The syndrome of hydatidiform H-mole: morphologic evolution of the complete and partial mole. *Am. J. Obstet. Gynecol.*, **132**, 20–7.
3. Grimes, D.A. (1984) Epidemiology of gestational trophoblastic disease. *Am. J. Obstet. Gynecol.*, **150**, 309–418.
4. Flam, F. and Rutgvist, L.E. (1992) Under registration of gestational trophoblastic disease in the Swedish Cancer Registry. *Eur. J. Epidemiol.*, **8**, 683–6.
5. Bracken, M.B. (1987) Incidence and aetiology of hydatidiform mole: an epidemiological review. *Br. J. Obstet. Gynaecol.* **94**, 1123–35.
6. Palmer, J.R. (1994) Advances in the epidemiology of gestational trophoblastic disease. *J. Reprod. Med.*, **39**, 155–62.
7. National Co-ordination Research Group of Chorioma (1980) Incidence of hydatidiform mole (a retrograde study of 2, 023, 621 women in 23 provinces). *Zhongua Yizne Zazhi*, **60**, 641–4.
8. Song, H. and Wu, P. (1987) Hydatidiform mole in China: a preliminary survey of incidence in more than three million women. *Bull. WHO*, **65**, 507.
9. Takeuchi, S. (1984) Incidence of gestational trophoblastic disease by regional registration in Japan. *Hum. Reprod.*, **2**, 729–34.
10. Rolon, P.A. and de Lopez, B.H. (1977) Epidemiologic aspects of hydatidiform mole in the Republic of Paraguay (South America). *Br. J. Obstet. Gynaecol.*, **84**, 862–4.
11. Marquez-Monter, H., de la Vega, G.A., Ridaura, C. and Röbles, M. (1968) Gestational choriocarcinoma in the general hospital of Mexico: analysis of forty cases. *Cancer*, **22**, 91–8
12. Hayashi, K., Bracken, M.B., Freeman, D.H., Jr and Hellenbrand, K. (1982) Hydatidiform mole in the United States (1970–1977): a statistical and theoretical analysis. *Am. J. Epidemiol.*, **115**, 67–77.
13. Bagshawe, K.D. and Dent, J. (1986) Hydatidiform mole in England and Wales 1973–1983. *Lancet*, **ii**, 673–7.
14. Yen, S. and MacMahon, B. (1968) Epidemiologic features of trophoblastic disease. *Am. J. Obstet. Gynecol.*, **101**, 126–32.
15. Matalon, M. and Modan, B. (1972) Epidemiologic aspects of hydatidiform mole in Israel. *Am. J. Obstet. Gynecol.*, **112**, 107-12.
16. Nielsen, N.H. and Hansen, J.P.H. (1979) Trophoblastic tumors in Greenland. *J. Cancer Res. Clin. Oncol.*, **95**, 177–86.

16a. Takeuchi, S. (1987) *Incidence of Hydatidiform Mole in Japan* (Abstract). Second World Congress in Trophoblastic Neoplasms, Singapore, p. 11.

17. Okudaira, Y. and Strauss, L. (1967) Ultrastructure of molar trophoblast: observations on hydatidiform mole and chorioadenoma destruens. *Obstet. Gynecol.*, **30**, 172–87.
18. Notake, Y. (1963) *Atlas of Tissue Culture in Obstetrics and Gynaecology*, Japan Obstetrics and Gynaecology Society, Tokyo.
19. Kajii, T. and Ohama, K. (1977) Androgenetic origin of hydatidiform mole. *Nature*, **268**, 633–4.
20. Teoh, E.S., Dawood, M.Y. and Ratnam, S.S. (1971) Epidemiology of hydatidiform mole in Singapore. *Am. J. Obstet. Gynecol.*, **110**, 415–20.
21. Stone, M., Dent, J., Kardana, A. and Bagshawe, K.D. (1976) Relationship of oral contraception to development of trophoblastic tumor after evacation of a hydatidiform mole. *Br. J. Obstet. Gynaecol.*, **83**, 913.
22. Bagshawe, K.D. and Lawler, S.D. (1982) Choriocarcinoma, in *Cancer Epidemiology and Prevention* (eds D. Schottenfeld and J.F. Fraumeni), Saunders, Philadelphia, pp. 909–24.
23. Song, H., Wu, B., Tang, M. and Wang, Y. (1981) *Trophoblastic Tumors: Diagnosis and Management*, Capital Hospital, Beijing, China.
24. Nakano, R., Sasaki, K., Yamoto, M. and Hata, H. (1980) Trophoblastic disease: analysis of 342 patients. *Gynecol. Obstet. Invest.*, **11**, 237–42.
25. Kim, S.J. (1995) Clinical management of benign and malignant trophoblastic disease in North-East Asia. *Curr. Obstet. Gynecol.*, **5**, 13–18.
26. Matsuura, J., Chiu, D., Jacobs, P.A. and Szulman, A.E. (1984) Complete hydatidiform

mole in Hawaii: an epidemiological study. *Genet. Epidemiol.*, **1**, 271.

27. Messerli, M.L., Lilienfeld, A.M., Parmley, T. *et al.* (1985) Risk factors for gestational trophoblastic neoplasia. *Am. J. Obstet. Gynecol.*, **153**, 294.
28. Sasaki, K., Yamoto, M., Hata, H. and Nakano, R. (1979) The relationship between maternal aging and the incidence of hydatidiform mole and malignant changes. *Acta Obstet. Gynecol. Jpn.*, **31**, 292–6.
29. La Vecchia, C.L., Franceschi, S., Parazzini, F. *et al.* (1985) Risk factors for gestational trophoblastic disease in Italy. *Am. J. Epidemiol.*, **121**, 457–64.
30. Brinton, L.A., Wu, B.Z., Wang, W. *et al.* (1989) Gestational trophoblastic disease: a case control study from the People's Republic of China. *Am. J. Obstet. Gynecol.* **161**, 121–7.
31. Berkowitz, R.S., Cramer, D.W., Berstein, M.R. *et al.* (1985) Risk factors for complete molar pregnancy from a case control study. *Am. J. Obstet. Gynecol.*, **152**, 1016–20.
32. Sand, P.K., Lurain, J.R. and Brewer, J.I. (1984) Repeat gestational trophoblastic disease. *Obstet. Gynecol.*, **63**, 140–4.
33. Bagshawe, K.D. (1969) *Choriocarcinoma.* Clowes, London.
34. Federschneider, J.M., Goldstein, D.P., Berkowitz, R.S. *et al.* (1980) Natural history of recurrent molar pregnancy. *Obstet. Gynecol.*, **55**, 457.
35. Kim, S.J. (1982) Difficult cases of trophoblastic disease and its classification and management. *Semin. Oncol.*, **9**, 234–8.
36. De George, F.V. (1981) Hydatidiform mole in other pregnancies of mothers of twins. *Am. J. Obstet. Gynecol.*, **108**, 369–71.
37. Parazzini, F., La Vecchia, C., Pampallona, S. and Francheschi, S. (1985) Reproductive patterns and the risk of gestational trophoblastic disease. *Am. J. Obstet. Gynecol.*, **152**, 866.
38. Olesnicky, G. and Quinn, M. (1984) Molar pregnancy after artificial insemination (donor). *Lancet*, **ii**, 1296.
39. Parsons, L. and Sommers, S.C. (1978) *Genetics of Hydatidiform Mole. Trophoblastic Disease. Gynecology*, 2nd Edn., Saunders, Philadelphia, pp. 534–5.
40. Chun, D., Braga, C., Chow, C. and Lok, L. (1964) Clinical observations on some aspects of hydatidiform moles. *J. Obstet. Gynec. Br. Commonw.*, **71**, 180–4
41. Ambani, L.M., Vaidya, R.A., Rao, C.S. *et al.* (1980) Familial occurrence of trophoblastic disease: report of recurrent molar pregnancies in sisters in three families. *Clin. Genet.*, **18**, 27–9.
42. Bagshawe, K.D., Rawlins, G., Pike, M.C. and Lawler, S.D. (1971) ABO blood-groups in trophoblastic neoplasia. *Lancet*, **i**, 553–6.
43. Tomoda, Y. *et al* (1981) Rh-D factor in trophoblastic tumor: a possible cause of high incidence in Asia. *Am. J. Obstet. Gynecol.*, **139**, 742–4.
44. Lawler, S.D., Fisher, R.A., Pickthall, V.J. *et al.* (1982) Genetic studies on hydatidiform moles: I. The origin of partial moles. *Cancer Genet. Cytogenet.*, **5**, 309–20.
45. Vassilakos, P., Riotton, G. and Kajii, T. (1977) Hydatidiform mole: two entities. A morphologic and cytogenetic study with some clinical considerations. *Am. J. Obstet. Gynecol.*, **127**, 167–70.
46. Wake, N., Takagi, N. and Sasaki, M. (1978) Androgenesis as a cause of hydatidiform mole. *J. Natl. Cancer Inst.*, **60**, 51–3.
47. Fisher, R.A. and Newlands, E.S. (1993) Rapid diagnosis and classification of hydatidiform moles with polymerase chain reaction. *Am. J. Obstet. Gynecol.*, **168**, 563–9.
48. Acosta-Sison, H. (1959) Observation which may indicate the etiology of hydatidiform mole and explain its high incidence in the Philippines and Asiatic countries. *Philippines J. Surg.* **14**, 209–97.
49. Marquez-Monter, H., Alfara de la Vega, G., Robles, M. and Bolio-Cicero, A. (1963) *Am. J. Obstet. Gynecol.*, **85**, 856.
50. Hsu, C., Chen, T.Y., Chiu, W.H. *et al.* (1964) Some aspects of trophoblastic disease peculiar to Taiwan. *Am. J. Obstet. Gynecol.*, **92**, 308–16.
51. Pour-Reza, M. *et al.* (1974) Serum creatine, urea and protein level changes in hydatidiform mole. *JAMA*, **230**, 580–1.
52. McCorriston, C.C. (1968) Racial incidence of hydatidiform mole. *Am. J. Obstet. Gynecol.*, **101**, 377–82.
53. Martin, P.M. (1978) High frequency of hydatidiform mole in native Alaskans. *Int. J. Gynaecol. Obstet.*, **15**, 395–6.

54. Parazzini, F., La Vecchia, C., Mangili, G. *et al.* (1988) Dietary factors and the risk of trophoblastic disease. *Am. J. Obstet. Gynecol.*, **158**, 93–9.

54a. Parazzini, F., Nangili, G., La Vecchia, C. *et al.* (1991) Risk factors for gestational trophoblastic disease: a separate analysis of complete and partial hydatidiform moles. *Obstet. Gynecol.*, **78**, 1039–45.

55. Palmer, J.R. (1991) Oral contraceptive use and gestational choriocarcinoma. *Cancer Detect. Prev.*, **15**, 45–8.

56. Constakle, J.D. and Hatch, M.C. (1985) Reproductive effects of herbicide exposure in Vietnam: recent studies by the Vietnamese and others. *Teratogenesis Carcinog. Mutagen.*, **5**, 231-50.

57. Ujeno, Y. (1985) Epidemiological studies of human fetal development in area with various doses of natural background radiation. *Arch. Environ. Health*, **40**, 181.

58. Baltazar, J.C. (1976) Epidemiologic features of choriocarcinoma. *Bull. WHO*, **54**, 523–32.

59. Walden, P.A. and Bagshawe, K.E. (1976) Reproductive performance in women successfully treated for gestational trophoblastic tumors. *Am. J. Obstet. Gynecol.*, **125**, 1108–14.

60. Paradinas, F.J. (1992) The histological diagnosis of hydatidiform mole. *Curr. Diagn. Pathol.*, **1**, 24–31.

61. Park, W.W. and Lee, J.C. (1950) Choriocarcinoma: a general review with analysis of 516 cases. *Arch. Pathol.*, **49**, 73–104, 205–41, 361.

62. Buckley, J.D., Henderson, B.E., Morrow, C.P. *et al.* (1988) Case-control study of gestational choriocarcinoma. *Cancer Res.*, **48**, 1004.

63. Cho, S. and Kim, S.J. (1993) Genetic study of hydatidiform moles by restriction fragment length polymorphisms (RFLPs) analysis. *J. Korean Med. Sci.*, **8**, 446–52.

64. Scott, J.S. (1962) Choriocarcinoma: observation on etiology. *Am. J. Obstet. Gynecol.*, **183**, 185–93.

65. Lawler, S.D. (1978) HLA and trophoblastic tumors. *Brit. Med. Bull.*, **34**, 305–8.

66. Yuen, B.H. and Cannon, W. (1981) Molar pregnancy in British Columbia: estimated incidence and post-evacuation regression patterns of the beta subunit of human chorionic gonadotrophin. *Am. J. Obstet. Gynecol.*, **139**, 316–19.

67. Takeuchi, S. (1987) *Incidence of Hydatidiform Mole in Japan* (Abstract). Second World Congress on Trophoblastic Neoplasms, Singapore, p. 11.

68. Mazzann, P., La Vecchi, C., Parazzini, F. *et al.* (1986) Frequency of hydatidiform mole in Lombardy, Northern Italy. *Gynecol. Oncol.*, **24**, 337–9.

69. Franke, H.R., Risse, E.K.J., Kenemans, P. *et al.* (1983) Epidemiologic features of hydatidiform mole in the Netherlands. *Obstet. Gynecol.*, **62**, 613–16.

70. Graham, I.H. and Fajardo, A.M. (1988) The incidence and morphology of hydatidiform mole in Abu Dhabi, United Arab Emirates 1978–1986. *Br. J. Obstet. Gynaecol.*, **95**, 391–5.

71. Ogunbode, O. (1978) Benign hydatidiform mole in Ibadan, Nigeria. *Int. J. Gynaecol. Obstet.*, **15**, 387–90.

72. Leighton, P.D. (1973) Trophoblastic disease in Uganda. *Am. J. Obstet. Gynecol.*, **117**, 341–4.

73. Jacobs, P.A., Szulman, A.E., Funkhouser, J. *et al.* (1982) Human triploidy: relationship between parental origin of the additional haploid complement and development of partial hydatidiform mole. *Ann. Hum. Genet.*, **46**, 223–31.

74. Wei, P.N. and Ouyang, P.C. (1963) Trophoblastic disease in Taiwan: a review of 157 cases in a 10 year period. *Am. J. Obstet. Gynecol.*, **85**, 844.

75. Kim, S.J. (1985) Gestational trophoblastic disease in Korea. *Korean J. Obstet. Gynecol.*, **28**, 1–17.

76. Poen, H.T. and Djojopranoto, M. (1965) The possible etiologic factors of hydatidiform mole and choriocarcinoma: preliminary report. *Am. J. Obstet. Gynecol.*, **92**, 510–13.

77. Ong, H.D., Lee, P.Y., Ng, T.K.F. and Chong, C.H. (1978) Clinical observation of hydatidiform mole in a Malaysian hospital. *Singapore Med. J.*, **19**, 33–6.

78. Javey, H. and Sajadi, H. (1978) Hydatidiform mole in southern Iran: a statistical survey of 113 cases. *Int. J. Gynaecol. Obstet.*, **15**, 390–4.

79. Di Fabio, C. and De Aloysio, D. (1976) Valutazione statistica di alcuri dati epidemiologici concernenti la mola indatea. *Riv. Ital. Ginecol.*, **57**, 187–93.

80. Steigrad, S.J. (1969) The incidence of neoplas-

tic trophoblastic disease in Australia. *Aust. NZ J. Obstet. Gynaecol.*, **9**, 100–2.

81. Sengupta, B.S., Persaud, V. and Wynter, H.N. (1977) Choriocarcinoma in Jamaica. *Int. Surg.*, **62**, 84–7.
82. Brisson, J. and Fabia, J. (1976) Incidence de la mole hydatidiforme et des maladies trophoblastique dans l'est du Quebec, 1969-1973. *Union Med. Can.*, **105**, 1238–40.
83. Ringertz, N. (1970) Hydatidiform mole, invasive mole and choriocarcinoma in Sweden 1958–1965. *Acta Obstet. Gynecol. Scand.*, **49**, 195–203.
84. Ayangade, O. (1979) Gestational trophoblastic disease in Nigeria: a 10 year review. *East Afr. Med. J.*, **56**, 278–82.
85. MacGregor, C., Ontiveros, E.C., Vargas, E.L. and Valenzuela, S. (1969) Hydatidiform mole analysis of 145 patients. *Obstet. Gynecol.*, **33**, 343–51.
86. Brewer, J.I. and Gerbie, A.B. (1967) Early development of choriocarcinoma, in *Choriocarcinoma: Transactions of a Conference of the International Union Against Cancer* (eds J.F. Holland and M.D. Hreshchyshyn), Springer-Verlag, Berlin, pp. 45–53.
87. Chan, D.P. (1962) Chorion epithelioma: a study of 41 cases. *BMJ*, **2**, 953–6.
88. Pai, K.N. (1967) A study of choriocarcinoma: its incidence in India and its aetiopathogenesis, in *Choriocarcinoma: Transactions of a Conference of the International Union Against Cancer* (eds J.F. Holland and M.M. Hreshchyshyn), Springer-Verlag, Berlin, p. 54–7.
89. Acosta-Sison, J. (1967) The chance of malignancy in a repeated hydatidiform mole. *Am. J. Obstet. Gynecol.*, **78**, 876.
90. Srivannaboon, S. *et al.* (1974) The incidence of trophoblastic disease in Siriraj hospital. *J. Med. Assoc. Thai.*, **56**, 537–42.
91. Matalon, M., Paz, B., Modan, M. and Modan, B. (1972) Malignant trophoblastic disorders: epidemiologic aspects and relationship to hydatidiform mole. *Am. J. Obstet. Gynecol.*, **112**, 101–6.

PATHOLOGY 4

Fernando J. Paradinas

4.1 INTRODUCTION

Trophoblastic tumors are fetal allografts in maternal tissues and present unique biological, immunological and pathological problems. One of the main functions of trophoblast is to gain access to the maternal circulation, and normal trophoblast infiltrates, invades vessels and can even be transported to the lungs[1–3] in a fashion which is otherwise only seen in malignant neoplasms. Invasion and metastases are criteria used to diagnose malignancy in other neoplasms but are not usually applicable to trophoblast. In addition, trophoblastic tumors are relatively rare and unfamiliar to both physician and pathologist in non-specialized centers and the frequent difficulties and potential dangers of obtaining adequate samples from deeply invasive and hemorrhagic lesions can make pathological diagnosis difficult or impossible. These facts justify the well-established approach of treating patients on the basis of clinical criteria and serological human chorionic gonadotropin (hCG) estimations. It also means that some patients will be treated and cured without our ever knowing whether the disease treated was an invasive hydatidiform mole (IM) or a choriocarcinoma (CC). Terms such as gestational trophoblastic disease (GTD) and persistent trophoblastic disease (PTD) accurately describe this situation[4, 5].

The increasing use of ultrasound in the diagnosis and management of abnormal pregnancies has resulted in earlier evacuation of moles[6,7] and earlier chemotherapy in PTD[5]. Early evacuation has meant a decrease in the number of molar pregnancies which present with the symptoms and signs of overgrowth of trophoblast and excessive hCG secretion, such as uterine size larger than dates, hyperemesis, toxemia or hyperthyroidism[8,9], and most complete hydatidiform moles (CHMs) present nowadays as abortions or terminations of abnormal anembryonic pregnancies towards the end of the first trimester in which a mole may or may not be suspected and when pathological criteria useful to diagnose older CHMs are no longer valid[6,7]. The success of chemotherapy has resulted in a marked reduction in the number of pathological specimens available for study and few pathologists can today claim to have seen an IM or a CC in a hysterectomy specimen. However, the aggressive behavior of trophoblastic tumors unchecked by chemotherapy is well known from earlier accounts[10–16]. In recent years, genetic studies have provided us with additional

Gestational Trophoblastic Disease.
Edited by B.W. Hancock, E.S. Newlands and R.S. Berkowitz.
ISBN 0 412 63100 8

information which has helped both to understand the nature of these abnormalities and to test and improve the morphological criteria which have so far been the basis of pathological diagnosis.

4.2 NORMAL TROPHOBLAST

Two morphologically distinct trophoblastic populations are seen at the implantation site: villous and extravillous trophoblast. Villous trophoblast covers chorionic villi (Figure 4.1) and consists of cytotrophoblast and syncytiotrophoblast. The rather primitive mononuclear cytotrophoblastic cells have a clear cytoplasm (which reflects their paucity of cellular organelles) and a high mitotic rate. They usually express cytokeratins but produce little or no hormones. Syncytiotrophoblast differentiates from cytotrophoblast and is composed of multinucleated cells with abundant dense cytoplasm. It secretes abundant hCG, some human placental lactogen (hPL) and placental alkaline phosphatase (PLAP) but has little capacity for further proliferation. Production of hCG decreases while hPL and PLAP increase as pregnancy advances[17] and the amounts of villous trophoblast in relation to the amounts of villous stroma (Figure 4.1) gradually decrease with increasing gestational age[18]. Trophoblast also synthesizes estrogen and progesterone[19]. Extravillous trophoblast forms trophoblastic columns in intervillous spaces and infiltrates decidua, spiral arteries and myometrium at the placental bed (placental site trophoblast or PST). It is composed of mononuclear and multinucleated cells with a dense eosinophilic cytoplasm (Figure 4.2), morphologically different from villous cytotrophoblast and syncytiotrophoblast and defined immunocytochemically by positive staining for hPL and cytokeratins, but containing scanty hCG and PLAP. Modern techniques[17,20,21] have therefore resolved the argument about the origin of these

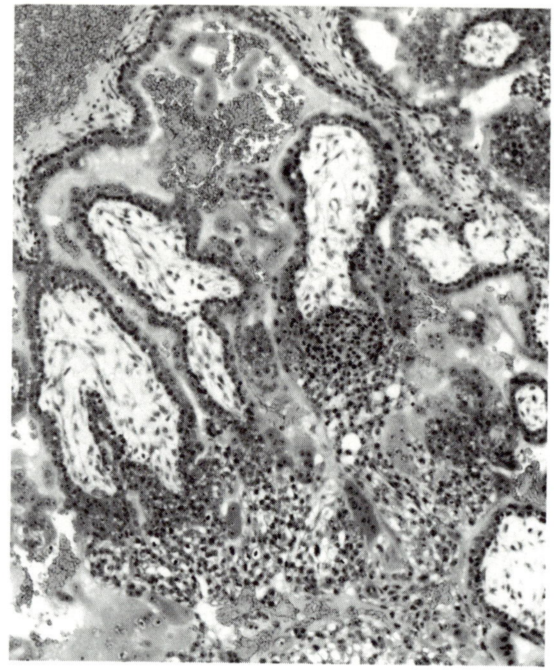

Figure 4.1 Villous trophoblast forming polar trophoblastic columns in early pregnancy. It consists of mononuclear cytotrophoblast and multinucleated syncytium. ×400.

cells[22,23] in favor of trophoblast and the term 'intermediate trophoblast' has been proposed. The functions and biological differences between the various types of trophoblast are under study and include the production of proteolytic enzymes which facilitate tissue invasion, thromboplastin and plasminogen activator, which control fibrin formation and may be important in maintaining vascular patency and expression of human lenkocyte antigen (HLA) type I, whose role in the success of the fetal allograft is still unknown[24–26].

4.3 CLASSIFICATION OF TROPHOBLASTIC LESIONS (TABLE 4.1)

The common pathology of these lesions is an excessive proliferation of trophoblast. In hydatidiform moles this essentially con-

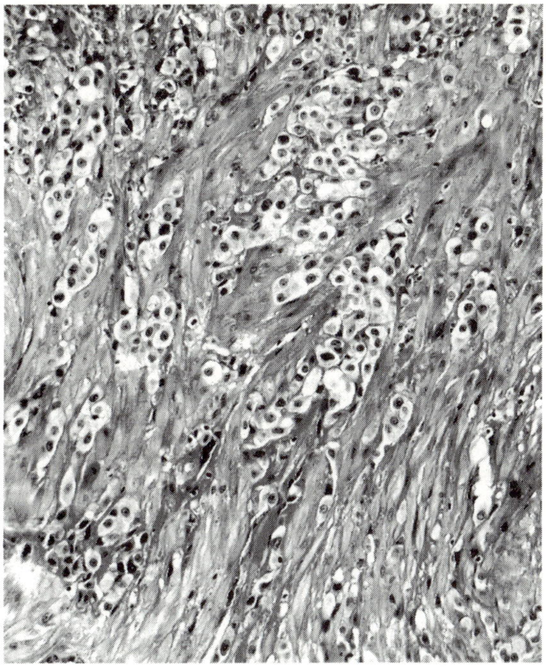

Figure 4.2 Placental site trophoblast infiltrating myometrium. In this area it is predominantly composed of mononuclear intermediate trophoblast. ×180.

sists of chorionic villi covered by villous trophoblast and variable amounts of intermediate trophoblast. This is known to occur in association with at least two distinct morphological and genetic abnormalities: CHM, a diploid, hyperdiploid or tetraploid conception in which all the nuclear genome is derived from the father[27,28]; and Partial Mole (PHM), a triploid and rarely tetraploid conception with at least two sets of paternal and one set of maternal chromosomes[29–31]. CHM is so named because when hydrops is fully developed it involves most or all the villi, whereas in fully developed PHM hydrops is characteristically focal. About 85% CHMs and 99% PHMs remit after one or more evacuations but a few can relentlessly progress, requiring chemotherapy. IM is usually a CHM and rarely a PHM which invades the myometrium and can even perforate the uterus.

In the typical and most common form of CC the tumor is composed predominantly of cells resembling villous cyto- and syncytiotrophoblast but, unlike in moles, there is no villous stroma. The tumor invades vessels and metastasizes in the most aggressive way, and without treatment the disease was nearly always fatal[13]. PST can also proliferate excessively. Exaggerated forms of placental site reaction may remit spontaneously or be cured by simple curettage, when the term placental site trophoblastic nodule (PSTN) or plaque has been used[32]. Rarely, they progress unchecked, invade adjacent organs and metastasize in a neoplastic fashion[33]; the term placental site trophoblastic tumor (PSTT) has been

Table 4.1 Abnormal trophoblastic proliferations

Abnormality	*Embryo*	*Hydrops*	*Trophoblast*
Of villous trophoblast			
Hydropic abortion	Yes	Mild	No excess
Partial hydatidiform mole (PHM)	Yes	Focal	Some excess
Complete and invasive HM (CHM)	No	Extensive	Marked excess
Choriocarcinoma	No	No villi	Neoplastic
Of placental site trophoblast			
Placental site trophoblastic nodule (PSTN)	No	No villi	Self-limiting
Placental site trophoblastic tumor (PSTT)	No	No villi	Neoplastic

generally accepted for this rare disease[34] which, being chemoresistant, is nowadays seen more often than typical CC in hysterectomy specimens.

4.4 MOLAR PREGNANCY

Hydatidiform moles were recognized by Greek and medieval physicians as abnormal conceptions[35–38] but the origin of CHMs from trophoblast was not generally accepted until the late nineteenth century. Observations in the ensuing 50 years culminated in the studies of Hertig[11,12,39], who regarded it as a disease which affected the conceptus in early gestation and which resulted, when fully developed, in a mass of hydropic chorionic villi and no fetus (Figure 4.3). He recognized a transitional mole (which he thought rare) in which hydrops was less extensive and a fetus was present (Figure 4.4). The term transitional implied an intermediate form between the fully developed classical mole and the frequent finding of microscopical hydrops in first-trimester abortions, which would then be the mildest expression of the disease when arrested in early pregnancy. The fact that classical moles were diagnosed and evacuated on average later than transitional moles and these later than hydropic abortions seemed to support this theory. Later studies, particularly by Park, emphasized that a common denominator to molar pregnancies was the excessive proliferation of trophoblast and dismissed hydropic placentas in which this was absent as malformations unrelated to classical mole[15]. Genetic studies in recent years have firmly established that CHM is almost always purely androgenetic, and transitional mole, now PHM, occurs when there are two or more paternally derived sets of chromosomes and at least one maternally derived set. First-trimester hydropic abortions (HA) are also often due to chromosomal abnormalities which include trisomies, monosomies, translocations and triploidy due to two maternal and one paternally derived set. Moles are therefore genetically determined and trophoblastic overgrowth in them appears associated with the presence of more than one paternal set of chromosomes, CHMs being diploid and PHMs triploid. In our experience exceptions to this rule are rare but diploid PHMs represent a significant proportion in many recent publications. The main reasons for this are probably pathological misdiagnoses due to the failure to update diagnostic criteria for the younger CHMs

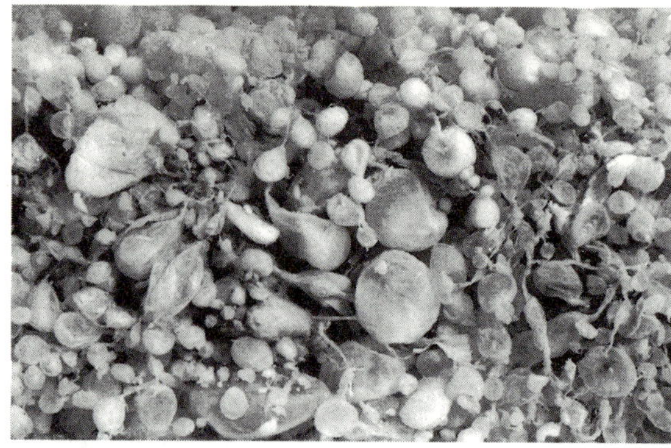

Figure 4.3 Complete mole evacuated in the second trimester. Hydropic change is generalized and no fetus is present (natural size).

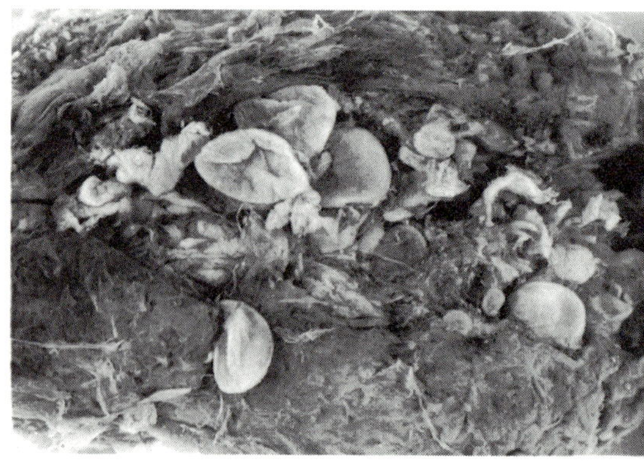

Figure 4.4 Partial mole evacuated in the second trimester. A malformed fetus was present and hydropic change involves only some of the villi (natural size).

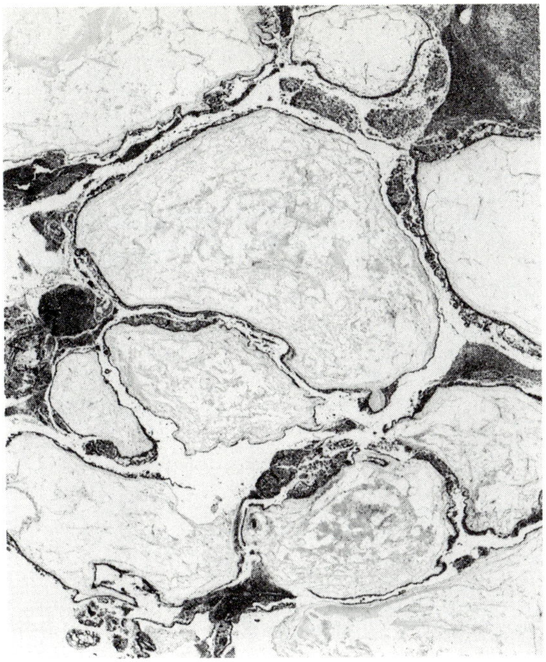

Figure 4.5 Hydrops and cistern formation in complete mole evacuated at 18 weeks gestation. Hydropic change is generalized and no residual vessels are present. ×20.

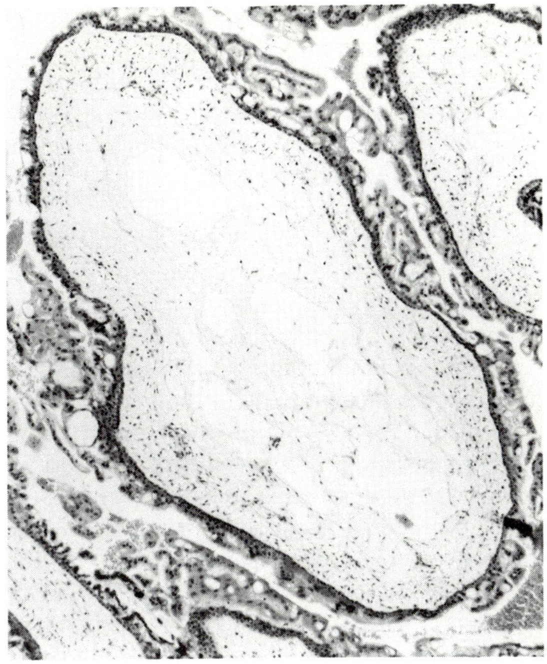

Figure 4.6 Complete mole. Fluid collects in the middle, forming cisterns, and the stroma is compressed against the trophoblastic layers which show circumferential hyperplasia. ×50.

seen nowadays and also to the morphological similarities between PHM and some trisomies which cause HA. Until better diagnostic criteria are generally applied, pathological diagnosis of moles and mole types will remain poor and much of the recently published genetic, flow cytometric clinical and prognostic data based on doubtful pathological diagnoses will also be of doubtful value. In the present account we have therefore made special emphasis on the pathological features which we and others have found useful in discriminating between the two types of mole and non-molar abortions.

4.5 COMPLETE HYDATIDIFORM MOLE

In the classical, fully developed CHM pathological examination shows swollen villi often completely surrounded by excessive circumferential villous trophoblast (Figure 4.5), in which nuclear pleomorphism is usually more intense than in normal pregnancy. Clusters of similar cyto- and syncytiotrophoblast and some intermediate trophoblast are often seen amongst villi. Fluid tends to collect in 'cisterns' in the middle of villi, resulting in compression of other components of villous stroma beneath the cytotrophoblastic layer (Figure 4.6), which shows few or no blood vessels, and this hydropic change tends to be generalized. This description is accurate for CHMs evacuated in the second trimester but CHMs are nowadays evacuated much earlier than before[7] at an average of 12 weeks gestational age (GA). The most useful features by which to recognize these young CHMs are as follows:

(a) Circumferential trophoblast excess is usually present and intense. Trophoblast excess is a constant finding in CHM when the sample is adequate and it is recognized by the presence of more than two layers of trophoblast forming sprouts or more extensive circumferential masses (Figure 4.7). Patients who eventually need chemotherapy have, on average, higher serum hCG values than those who do not[7] and, initially, Hertig[12,40] reported a direct correlation between more abundant and more pleomorphic trophoblast and a worse prognosis; this has not been confirmed by further studies[41–43] and is probably explained by the fact that excess trophoblast is only loosely attached to villi and the amounts in the sample may not be representative of the whole, or indeed, of what is left *in utero*. Serial hCG estimations are a better indication of what residual trophoblast is doing than any form of histological grading system, but although these have now been abandoned in specialized centers, claims to their value are published from time to time and some as recently as 1988[43]. In our experience, excess trophoblast is, if anything, easier to detect in younger than in older CHMs, since fully developed hydrops in older moles is sometimes associated with attenuation of trophoblastic layers. It is not unusual for older CHMs with hydrops and no detectable excess trophoblast in the sample to be misdiagnosed as HAs. This should not occur if it is remembered that in HA hydrops is usually microscopical and seldom exceeds 3 mm and, except in rare circumstances, molar pregnancy should be suspected when hydrops is intense or generalized even in the absence of excess trophoblast, which may not be present because of sampling error.

(b) Complete (generalized) hydrops is not fully developed in young CHMs. It is important to stress that complete hydrops, from which CHM derives its name and which results in the characteristic 'bunch of grapes' of classical mole (Figure 4.3) does not occur overnight. Time is required for this to happen and whereas most CHMs had generalized hydrops when they were evacuated at around 16–20 weeks GA, nowadays, with CHM evacuated on average at about 12 weeks, hydrops in most specimens is only partial. Many CHMs referred to our institution have been erroneously called PHMs initially on this account. With today's modern ultrasound techniques, it is not uncommon for anembryonic pregnancies to be terminated at six to eight weeks gestation and sometimes CHMs spontaneously abort about this time, when hydrops is inconspicuous, very focal or only microscopical (Figure 4.7). The pathological criteria for recognizing these

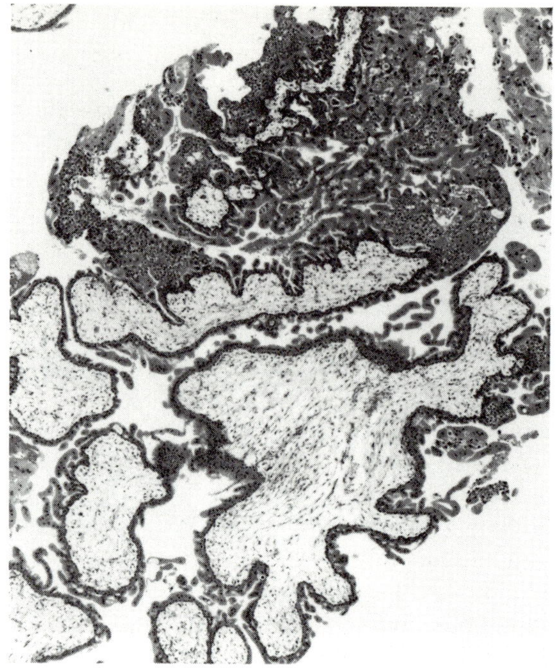

Figure 4.7 Complete mole evacuated at seven weeks gestation. There is budding of the trophoblastic layers mimicking the secondary villi of early placental development but excess trophoblast is present both on villi and between villi. These polyploid villi are very characteristic of young complete moles. Stromal vessels are a constant finding at this stage. ×70.

pregnancies as molar are already present in Szulman's publications[44,45], but without stressing enough their younger GA. However, a comparison between young and old CHMs is made by Kajii *et al.*[46] in a publication which is already 11 years old; we have been using these criteria for some 10 years and successfully separated CHMs with high risk and PHMs with low risk of GTD[7].

(c) In young CHM most villi have stromal blood vessels. The presence of vessels in CHM is a major source of diagnostic confusion. It is true to say that when CHMs were evacuated late, most had no vessels, although Elston found them in 16% of his material with an average GA of 17 weeks[47]. Indeed, Hertig believed that the lack of fetus and fetal vasculature was the main reason for the accumulation of fluid in molar villi. This view is no longer tenable and more modern publications describe the frequent presence of vessels in androgenetic CHMs, particularly young CHMs[6,7,44–46]. In our experience it is rare to see avascular CHMs before the 12th week of gestation[7]; in most cases the vessels are collapsed and empty, although occasionally they are open and rarely may contain nucleated red cells (see below for discussion of this unusual finding). Some textbooks and publications[48] still state that CHMs are avascular and many pathologists diagnose moles with vessels as PHMs when in fact they are seeing younger CHMs. In our experience whether a mole has vessels or not depends purely on its GA and – if a fetus is present – on the time lapsed since fetal death occurred. In a large study we found a higher proportion of avascular PHMs than avascular CHMs, reflecting the longer GA of PHMs[7].

(d) In CHM stromal karyorrhexis is very common before hydrops develops. Karyorrhexis (nuclear debris) in villous stroma of otherwise well-preserved villi is almost always seen in young CHMs in some villi before hydrops develops and is useful in diagnosis. This observation of Szulman[44, 45] is already incorporated in the diagnostic criteria of the WHO report on gestational trophoblastic diseases of 1983[4] but is not sufficiently stressed in later publications[26]. It should not be confused with cell necrosis in vessel walls, which is also common in PHMs and HAs after fetal death and it should not be considered in isolation as an absolute diagnostic criterion, since necrosis of stromal cells is possible in other circumstances but it is so common and intense in CHM and so rare and slight in PHM and HAs that its presence should make us think of the possibility of CHM, particularly when the material available is scanty and likely to be unrepresentative.

(e) Irregularly shaped villi with secondary budding (Figure 4.7) **are common and very characteristic of young CHMs.** The fact that in young CHMs cistern are rare and secondary villi sprout from primary villi in a fashion resembling that of early placentations is already mentioned by Szulman and Surti[44,45] and Kajii *et al.*[46]. Unlike in normal placentation, where villi are regular in size, radiate from a central cavity and have polar trophoblast, the secondary villi of CHM are irregular in size and distribution and have circumferential excess trophoblast. These irregular villi are often mistaken for the scalloped villi of a PHM and, although the differences between them are lengthy to describe, they can be readily appreciated by comparing Figure 4.7 with Figure 4.10 and 4.11.

(f) Transverse sectioning of irregular villi in CHM often results in oval or irregular pseudoinclusions of trophoblast (Figure 4.8). These are often cystic and large and very different from the more round inclusions seen in PHM (see Figure 4.11).

(g) The stroma of a CHM is usually mucoid and has little reticulin. There is no progressive fibrosis with increasing molar age. Before the development of hydrops, villous stroma in CHM contains only a little

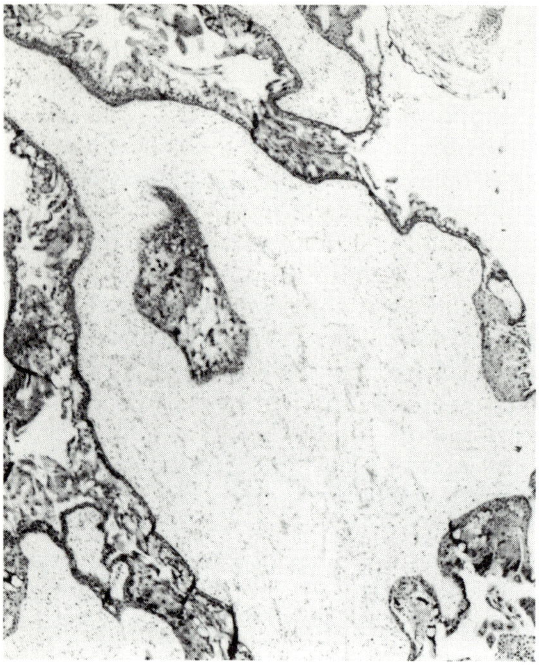

Figure 4.8 Irregular trophoblastic inclusion in complete mole. Trophoblastic invaginations often result in pseudoinclusions but these are irregular or oval and different from those seen in partial mole (see Figure 4.11). ×50.

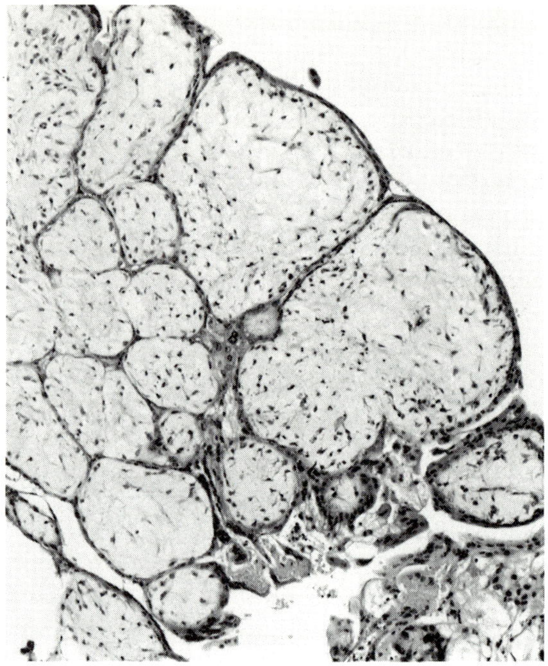

Figure 4.9 Complete mole in early gestation. Trophoblastic invaginations and budding occasionally result in a characteristic lobulated appearance. ×100.

reticulin around blood vessels[6,7]. With development of hydrops a little collagen may be seen in the condensed stroma at the periphery of cisterns but, unlike in PHM, fibrosis is not a feature of villous stroma in older moles, and even in necrotic CHMs retained for long periods the correct diagnosis may be inferred from the lack of fibrous stroma and the generalized hydrops usually present at this stage. In young CHMs the combination of basophilic mucoid stroma and invaginations of trophoblast from secondary villi may result, in cross-sections, in a characteristic lobulated appearance superficially resembling a fragmented intracanalicular breast fibroadenoma (Figure 4.9).

(h) In most CHMs no evidence of embryonic development is found. CHMs, which result from a double dose of purely paternally derived genes, form excess trophoblast but no embryo, whereas in contrast a proliferation derived from a double dose of purely maternal genes results in a benign ovarian cystic teratoma which contains a mixture of embryonic tissues but no trophoblast (see Chapter 2). This different behavior of male and female derived genes is an example of the biological phenomenon of genomic imprinting which appears to apply in most cases of CHM. However, we and others[6,7,49] have very rarely found nucleated fetal red cells, amnion or other embryonic tissues in specimens which are morphologically typical CHMs and genetically androgenetic[50]. Some of these are probably examples of CHM with unsuspected twin pregnancies but in others the presence of fetal red cells in molar villi remains unexplained and the possibility that some embryonic development may rarely occur in CHM has not yet been adequately excluded. For practical purposes the presence of embryo, amnion or fetal red cells in mole is strongly suggestive of PHM but CHM is not excluded absolutely and the latter should be considered if other histological features suggest it, or if the mole is diploid on flow cytometry (FC).

Ideally, a morphological diagnosis of CM based on these macroscopical and microscopical features should be confirmed by genetic studies but this is seldom possible, or indeed necessary; additional support for diagnosis of CHM rather than PHM can be derived from the finding of a diploid DNA complement by FC[51–54] and by finding a hyperdiploid fraction significantly higher than that of normal placentas[55]. This can now be done in fixed or paraffin-embedded material[56].

4.6 THE MORPHOLOGY OF GENETICALLY UNUSUAL COMPLETE HYDATIDIFORM MOLE

No morphological differences have been found between XX and XY CHMs[46]. Most CHMs have a diploid karyotype but some are tetraploid[57,58] and very rarely triploid but androgenetic[54,59]. Examination by FC and interphase cytogenetics of large numbers of cells from CHMs[7,60–62] has shown hyperdiploid and tetraploid fractions not easily explained by cells in division and which may represent aneuploid cell populations in about 40% of CHMs. This fits well with the common observation of large pleomorphic nuclei in molar trophoblast and has been confirmed by *in situ* hybridization studies[60,61] but it does not mean that all the cells in the CHM are tetraploid and does not conflict with earlier cytogenetic studies which showed diploid karyotypes in most CHMs. In fact, the criteria for diagnosis of tetraploidy by FC are not generally agreed[63] and caution should be exercised before concluding that a mole is tetraploid when using FC, since molar diploid cell populations are usually masked by maternal tissues used as internal diploid control by most workers[7]. We have not noted any significant morphological differences between CHMs with high and low hyperdiploid fractions but this deserves further study. Very rarely, moles with morphology indistinguishable from that of androgenetic CHM are found to have a normal diploid biparental genetic make-up[49,64]. Fetal red cells have occasionally been seen in vessels of such biparental diploid moles[49,64] and we have seen two such moles in the same patient[64]. We do not know if the diploid moles with normal karyotype seen in the same patient by Vejerslev *et al.*[65] also represent examples of the same condition, but most were diagnosed as PHM and had significant fetal development. These unusual moles are very rare and their prognosis is not yet known but represent an interesting group which may hold clues to the mechanisms of molar change and trophoblast growth; they merit further study.

4.7 PARTIAL HYDATIDIFORM MOLE

The presence of swollen villi in triploid conceptuses has been known for a number of years[66,67] but in a systematic study, Vassilakos *et al.*[29] pointed out that characteristically this change affected only part of the placenta; a fetus, often with congenital malformations, was frequently found and excessive trophoblastic proliferation was either absent or very mild. They included specimens with microscopical hydrops and no trophoblastic excess and karyotypes showed triploid, tetraploid and trisomic conceptions, the group being genetically heterogeneous and corresponding morphologically to molar types I and II of Hertig, i.e. to HA and transitional mole[12]. The authors suggested that PHM was not followed by PTD but, soon after, cases of PTD and CC following PHM were reported[68–70]. Subsequent studies including only specimens in which trophoblastic excess was present[31,45,71,72] indicated that PHM was almost always due to triploidy when two chromosome sets came from the father and one from the mother. These studies also showed that paternally derived triploidy (83%) was considerably commoner than maternally derived triploidy (17%) and that maternal triploids usually aborted earlier than PHM. When present, the fetus in triploidy was often abnormal and malformations included cranial, cardiac, urogenital and limb abnormalities[73] but in some cases, particularly in live-born fetuses or those aborted late in pregnancy, both fetus and placenta were apparently normal. Triploidy is a commoner genetic abnormality than androgenetic CHM[49] and if 83% of triploids are paternally derived (i.e. PHMs), PHM should be at least twice as common as CHM. However, in a survey done in 1986–1987 Paradinas *et al.*[74] found that only a third of histologically confirmed moles registered in one year were PHMs, suggesting underdiagnosis of PHM in the UK. In specialized centers the association of PHM with triploidy has been well over 90%[7,49,53,54]; tetraploid PHMs are rare[58] but most FC studies include a small proportion of diploid specimens morphologically diagnosed as PHMs. Reports from non-specialized centers have included high proportions of diploid PHMs, reaching 31% in one study[55] and 83% in another[75]. In a study of GTD following PHM Bagshawe *et al.*[76] found that only five of 11 patients referred with a diagnosis of PHM who developed GTD were true PHMs; after reviewing some 2000 specimens initially diagnosed as PHM in patients referred for follow-up in the last 10 years it was found that nearly half of them are in fact either CHMs or HAs. This is also the experience of others[77].

Confusion between CHM and PHM results from the failure to update diagnostic criteria for the younger CHMs seen today. A diagnosis of PHM based exclusively on the presence of blood vessels or partial hydrops is often wrong and a diagnosis of PHM based on the presence of fetal tissues or amnion is occasionally wrong and due to either twin pregnancy or to the rare androgenetic CHMs with fetal red cells, discussed earlier. It is not surprising that studies set to test intra- and inter-observer variations using old criteria[48] found total confusion. The confusion between PHM and HA is both conceptual and morphological. HAs include trisomies, monosomies, translocations and maternally derived triploids[78,79] and some of these were regarded as PHMs by Vassilakos *et al.*[29]. Trophoblast in them is abundant because they abort early and some have morphological similarities with PHM. There is no evidence that they present a risk of GTD greater than a normal pregnancy but they may be difficult to differentiate from PHM in inadequate samples[6,7]. As a group they are more frequent than PHM and at present represent some 10% of cases initially registered as PHMs[7].

Because of these diagnostic problems, and until modern criteria are more generally applied, we are suspicious of any reports of diploid PHMs and of high incidences of GTD after PHM, since such reports may include misdiagnosed CHMs. Whether the diploid moles with biparental contribution mentioned earlier should be called PHMs or CHMs depends on whether they resemble CHMs or PHMs in morphology and behavior; the few we have seen resembled CHM morphologically but are too few to assess their incidence of GTD.

The main features useful in diagnosing PHMs are as follows:

(a) Trophoblastic excess is usually present in PHM but it is seldom intense and may not be detected if the specimen is not extensively

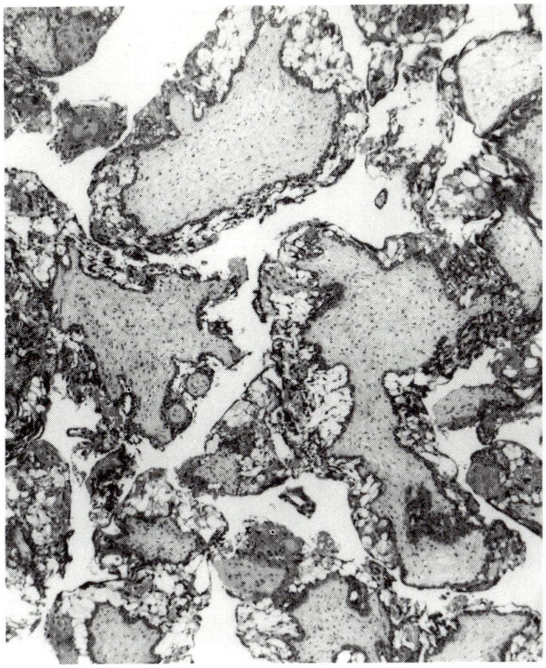

Figure 4.10 Partial mole. Circumferential hyperplasia is in this case striking but consists mainly of syncytiotrophoblast. This hyperplasia can be very focal and may not be detected unless sampling is extensive. ×50.

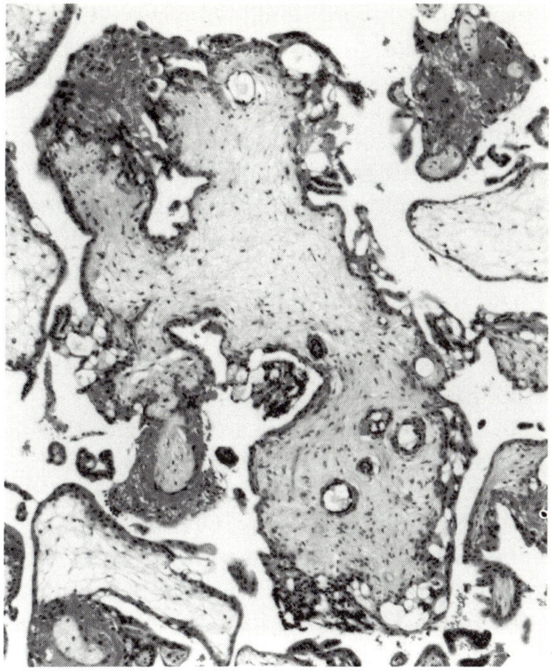

Figure 4.11 Partial mole. The irregular outline of villi has sharp angulations and the inclusions caused by trophoblast invaginations are rounded. ×80.

sampled. Most PHMs are evacuated in the second trimester when excessive trophoblast is usually predominantly syncytiotrophoblast projecting from the surface of villi (Figure 4.10) or invaginating into villous stroma to form pseudoinclusions (Figure 4.11); this excess may be present in both hydropic and non-hydropic villi. Clusters of cyto and syncytiotrophoblast and intermediate trophoblast such as those seen in CHM are rare but may be seen in PHMs evacuated unusually early (8–10 weeks). As in CHM, there are no generally agreed criteria of how to measure excess trophoblast in PHM but it should exclude the polar trophoblastic columns so common in early pregnancy (Figure 4.1) and first-trimester HAs. In many PHMs the abnormal distribution of trophoblast is more striking than its excess. This is particularly so if the sample is poor. Indeed, some of the patients with triploid PHMs who required chemotherapy in our institution had no appreciable excess trophoblast in inadequate samples[6] and at present we do not insist on excess trophoblast if other morphological features seen in association with triploidy are present. It has been claimed that proliferative activity of trophoblast in PHMs is less intense than that in HA[80], but there is conflicting evidence for this[81,82] and none of the studies compare specimens of similar GA. In our experience hCG in PHM is usually higher and remains elevated after evacuation for longer than after HA[7], and this is also reflected in a higher tendency for PTD. As a rule there is no excess circumferential trophoblast in HA but occasional sprouts of trophoblast round small villi may be seen; however, polar trophoblast is very common in HA, whereas it is rare to find it in PHM. In PHM the amounts of trophoblast, its proliferative activity, its aneuploid fractions on FC and the persistence of elevated hCG after evacuation are significantly less intense than in CHM[7,55,80–82]. The fact that syncytiotrophoblast in PHM expresses more PLAP and hPL and less hCG than CHM[83] probably reflects the older GA of PHMs, since PLAP and hPL are usually higher in later pregnancy.

(b) In PHM hydrops and cisterns characteristically involve only some of the villi. This is clearly seen in PHMs evacuated late in the second trimester, when CHMs would be expected to have generalized hydrops. This focal hydrops and presence of a fetus permits sometimes a correct ultrasound diagnosis of PHM, but on rare occasions ultrasound diagnoses of PHM turn out to be CHM with a non-molar twin pregnancy or focal placental hydrops in rare congenital abnormalities unrelated to molar pregnancy[84,85]. The diagnostic confusion resulting from interpreting partially developed hydrops in young CHMs as evidence of PHMs has already been discussed. In a small proportion of PHMs hydrops is mild and cisterns may be small or absent in the sample; sampling error is a possible explanation for this but in some PHMs early fetal death may result in extensive fibrosis of villi rather than marked hydrops and the uterus may be characteristically smaller than expected for dates[86]. In most cases, however, hydrops increases with GA and is more intense than in HA[7]. In most HAs cisterns are absent and hydrops seldom exceeds 3 mm in size but occasional 1–3 mm cisterns do not rule out HA. A common pitfall is to interpret in HA fragments of a gestational sac which has lost its amnion as villi with large cisterns, but as a rule the wall of the gestational sac contains more collagen than surrounding villi and the possibility of HA should always be considered when the

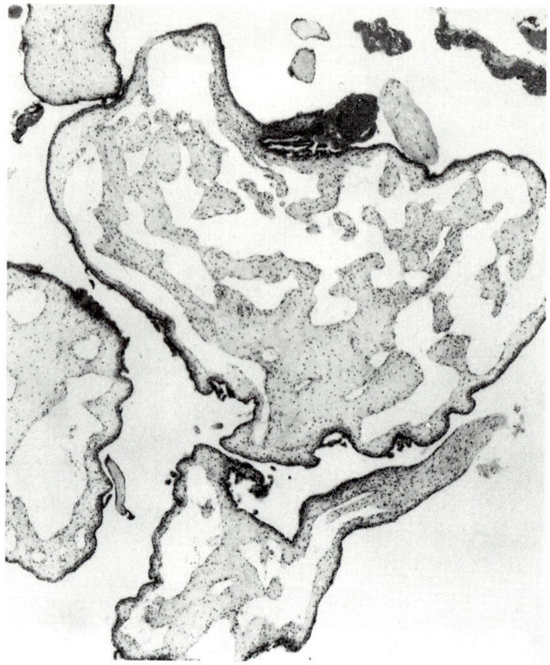

Figure 4.12 Angiomatoid vessels in partial mole. These are commoner in older moles, and although not pathognomonic of partial mole they are present in about a third of cases. ×50.

suspected cisterns are few and surrounded by smaller villi, particularly when the placental material obtained is scanty.

(c) Vessels, often containing nucleated fetal red cells, are a common finding in PHM but old PHMs can be avascular. Whereas the vessels of a CHM are often collapsed and inconspicuous, those of a PHM are often open but they gradually decrease in numbers with increasing GA; in one study[7] we found no vessels in 30 of 146 (20%) PHMs, whereas only 12% of our CHMs were avascular. The mean GA of avascular PHMs was significantly older than that of PHMs with vessels and a fetus was seldom found with them, suggesting that early fetal death could be a factor in the loss of vessels. In some PHMs avascularity of some villi is associated with angiomatoid vessels in others (Figure 4.12). These abnormal vessels, mistaken in

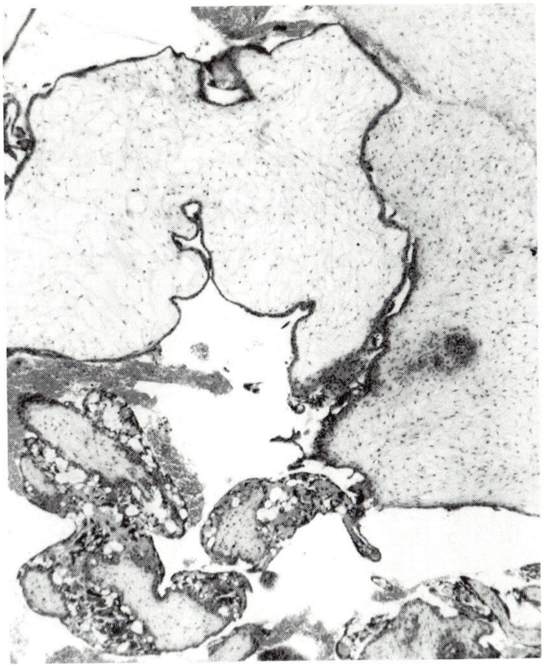

Figure 4.13 Non-hydropic villi in a partial mole are often referred to as normal, but some can be very abnormal and show excess trophoblast and irregular outline. ×50.

early publications for maze-like cisterns[45], are commoner in older PHMs[7,45] and are seldom seen before 12 weeks GA. It is possible that in some PHMs loss of vessels in some villi precedes fetal death and is compensated by increased and malformed vessels in others. More often than not, angiomatoid vessels are empty, suggesting fetal death long before evacuation. Very rarely we have seen similar abnormal vessels in diploid non-molar abortions and in CHM, but their presence in nearly 30% of PHMs makes them a useful if not pathognomonic feature.

(d) Karyorrhexis in villous stroma is seldom present or intense in PHM. This excludes nuclear debris found within and in the wall of vessels and villi in which the covering trophoblastic layers are already necrotic. The reluctance of some publications to emphasize this as a useful diagnostic criterion for CHM is understandable, since karyorrhexis is such a non-specific histological abnormality, but its correlation with CHM is very high[7,44,45], although its significance has not yet been explained.

(e) PHMs have abnormally shaped villi often described as scalloped or dentate (Figures 4.10 and 4.11) **and invaginations of trophoblast result in rounded inclusions.** Unlike the abnormally shaped villi of CHM (Figure 4.7) the irregularities in outline are sharp and angulated and appear in cross-section as rounded inclusions which may be solid or cystic and which contrast with the more oval or irregular inclusions of CHM. Infolding of trophoblastic layers in the hydropic villi of a PHM may also result in pseudoinclusions similar to those of CM, which are therefore less useful in differential diagnosis. Scalloping and round inclusions can be seen in both hydropic and non-hydropic villi, and although the small villi of PHM are often described as normal some can in fact be very abnormal and may show excess trophoblast (Figure 4.13). Unfortunately, irregular villi and round inclusions may also occur in non-molar HAs, particularly in trisomies, including the two commonest forms trisomy 16 and 18, and in monosomy 45XO[87], but in these conditions hydrops is absent or mild and there are usually no cisterns and no excess trophoblast. Nevertheless, these are a common source of diagnostic errors, even in experienced hands. Some of these conditions were initially regarded as part of the syndrome of PHM[29] but there is no evidence that they represent an increased risk of PTD. The irregular villi in these specimens (Figure 4.14) are less sharp and angulated than in PHM and the round inclusions are few and small. In addition, if the specimen is adequate, villi with polar trophoblastic columns may be found in HAs and single cell trophoblastic inclusions (Figure 4.15) of the type described in trisomies may be numerous, although the fact that they also occur in about 10% of

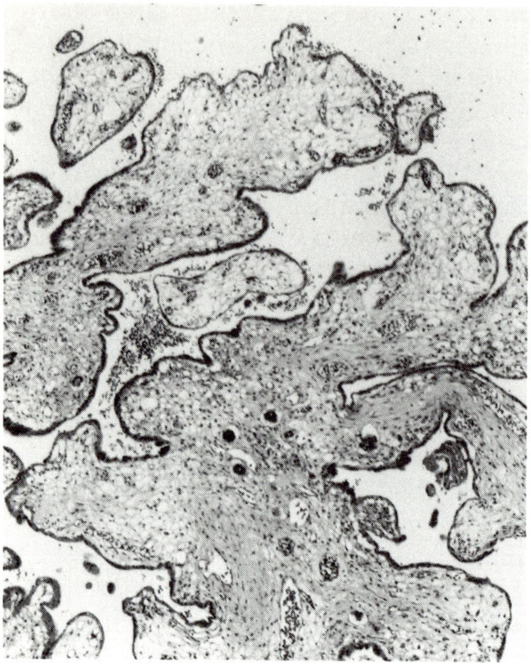

Figure 4.14 Irregular villi and rounded trophoblastic inclusions in monosomy XO. The inclusions are few and small. The irregular outline is less angular than in partial mole, there is no excess trophoblast and hydrops is often minimal or absent. ×70.

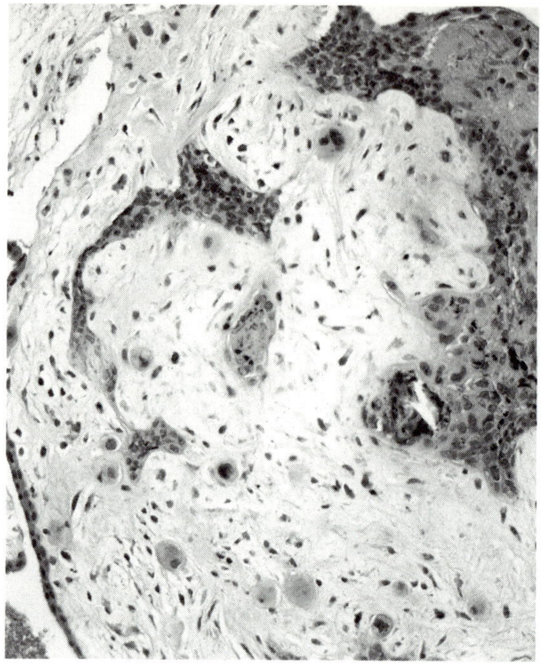

Figure 4.15 Trophoblastic inclusions consisting of single cells resembling intermediate trophoblast are common in trisomies and rare in partial mole. ×150.

PHMs and in CHMs[7,45] makes them less useful in differential diagnosis.

(f) In PHM villous stroma contains abundant collagen and this increases with GA. In PHMs evacuated very early (eight weeks) the stroma may be more immature and mucoid, scalloping less intense and trophoblast more abundant, so that they may resemble CHMs, but as a rule there is a fine mesh of reticulin fibers in non-hydropic villi, with stromal cells often present in this mesh. Fibrosis increases with GA and is present at the periphery of cisterns. Unlike CHMs, PHMs retained for long periods are often very fibrous.

(g) An embryo or fetus, often malformed, probably always develops in PHM but frequently dies in early pregnancy and may not be identifiable in the specimen. Fetal tissues were only present in 20% of a series of PHMs reviewed by us[7], but there were fetal red cells in molar villi in nearly 50% and chorioamniotic membranes in 40% of them. Fetal red cells may persist in vessels long after fetal death and are sometimes seen together with a necrotic embryo. The finding of fetal tissues with a mole is often interpreted as proof of PHM and although in most cases this is true, the possibilities of androgenetic CHM with twin pregnancy and CHM with unexplained fetal red cells in molar villi (see section 4.5) should be considered if the features of the mole are not those of a PHM and particularly if the mole is diploid.

As in CHM, cytogenetic, molecular genetic and interphase cytogenetic studies[61,88,89] can be helpful for accurate diagnosis. In their absence FC is helpful for differentiating between diploid CHMs and triploid PHMs and between the latter and non-molar diploid HAs, particularly when placental material is scanty. Maternal age and GA at evacuation can be helpful in making a decision as to whether to start hCG follow-up or not when morphology does not discriminate well between PHM and HA. PHMs are usually evacuated in the second trimester and are not more common in older women, whereas HAs abort in the first trimester and increase dramatically with maternal age[7], so a miscarriage before 10 weeks in a woman over 35 is more likely to be due to an HA than a PHM.

4.8 INVASIVE MOLE

The majority of CHMs remit after evacuation and curettage, but the tendency in some instances to invade the myometrium resulting in uterine perforation and extension to adjacent organs is well known and approximately 16% of CHMs behaved in this way[12,15,16]. Histologically the appearance of the chorionic villi is similar to that of other CHMs, but swelling of villi is less often seen in deeply implanted invasive moles and histological diagnosis is based on the excessive trophoblastic proliferation, markedly irregular shape of villi and their invasive nature (Figure 4.16). Some degree of myometrial invasion is probably present in most moles; indeed, myometrial invasion is not exclusive to molar pregnancies and Hertig[12], borrowing the terminology used for myometrial placentation, classified invasive moles into accreta, increta and percreta. Since hysterectomy is nowadays rarely necessary in the treatment of invasive moles, the few specimens seen are usually in unmonitored and often unsuspected pregnancies and, sometimes, are paradoxically percreta moles (the rarest form) presenting as acute abdomen due to uterine perforation (Figure 4.17) and consisting of a hematoma with molar villi often implanted on a pelvic organ such as the ovary, tube or broad ligament, or on a loop of intestine. In the last two years we have seen several invasive CHMs in perimenopausal patients on hormone replacement therapy (HRT). This may be coincidental, but a relationship is possible if HRT stimulates ovulation, since the risk of CHM at this age is markedly increased.

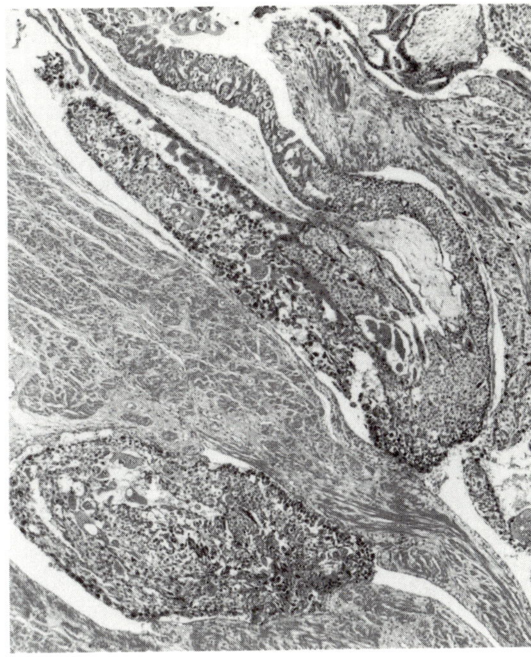

Figure 4.16 Invasive mole in myometrial vessels. There is abundant excess trophoblast but hydrops is not conspicuous. ×50.

IM after PHM is very rare. All but one of the IMs in hysterectomy specimens in our archival material are CHMs but rare invasive triploid PHMs requiring hysterectomy have been reported[70,90] and we have seen a PHM which required three curettages, the last under ultrasound control, for removal of deeply implanted myometrial villi.

4.9 MOLAR METASTASES

CHMs can spread to the cervix, vaginal wall and vulva[47,91,92] but with modern chemotherapy this does not imply a worse prognosis[47]. In the past, up to 10%

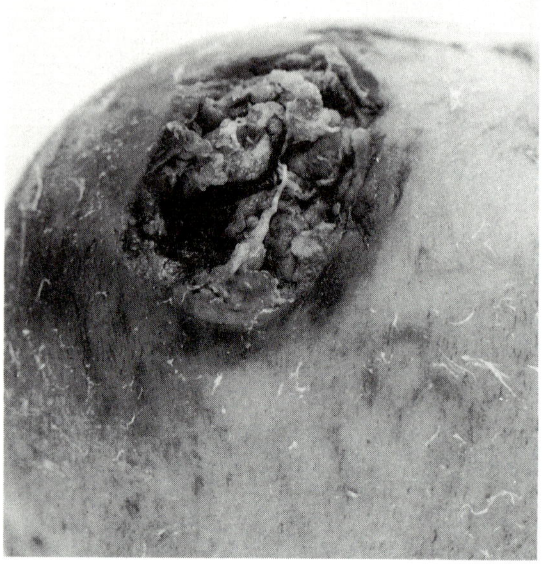

Figure 4.17 Fundal perforation in unsuspected invasive mole. The patient was unaware of her pregnancy, which was not monitored. ×4.

of patients with CHM had radiological lung opacities which were interpreted as metastases[93] and this was confirmed histologically in some cases[94,95]. With early diagnosis and early chemotherapy the number of patients with metastases has been reduced and the disease is usually limited to the uterus and parametrial tissues. Exceptionally, tissue from CHMs has been found in other sites, including brain, retroperitoneum and inguinal lymph nodes[15]. In pre-chemotherapy days lung metastases sometimes regressed after evacuation or eradication of the mole[96], but the appearance or persistence of metastases long after evacuation of a CHM may indicate PTD or CC. We have not seen tissue from PHMs outside the uterus.

4.10 ECTOPIC MOLES

Ober and Maier[97] accepted only four of 22 cases of tubal mole reported in the literature[98] as possible examples of ectopic CHM. We have only seen three acceptable examples of tubal CHM amongst 28 cases referred with that diagnosis in the last 10 years, most cases turning out to be non-molar specimens with abundant polar trophoblast in early gestation. It appears that tubal moles are considerably rarer than tubal CC and we have found no reliable reports of tubal mole followed by CC, although PTD after tubal pregnancy does occur. We have not seen tubal PHMs but cases have been reported[99, 100]. Ectopic pregnancies are sometimes diagnosed before eight weeks GA and there is no information of what a PHM looks like at that stage.

4.11 HYDATIDIFORM MOLES WITH TWIN PREGNANCY

The fact that CHMs can coexist with a twin pregnancy has already been mentioned as a possible cause of confusion in the ultrasound and histological diagnosis of PHM and as one of the possible explanations of the finding of fetal red cells in the vessels of a CHM. Twin molar pregnancies have been reported from time to time and in a review of 82 reported cases of mole with fetus Beischer *et al.*[67] found that 52 had a single placenta (probably PHMs) and 30 were dizygotic. Evidence of dizygosity can be obtained by cytogenetic[101], molecular genetic[102] and interphase cytogenetic studies[103]; the last two can be performed in paraffin-embedded tissues. The frequency of dizygotic twin pregnancy in the general population is one in about 110[101]. We see CHMs with evidence of a twin – or a second population of non-molar villi suggestive of a twin – in about one in 200 histologically confirmed CHMs, but our CHMs are referred cases sampled elsewhere and the incidence may in fact be higher and similar to that of dizygosity in general. Many of our cases were early abortions, but some were mid-trimester terminations and a few had progressed into the third trimester, resulting in the delivery of a normal infant and very necrotic molar tissue. Very rare cases of CHM with two twins have been reported[104] and we have seen one such case. A rare combination of CHM and PHM is also on record[105]. Combinations of PHM with a normal twin are considerably rarer and we have only seen two examples: one possible reason is that it may be more difficult to detect morphologically, particularly in early abortions, and another that at least some of the molar pregnancies with a twin occur in *in vitro* fertilization programs[106], when abnormal triploid embryos may be easier to detect than diploid androgenetic embryos before implantation. The incidence of GTD in CHM with a twin is similar to that of CHM on its own[103,107,108].

4.12 PROGNOSIS OF MOLES

No immortal cell lines or long-term growth in nude mice have yet been achieved with trophoblast of moles[109], whereas this can be readily done with CCs. This supports the view that the excessive trophoblastic proliferation in moles lacks features of malignancy. Nevertheless, molar trophoblast can continue to grow and invade, needing active intervention to preserve the uterus or to avoid a catastrophic hemorrhage. Exceptionally, molar trophoblast can survive for over a year and the immediately preceding pregnancy may not be that causing CC[110,111]; however, most complications due to persistent or invasive moles occur in the six months following a molar evacuation[112–114]. The reported incidence of CHMs needing treatment varies according to the criteria for diagnosis of PTD and to whether PHMs and HAs have been reliably excluded in the series. The low figure of 8% for all moles reported from our institution[76,112,113] did not include histological confirmation in all cases and a figure of 14% for CM is probably more accurate. Figures of up to 30% reported from the USA[115,116] result from less stringent diagnostic criteria for GTD and many such patients would not have been treated in our institution. A higher incidence of PTD was suggested in heterozygous (dispermic) moles[116,117], which comprise about 20% of CHMs[28], but this has not been supported by more recent studies[26,28,118]. The lack of relationship between the amounts of trophoblast in the sample and the incidence of GTD has already been discussed. Although as a group CHMs with higher hyperdiploid fractions have higher incidences of GTD[55] this does not predict outcome in individual patients. Neoplastic transformation of a mole is recognized when villous stroma is no longer formed but nothing is known of the factors which control this change in behavior. In the past, approximately 3% of CHMs became CCs[11,12]. Because of early chemotherapy in CHM, the figure now is probably lower, but the real incidence is not known, since histological confirmation in GTD is nowadays seldom available.

The incidence of GTD after PHM is considerably lower than after CHM. High incidences of 18% and 20%[75,81] include many diploid PHMs which could be misdiagnosed CHMs. Using American criteria for diagnosis of GTD, 5.5% of patients with PHMs were treated in the New England Trophoblastic Disease Center[119], but they included two diploid PHMs which required more intensive chemotherapy than triploid PHMs. If these two are excluded the incidence would be 4.8%. We have seen GTD following PHM in about 1% of histologically reviewed PHMs[6] but since many PHMs go unrecognized the real incidence could be even lower and an estimate of 0.5% in one study[76] may not be far from the truth. The incidence of CC after PHM is not known. We have seen five histologically confirmed cases, but have failed to date to demonstrate by FC or genetic studies origin of the tumor from the preceding PHM. This is not surprising, since malignant transformation is often associated with aneuploidy and loss of polymorphisms and this can complicate the picture. We have not observed more trophoblast in PHMs which develop GTD than in PHMs which do not, but trophoblastic excess in PHM can be very focal and the potential for sampling error is great.

4.13 CHORIOCARCINOMA

This is a malignant neoplasm in which differentiation towards villous cytotrophoblast and syncytiotrophoblast is seen (Figure 4.18). It can occur after CHM, PHM, normal pregnancy, stillbirth, abortion or ectopic pregnancy. In some cases there is no known preceding pregnancy and the theory that CC can develop from a conceptus *ab initio* has been proposed[120]. The incidence of CC after CHM is about a thousand times greater than after a normal pregnancy. The proportion of CCs preceded by moles in reported series varies between 39% and 78%[4]. It is generally assumed that the immediate antecedent pregnancy is responsible for the tumor and although in most cases it may be so, it is not necessarily so[110,111]. As in the case of hydatidiform mole, there are remarkable differences in the incidence of CC in various parts of the world[4,26,121]. These are not always explained by an increase in preceding moles but a serious epidemiological study of the problem is hindered by variations in the way in which the information is recorded, bias in the selection of reported cases and the very success of therapy, which all too often nowadays precludes us from knowing the true nature of the trophoblastic disease treated.

Macroscopically, uterine CC appears as a hemorrhagic nodule which may be in contact with the lining of the uterine cavity or may lay in the myometrium (Figure 4.19). Microscopically, viable tumor is usually seen only at the periphery of the nodule and within vascular spaces in adjacent myometrium and as a rule no intrinsic vasculature can be demonstrated. The characteristic bilaminar structure of villous trophoblast is usually easily identifiable but in some cases most of the tumor is either predominantly syncytiotrophoblastic (Figure 4.20) or predominantly cytotrophoblastic (Figure 4.21). A direct correlation between the intensity of the surrounding inflammatory reaction and a better prognosis has been demonstrated[122] and some relationship between the degree of anaplasia and prognosis has been suggested[123]; these studies have less relevance today because of the good therapeutic response seen in most patients.

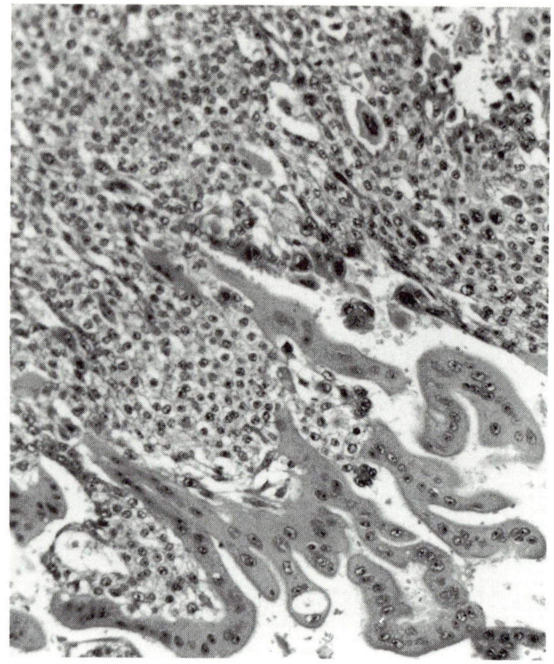

Figure 4.18 The typical form of choriocarcinoma forms cyto- and syncytiotrophoblast similar to that of villous trophoblast. ×180.

Some predominantly cytotrophoblastic tumors secrete smaller amounts of hCG[124]. This is not surprising, since synthesis of hCG occurs mainly in syncytiotrophoblast. Some hPL is usually demonstrable in syncytiotrophoblast but, unlike placental site

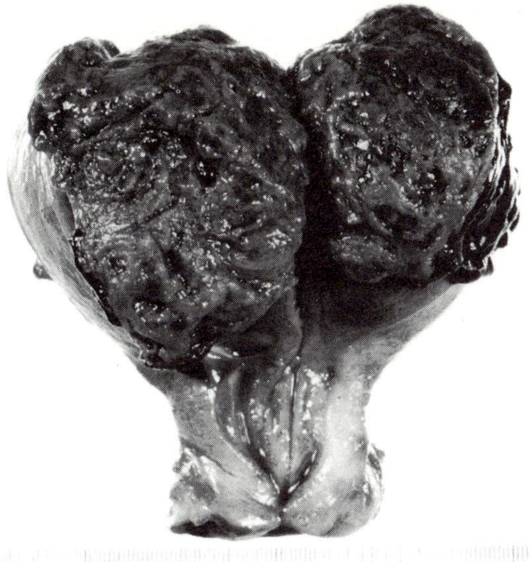

Figure 4.19 Choriocarcinoma grows by invading maternal vessels and viable tumor is usually only found at the periphery of a hemorrhagic mass. Reduced from natural size.

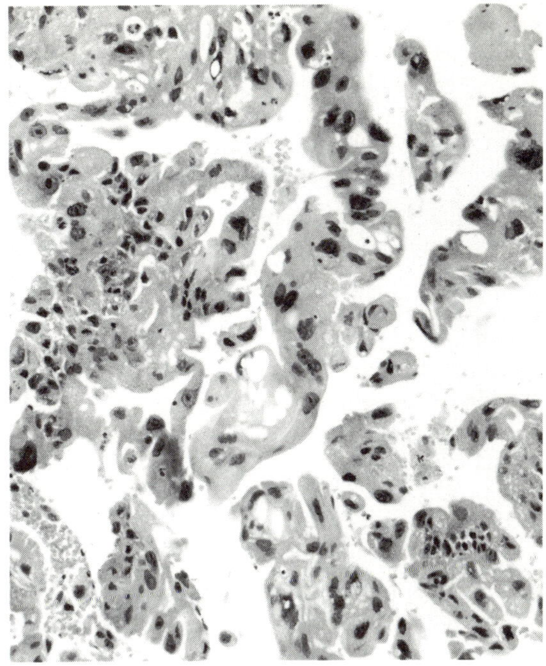

Figure 4.20 Predominantly syncytiotrophoblastic choriocarcinoma in endometrial curettings. ×180.

trophoblast, villous cytotrophoblast does not contain significant amounts of hPL. The morphology of CC is sometimes changed after chemotherapy, and when therapy-resistant metastases are removed they are often composed of bizarre mononuclear cells[125] which probably represent therapy-resistant clones. These atypical CCs are sometimes difficult to differentiate from PSTT but unlike PSTT (p. 64) they form hemorrhagic nodules, readily infiltrate vessels, have a high mitotic rate and express more hCG than hPL[126].

CC metastasizes readily and it is not uncommon to find secondary nodules in the cervix or vagina on presentation. The lungs, brain and liver are the distant organs more often involved and sometimes metastases dominate the clinical picture and patients may rarely present with intracerebral hemorrhage or with acute cor pulmonale due to extensive intravascular lung disease[127,128]. Unexplained intracerebral hemorrhage or acute cor pulmonale in a woman of childbearing age should prompt suspicions of CC. Failure to consider this possibility has led in the past to CC developing in immunosuppressed organ recipients[129]. Melena or hematuria from metastases to intestine or kidney are less common[128]. In contrast, lymph nodes are rarely the site of metastasis and the finding of a tumor with apparent trophoblastic differentiation in lymph nodes without evidence of a gestational primary should raise doubts about the gestational origin of the tumor, which could be of germ cell origin or a carcinoma with trophoblastic metaplasia. CC following a normal term pregnancy is sometimes the result of malignant transformation in an otherwise normal placenta (Figure 4.22) but the primary tumor may be microscopical and may not be detected, since pathological examination of apparently normal placentae in nor-

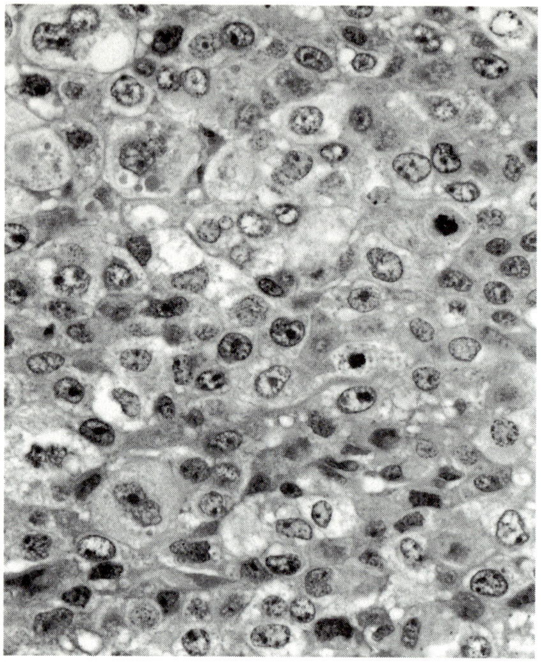

Figure 4.21 Some choriocarcinomas are predominantly cytotrophoblastic and secrete less hCG but retain a predominantly intravascular mode of invasion; unlike placental site tumor they contain little hPL, are composed of cells with less dense cytoplasm and have numerous mitoses. ×450.

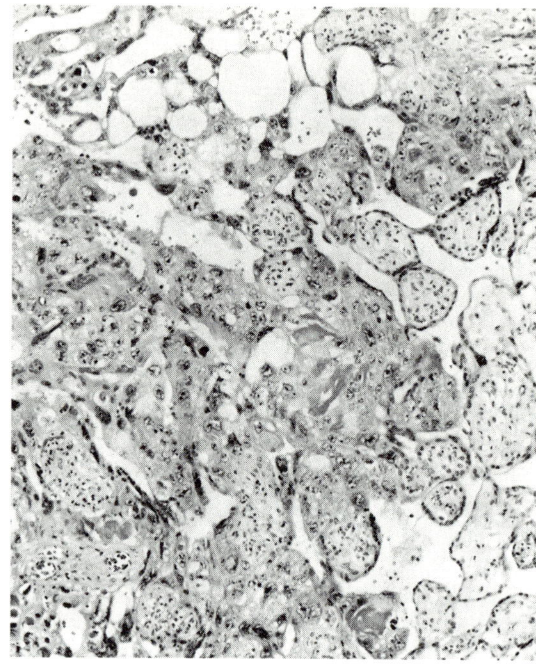

Figure 4.22 Choriocarcinoma in third-trimester placenta. The patient developed lung metastases soon after delivery of a stillborn infant. ×100.

mal births is seldom carried out. Origin from specific pregnancies can nevertheless be demonstrated genetically[110]. It should be remembered that placental CC can metastasize to the child as well as the mother[130,131].

A common problem is the differential diagnosis between CC and trophoblast from an early pregnancy or that of a mole. A curettage in an early pregnancy may yield abundant cyto- and syncytiotrophoblast only. As a rule, normal young trophoblast is less pleomorphic than that of CC and its polar arrangement may still be discernible. It is exceptional to find villi when CC develops. The presence of villi and abundant trophoblast in endometrial curettings is suggestive of a recent early abortion rather than CC, which has in the past been overdiagnosed by pathologists[132], but in a few cases residual degenerate villi may often be seen[124], and Ober[97] describes a CC in the fallopian tube with chorion in the middle. The diagnosis was made on the basis of extensive trophoblastic infiltration of the tubal wall without infiltration by the villi and it was confirmed when the patient died with liver metastases. The presence of CC in term or near-term placentae is another example of coexistence of CC and villous stroma. The pleomorphic trophoblast from a mole, particularly a CHM, can be morphologically indistinguishable from that of CC, although it has a different biological behavior. Selective sampling of a second curettage after evacuation of a CHM may yield trophoblast without villous stroma, when a diagnosis of persistent trophoblast should be made and its significance judged together with clinical ultrasound and serological data. As a rule, the longer the period between evacuation of a known pregnancy and the finding of trophoblast in curettings, the more likely its pathological significance, provided a new pregnancy can be ruled out[132].

4.14 ECTOPIC CHORIOCARCINOMA (Figure 4.23)

Ober and Maier[97] found 58 acceptable examples of primary CC of the fallopian tube amongst 93 reported cases and added 18 cases of their own. About 60% of patients presented with acute symptoms simulating an ectopic pregnancy and the rest had a pelvic mass indistinguishable from an ovarian tumor. In no case was there evidence of a preceding ectopic mole but in two instances there were residual chorionic villi and evidence of a gestational sac, an unusual finding in uterine CC. In all other aspects (distribution of metastases, mortality, response to chemotherapy) the tumors behaved like uterine CCs and only five of 47 patients survived before the advent of chemotherapy; in contrast 15 of 16 patients given chemotherapy survived. Tubal CC may also present with metastases[99] and has been described following fertility treatment[133].

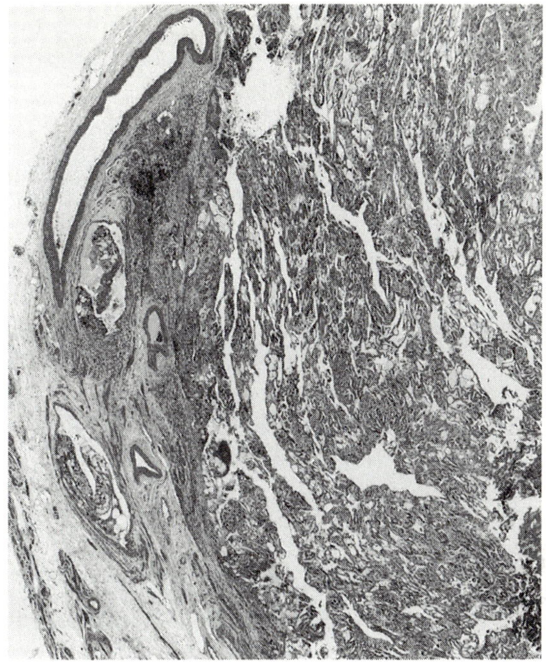

Figure 4.23 Choriocarcinoma in the fallopian tube. Tumor is obliterating the lumen and invading the wall, including vessels on the left. Choriocarcinoma does not have intrinsic vasculature. ×20.

Although cases of gestational CC of the ovary and peritoneal cavity have been reported[15,134,135] reliable evidence of their gestational rather than germ cell or metaplastic origin can only be obtained by genetic fingerprinting of the tumor, the patient and the patient's partner. Trophoblastic metaplasia and hCG production can occur in many carcinomas[136] including ovarian and endometrial carcinomas[137,138]. Histological differentiation from CCs is not always easy, since they can mimic the pattern of vascular invasion and the bilaminar structure of villous trophoblast (Figure 4.24). In some cases there is a second pattern, such as adenocarcinoma, squamous carcinoma or transitional cell carcinoma which gives away the diagnosis, but in others tumors are undifferentiated but for the presence of syncytiotrophoblast or hCG production: suspicions that the tumor may not be gestational should arise if the tumor is producing little hCG for its bulk, if it has a vascular stroma on histology and if it is resistant to chemotherapy. Confirmation is nowadays possible by comparing genetic polymorphisms of the tumor with those of the patient and her partner, and modern techniques can give a quick answer which can influence clinical decisions[139,140]. The problem is not just academic since in carcinomas with trophoblastic metaplasia

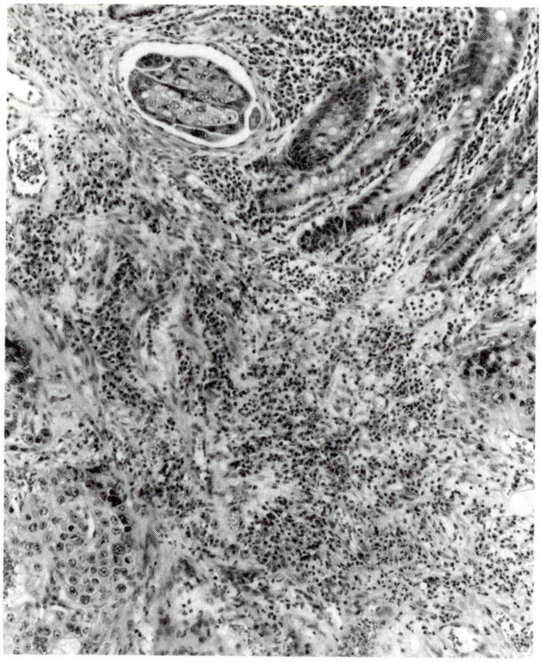

Figure 4.24 Carcinoma of the colon with trophoblastic metaplasia. The patient was a 64-year-old woman and in places the tumor was an adenocarcinoma, but in places (see intravascular tumor in the lamina propria) was differentiating towards trophoblast with hCG production. ×100.

surgical eradication offers the only hope of a cure. Carcinomas with trophoblastic metaplasia probably account for the majority of so-called 'primary choriocarcinomas', reported in viscera, including lungs, breast, stomach, intestine, liver, adrenal, pancreas, bladder and kidney[136,141–151].

4.15 PLACENTAL SITE TROPHOBLASTIC TUMOR

This is the tumorous counterpart of the non-villous trophoblast which infiltrates the placental site in normal pregnancy. Tumors of this type have been recognized for many years and have been variously named 'atypical chorioepitheliomas', 'syncytiomas' and 'corionepitheliosis'[16]. More recently, Kurman *et al.*[152] described 12 cases in which the lesion remained localized and was sometimes eradicated by simple curettage. They proposed the term 'trophoblastic pseudotumor' but within a few years it was clear that, on occasion, this lesion behaved in a locally aggressive way and could metastasize[33,34,153,154]. Although recognizing that this tumor is an atypical form of CH, we prefer to use the name 'placental site trophoblastic tumor'[34], which reflects the morphological similarities with placental site trophoblast.

PSTT presents with amenorrhea or irregular vaginal bleeding months or years after a normal pregnancy, an abortion or, rarely, a hydatidiform mole[33,154,155] and origin from both moles and normal pregnancy has been demonstrated genetically[156,157]. Occasionally, the patient may be peri- or postmenopausal[157–159]. The uterus is usually enlarged and pregnancy proteins such as hCG, hPL and β_1-glycoprotein (SP-1) are elevated although hCG is seldom as high as in CC. In five instances (less than 10% of reported cases) PSTT has been associated with the nephrotic syndrome, which has remitted after eradication of the tumor[33,160]. Fibrin and immunoglobulin M (IgM) have been found in glomerular intracapillary deposits and disseminated intravascular coagulation (DIC) postulated as the main pathogenetic mechanism. A report of virilization and testosterone production by a PSTT appears exceptional[161].

A curettage may yield decidua or myometrium infiltrated by trophoblastic cells with dense eosinophilic cytoplasm and pleomorphic nuclei (Figure 4.25); they can be mononuclear or multinucleated and they often form clusters or cords and separate smooth muscle fibers. It may be difficult, or even impossible, to differentiate between an exaggerated placental site reaction and PSTT in endometrial curettings, since there may be

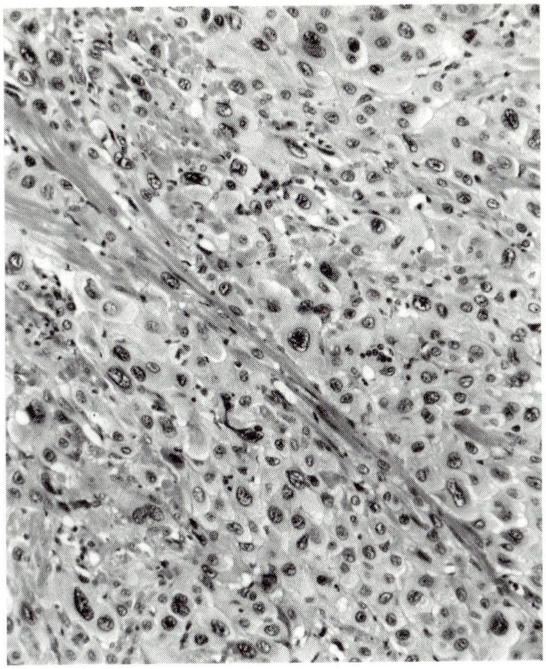

Figure 4.25 Placental site trophoblastic tumor infiltrating myometrium. Cells are predominantly mononuclear and mitoses are rare. Infiltration is predominantly interstitial and tumors express more hPL than hCG. ×180.

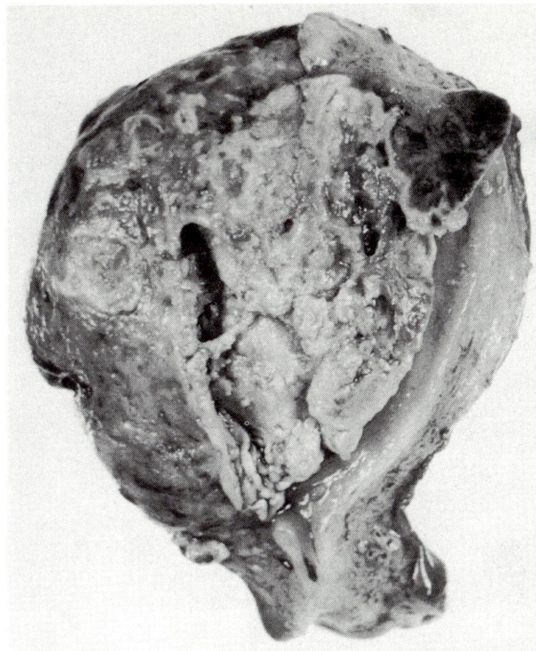

Figure 4.26 In placental site trophoblastic tumor necrosis is often extensive but unlike choriocarcinoma hemorrhage is less conspicuous. Reduced from natural size.

scanty material or this may be extensively necrotic[162]; also less confluent PSTT at the periphery of the mass may look identical to placental site reaction[163]. The formation of large clusters of trophoblastic cells appears to be a reliable criterion of neoplasia but in many instances it may only be possible to say that there is persistent placental site trophoblast and judge whether it is physiological or pathological in the light of clinical, ultrasound and serological observations. In PSTT aneuploidy seems to be less common than in CC and tumors are often diploid on FC[155,164,165].

Examination of hysterectomy specimens shows clear differences between PSTT and CC. PSTT forms masses in which necrosis is marked, but hemorrhage is less conspicuous (Figure 4.26). This reflects a lesser tendency to vascular invasion, infiltration being predominantly interstitial. Necrosis can be very extensive in long-standing tumors and dystrophic calcification can occur in areas of necrosis[126], tumor surviving only around vessels (Figure 4.27). In our experience these long-standing tumors express more PLAP than hPL or hCG[126]. There are good descriptions of the electron microscopy of PSTT and CC[26,166] but this seldom helps in diagnosis.

PSTT can infiltrate relentlessly and extend into adjacent organs such as the ovary, parametrium, rectum or bladder. Distant metastases can occur in lungs, peritoneum, liver, pancreas and brain, and we have observed retroperitoneal and supraclavicular lymph node metastases in a tumor with long evolution. It appears that mitotic counts

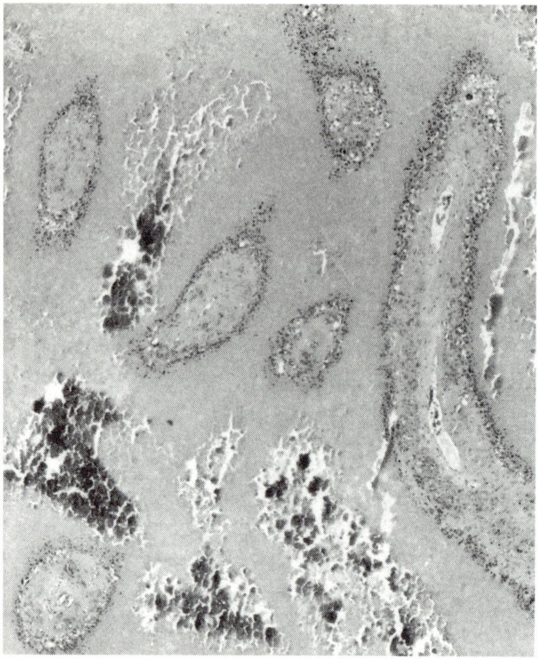

Figure 4.27 Calcification and necrosis in placental site tumor presenting after the menopause in a woman 14 years after the last known pregnancy. Viable tumor is only present around blood vessels. Long-standing tumors often express more PLAP than hPL or hCG. ×50.

(more than five mitoses per 10 high-power fields) may predict tumors with metastasizing potential[126,154,167,168]; even this may not prove reliable in some cases and we have seen a tumor with 11 mitoses per 10 high-power fields in curettings which apparently regressed, the patient refusing hysterectomy and being delivered of a normal infant two years later[126].

The importance of recognizing PSTT lies on the one hand in its lesser metastasizing potential, which makes it amenable to surgery, and on the other hand in its higher resistance to chemotherapy, which accounts for therapeutic failures when surgery is no longer able to arrest its progress. In our experience extrauterine pelvic extensions have been more difficult to manage than lung metastases[126]. Immunocytochemistry for hCG, hPL and PLAP is helpful in diagnosis. As a rule PSTT contains more positive cells for hPL than hCG and finding more hCG than hPL in a tumor may mean that the tumor is not PSTT but predominantly cytotrophoblastic CC. These tumors are predominantly mononuclear but have an intravascular rather than interstitial mode of infiltration. They tend to form hemorrhagic masses and metastasize early[126], so that they behave like CC in all but the fact that they tend to be chemoresistant like PSTT. Sometimes, there are great variations in the amounts of hCG detected serologically during treatment which are not always explained by tumor bulk, and we have observed tumors with morphology of PSTT in the uterus and morphology of CC in the metastases, as well as tumors with areas indistinguishable from PSTT and areas looking like cytotrophoblastic CC; it is therefore possible that CC and PSTT may not arise from different progenitor cells, and whether differentiation occurs towards villous trophoblast or placental site trophoblast could depend on environmental factors, including prior chemotherapy which could select chemoresistant clones[162]. In favor of this is the fact that a common form of presentation of PSTT is as a chemoresistant trophoblastic tumor, but there is no doubt that some PSTTs have their characteristic morphology even before chemotherapy is given.

A second area of difficulty arises in the differential diagnosis of PSTT from trophoblastic proliferations which regress spontaneously[32,169–172]. The term 'placental site trophoblastic nodule or plaque' has been proposed for these self-limiting lesions[32]. In our experience and that of others, regressing lesions often show marked hyalinization or central necrosis (Figure 4.28) and, occasionally, there is difficulty in demonstrating cytoplasmic hPL or hCG, although the epithelial nature of the

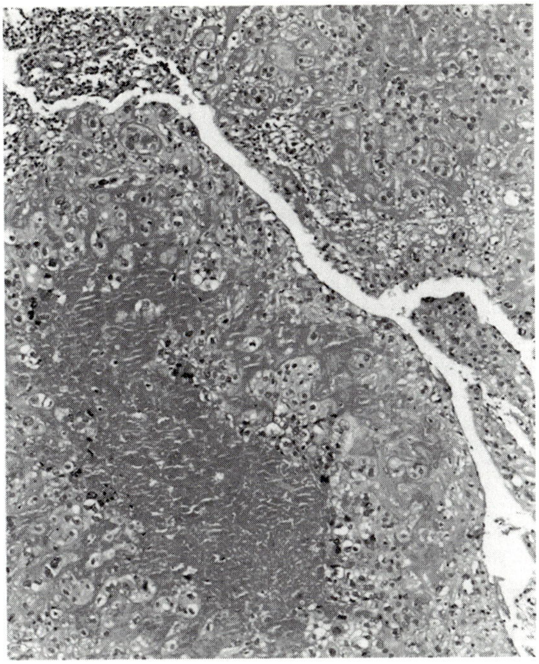

Figure 4.28 Regressing placental site nodule. There is often central necrosis and hyalinization around individual cells, and cells may not express any hormones, although they are usually positive for cytokeratin structural antigens. ×100.

trophoblastic cells can be demonstrated with cytokeratin antisera[126,169 172]. Some of these regressing nodules express more PLAP than hPL[170] but as in PSTT this may be a reflection of their age. As a rule, regressing PSTNs are not associated with elevated urinary or serum hCG but we have seen PSTNs persist for up to one year after the last known pregnancy.

4.16 PATHOLOGICAL LESIONS ASSOCIATED WITH TROPHOBLASTIC TUMORS

The increased pelvic and uterine vascularity associated with moles and CC is well known and sometimes persists even after hCG has returned to normal. It may be a source of life-threatening hemorrhage which may need either hysterectomy or uterine artery embolization when the uterus needs to be preserved.

Luteal ovarian cysts used to accompany hydatidiform mole and CC in a variable number of patients and an incidence of 94% in one report is quoted by Park[15]. They are nowadays less common. Luteinization of granulosa and theca cells may occur throughout both ovaries but its intensity varies in different patients and does not appear related to hCG levels in serum. Rupture can occur[173] and needle aspiration of the cysts has been recommended to prevent this. It is important not to confuse these ovarian lesions with metastatic CC.

REFERENCES

1. Marcuse, P.M. (1954) Pulmonary syncytial giant cell embolism: report of maternal death. *Obstet. Gynecol.*, **3**, 210–13.
2. Attwood, H.D. and Park, W.W. (1961) Embolism to the lungs by trophoblast. *Journal of Obstetrics and Gynaecology of the British Commonwealth*, **68**, 611–17.
3. Covone, A.E., Mutton, D., Johnson, P.M. and Adinolfi, M. (1984) Trophoblast cells in peripheral blood from pregnant women. *Lancet*, **ii**, 841–3.
4. World Health Organization Scientific Group (1983) Gestational trophoblastic diseases. *Technical Report Series 692.*
5. Newlands, E.S. (1995) Clinical management of trophoblastic disease in the United Kingdom. *Curr. Obstet. Gynaecol.*, **5**, 19–24.
6. Paradinas, F.J. (1994) The histological diagnosis of hydatidiform moles. *Current Diagnostic Pathology*, **1**, 24–31.
7. Paradinas, F.J., Browne, P., Fisher, R.A. *et al.* (1996) A clinical, histopathological and flow cytometric study of 149 complete moles, 146 partial moles and 107 non-molar hydropic abortions. *Histopathology*, **28**, 101–9.
8. Goldstein, D., Soto-Wright, V., Bernstein, M. and Berkowitz, R. (1994) The clinical presentation of complete molar pregnancy in present years. *Abstracts of the VII World*

Congress on Gestational Trophoblastic Diseases, Hong Kong, p. 10.

9. Johnson, I.R. (1995) Trophoblastic disease. *Current Obstetrics and Gynaecology* **5**, 1.
10. Park, W.W. and Lees, J.C. (1950) Choriocarcinoma: a general review, with analysis of 516 cases. *Archives of Pathology*, **49**, 73–104, 205–41.
11. Hertig, A.T. (1950) Hydatidiform mole and chorionepithelioma, in *Progress in Gynecology*, Vol. 2 (eds J.B. Meigs and S.H. Sturgis), Grune & Stratton, New York, pp. 372–94.
12. Hertig, A.T. and Mansell, H. (1956) Tumours of the female sex organs. Part 1. Hydatidiform mole and choriocarcinoma, in *Atlas of Tumour Pathology*, Sect. 9, Fasc. 33, Armed Forces Institute of Pathology, Washington, DC.
13. Brewer, J.I. (1959) The Albert F. Mathieu Chorionepithelioma Registry. *Annals of the New York Academy of Sciences*, **80**, 140–2.
14. Ober, W.B., Edgcomb, J.H. and Price, E.B. (1971) The pathology of choriocarcinoma. *Annals of the New York Academy of Sciences*, **172**, 299-426.
15. Park, W.W. (1971) *Choriocarcinoma: A Study of its Pathology*, Heinemann, London.
16. Elston, C.W. (1976) The histopathology of trophoblastic tumours. *Journal of Clinical Pathology* **29** (Supplement of the Royal College of Pathologists), **10**, 111–31.
17. Kurman, R.J., Young, R.H., Norris, H.J. *et al.* (1984) Immunocytochemical localization of placental lactogen and chorionic gonadotropin in the normal placenta and trophoblastic tumours, with emphasis on intermediate trophoblast and the placental site trophoblastic tumour. *International Journal of Gynecological Pathology*, **3**, 101-21.
18. Hamilton, W.J. and Boyd, J.D. (1960) Development of the human placenta in the first three months of gestation. *Journal of Anatomy*, **94**, 297-328.
19. Pattillo, R.A., Hussa, R.O., Yorde, D.E. and Cole, L.A. (1983) Hormone synthesis by normal and neoplastic human trophoblast, in *Biology of Trophoblast* (eds Y.W. Loke and A. Whyte), Elsevier, New York, pp. 283–316.
20. Heyderman, E., Gibbons, A.R. and Rosen, A.W. (1953) Immunoperoxidase localisation of human placental lactogen: a marker for placental origin of the giant cells in 'syncytial endometritis' and pregnancy, *Journal of Clinical Pathology*, **34**, 303–7.
21. Yeh, I.T., O'Connor, D.M. and Kurman, R.J. (1990) Intermediate trophoblast: further immunocytochemical characterization. *Modern Pathology*, **3**, 282–7.
22. Park, W.W. (1959) Disorders arising from the human trophoblast, in *Modern Trends in Pathology* (ed. D.H. Collins), Butterworth, London, pp. 180-211.
23. Boyd, J.D. and Hamilton, W.J. (1960) The giant cells of the pregnant human uterus. *Journal of Obstetrics and Gynaecology of the British Empire*, **67**, 208–18.
24. Dearden, L., Ockleford, C.D. and Gupta, M. (1983) Structure of human trophoblast: correlation with function, in *Biology of Trophoblast* (eds Y.W. Loke and A. Whyte), Elsevier, New York, pp. 70-110.
25. Wells, M. and Bulmer, J.N. (1988) The human placental bed: histology, immunohistochemistry and pathology. *Histopathology*, **13**, 483–98.
26. Silverberg, S.G. and Kurman, R.J. (1992) Tumours of the uterine corpus and gestational trophoblastic disease, in *Atlas of Tumour Pathology*, Third Series, Fasc. 3, Armed Forces Institute of Pathology, Washington, DC, pp. 219–85.
27. Kajii, T., and Ohama, K. (1977) Androgenetic origin of hydatidiform mole. *Nature*, **268**, 633–4.
28. Fisher, R.A., Povey, S., Jeffreys, A.J. *et al.* (1989) Frequency of heterozygous complete hydatidiform moles estimated by locus-specific minisatellite and Y chromosome-specific probes. *Human Genetics*, **82**, 259–63.
29. Vassilakos, P., Riotton, G. and Kajii, T. (1977) Hydatidiform mole: two entities. A morphologic and cytogenetic study with some clinical considerations. *American Journal of Obstetrics and Gynecology*, **127**, 167–70.
30. Szulman, A.E., Phillippe, E., Boué, G.J. and Boué, A. (1981) Human triploidy: association with partial hydatidiform moles and nonmolar conceptuses. *Human Pathology*, **12**, 1016–21.
31. Jacobs, P.A., Szulman, A.E., Funkhouser, J. *et al.* (1982) Human triploidy: relationship between parental origin of the additional

haploid complement and development of partial mole. *Annals of Human Genetics*, **46**, 223–31.
32. Young, R.H., Kurman, R.J. and Scully, R.E. (1990) Placental site nodules and plaques: a clinicopathologic analysis of 20 cases. *American Journal of Surgical Pathology*, **14**, 1001–9.
33. Eckstein, R.P., Paradinas, F.J. and Bagshawe, K.D. (1982) Placental site trophoblastic tumour (trophoblastic pseudotumour): a study of four cases requiring hysterectomy including one fatal case. *Histopathology*, **6**, 211–26.
34. Scully, R.E. and Young, R.H. (1981) Trophoblastic pseudotumour: a reappraisal. *American Journal of Surgical Pathology*, **5**, 75–6.
35. Ober, W.B. and Fass, R.O. (1951) The early history of choriocarcinoma. *Journal of History of Medicine and Allied Sciences*, **16**, 49–73.
36. Steven, D.H. (1983) Historical introduction: concepts of the trophoblast and its role in placentation, in *Biology of Trophoblast* (eds Y.W. Loke and A. Whyte), Elsevier, New York, pp. 3–21.
37. Elston, C.W. (1983) Development and structure of trophoblastic neoplasms, in *Biology of Trophoblast* (eds Y.W. Loke and A. Whyte), Elsevier, New York, pp. 188–232.
38. Lawler, S.D. (1984) Genetic studies on hydatidiform moles, in *Human Trophoblastic Neoplasms* (eds R.A. Pattillo and R.O. Hussa), Plenum, New York. pp. 147–61.
39. Hertig, A.T. and Edmonds, H.W. (1940) Genesis of hydatidiform mole. *Archives of Pathology*, **30**, 260–91.
40. Hertig, A.T. and Sheldon, W.H. (1947) Hydatidiform mole: a pathologico clinical correlation of 200 cases. *American Journal of Obstetrics and Gynecology*, **53**, 1–36.
41. Coppleson, M. (1958) Hydatidiform mole and its complications. *Journal of Obstetrics and Gynaecology of the British Empire*, **65**, 238–52.
42. Elston, C.W. and Bagshawe, K.D. (1967) The value of histological grading in the management of hydatidiform mole. *Journal of Obstetrics and Gynaecology of the British Commonwealth*, **79**, 717–24.
43. Genest, D.R., Laborde, O., Berkowitz, R.S. *et al.* (1991) A clinicopathologic study of 153 cases of complete hydatidiform mole (1980–1990): histologic grade lacks prognostic significance. *Obstetrics and Gynecology*, **78**, 402–9.
44. Szulman, A.E. and Surti, U. (1978) The syndromes of hydatidiform mole. I. Cytogenetic and morphological correlations. *American Journal of Obstetrics and Gynecology*, **131**, 665–71.
45. Szulman, A.E. and Surti, U. (1978) The syndromes of hydatidiform mole. II. Morphologic evolution of the complete and partial mole. *American Journal of Obstetrics and Gynecology*, **132**, 20–7.
46. Kajii, T., Kurashige, H., Ohama, K. and Uchino, F. (1984) XY and XX complete moles: clinical and morphological correlations. *American Journal of Obstetrics and Gynecology*, **150**, 57–64.
47. Elston, C.W. (1970) A histopathological study of trophoblastic tumours: with special reference to the cellular reaction to choriocarcinoma. MD Thesis, London University, pp. 71–2.
48. Howat, A.J., Beck, S., Fox, H. *et al.* (1993) Can histopathologists reliably diagnose molar pregnancy? *Journal of Clinical Pathology*, **46**, 599–602.
49. Jacobs P.A., Hunt, P.A., Matsuura, J.S. *et al.* (1982) Complete and partial hydatidiform mole in Hawaii: cytogenetics, morphology and epidemiology. *British Journal of Obstetrics and Gynaecology*, **89**, 258–66.
50. Fisher, R.A. and Paradinas, F.J. (unpublished observations).
51. Fisher, R.A., Lawler, S.D., Ormerod, M.G. *et al.* (1987) Flow cytometry used to distinguish between complete and partial hydatidiform moles. *Placenta*, **8**, 249–56.
52. Lage, J.M., Driscoll, S.G., Yavner, D.L. *et al.* (1988) Hydatidiform moles: application of flow cytometry in diagnosis. *American Journal of Clinical Pathology*, **89**, 596–600.
53. Lawler, S.D., Fisher, R.A. and Dent, J. (1991) A prospective genetic study of complete and partial hydatidiform moles. *American Journal of Clinical Pathology*, **164**, 1270–7.
54. Lage, J.M., Mark, S.D., Roberts, D.J. *et al.* (1992) A flow cytometric study of 137 fresh hydropic placentas: correlation between types of hydatidiform moles and

nuclear DNA ploidy. *Obstetrics and Gynecology*, **79**, 403–10.

55. Hemming, J.D., Quirke, P., Womak, C. *et al.* (1987) Diagnosis of molar pregnancy and persistent trophoblastic disease by flow cytometry. *Journal of Clinical Pathology*, **40**, 615–20.
56. Hedley, D.W., Friedlander, M.L., Taylor, L.W. *et al.* (1983) Method for analysis of cellular DNA content of paraffin-embedded pathological material using flow cytometry. *Journal of Histochemistry and Cytochemistry*, **31**, 1333–5.
57. Vejerslev, L.O., Fisher, R.A., Surti, U. and Wake, N. (1987) Hydatidiform mole: cytogenetically unusual cases and their implications for the present classification. *American Journal of Obstetrics and Gynecology*, **157**, 180–4.
58. Lage, J.M., Weinberg, D.S., Yavner, D.L. and Bieber, F.R. (1989) The biology of tetraploid hydatidiform moles: histopathology, cytogenetics and flow cytometry. *Human Pathology*, **20**, 419–25.
59. Vejerslev, L.L., Dissing, J., Hansen, H.E. and Poulsen, H. (1987) Hydatidiform mole: genetic origin in polyploid conceptuses. *Human Genetics*, **76**, 11-19.
60. Van de Kaa, C.A., Hanselaar, A.G.J.M., Hopman, A.H.N. *et al.* (1993) DNA cytometric and interphase cytogenetic analyses of paraffin-embedded hydatidiform moles and hydropic abortions. *Journal of Pathology*, **170**, 229-38.
61. Cheville, J.C., Greiner, T., Robinson, R.A. and Benda, J.A. (1995) Ploidy analysis by flow cytometry and fluorescence *in situ* hybridization in hydropic placentas and gestational trophoblastic disease. *Human Pathology*, **26**, 753–7.
62. Jeffers, M.D., Michie, B.A. and Oakes, S.J. (1995) Comparison of ploidy analysis by flow cytometry and image analysis in hydatidiform mole and non-molar abortion. *Histopathology*, **27**, 415–21.
63. Wersto, R.P., Liblit, R.L. and Koss, L.G. (1991) Flow cytometric DNA analysis of human solid tumours: a review of the interpretation of DNA histograms. *Human Pathology*, **22**, 1085–98.
64. Fisher, R.A., Paradinas, F.J. (unpublished observations).
65. Vejerslev, L.O., Sunde, L., Hansen, B.F. *et al.* (1991) Hydatidiform mole and fetus with normal karyotype: support for a separate entity. *Obstetrics and Gynecology*, **77**, 868–74.
66. Szulman, A.E. (1965) Chromosomal aberrations in spontaneous human abortions. *New England Journal of Medicine*, **272**, 811–18.
67. Beischer, N.A., Fortune, D.W. and Fitzgerald, M.G. (1967) Hydatidiform mole and coexistent foetus, both with triploid chromosome constitution. *British Medical Journal*, **3**, 476–8.
68. Szulman, A.E., Surti, U. and Berman, M. (1978) Patient with partial mole requiring chemotherapy. *Lancet*, **ii**, 1099.
69. Loi, L.M. and Sivanesaratnam, V. (1981) Malignant evolution with fatal outcome in a patient with partial hydatidiform mole. *Australia and New Zealand Journal of Obstetrics and Gynaecology*, **21**, 51–2.
70. Szulman, A.E., Wong, L.C. and Hsu, C. (1981) Residual trophoblastic disease in association with partial hydatidiform mole. *Obstetrics and Gynecology*, **57**, 392–4.
71. Lawler, S.D., Pickhall, V.J., Fisher, R.A. *et al.* (1979) Genetic studies of complete and partial hydatidiform moles. *Lancet*, **ii**, 580.
72. Lawler, S.D., Fisher, R.A. Pickhall, V.J. *et al.* (1986) Genetic studies on hydatidiform moles. I. The origin of partial moles. *Cancer Genetics and Cytogenetics*, **5**, 309-20.
73. Doshi, N., Surti, U. and Szulman, A.E. (1983) Morphologic anomalies in triploid liveborn fetuses. *Human Pathology*, **14**, 716–23.
74. Paradinas, F.J., Browne, P., Dent, J. *et al.* (1991) Problems in the histological diagnosis of hydatidiform mole: a survey from the UK. *Journal of Pathology*, **163**, 168A.
75. Davis, J., Kerrigan, D.P., Way, D.L. and Weiner, S.A. (1987) Partial hydatidiform moles: deoxyribonucleic acid content and course. *American Journal of Obstetrics and Gynecology*, **157**, 969–73.
76. Bagshawe, K.D., Lawler, S.D., Paradinas, F.J. *et al.* (1990) Gestational trophoblastic tumours following initial diagnosis of partial hydatidiform mole. *Lancet*, **335**, 1074–6.
77. Fukunaga, M., Ushigome, S. and Endo, Y. (1995) Incidence of hydatidiform mole in a Tokyo hospital: a 5-year (1989 to

1993) prospective, morphological and flow cytometric study. *Human Pathology*, **26**, 758–64.
78. Honoré, L.H. Dill, F.J. and Poland, B.J. (1976) Placental morphology in spontaneous human abortuses with normal and abnormal karyotypes. *Teratology*, **14**, 151–66.
79. Boué, J. Phillipe, E., Giroud, E. and Boué, A. (1976) Phenotypic expression of lethal chromosomal abnormalities in human abortuses. *Teratology*, **14**, 3–13.
80. Suresh, U.R., Hale, R.J., Fox, H. and Buckley, C.H. (1993) Use of proliferation cell nuclear antigen immunoreactivity for distinguishing hydropic abortions from partial hydatidiform moles. *Journal of Clinical Pathology*, **46**, 48–50.
81. Cheung, A.N.Y., Ngan, H.Y.S., Chen, W.Z. *et al*. (1993) The significance of the proliferating cell nuclear antigen in human trophoblastic disease: an immunohistochemical study. *Histopathology*, **22**, 565–8.
82. Jeffers, M.D., Grehan, D. and Gillan, J.E. (1994) Comparison of villous trophoblast proliferation rate in hydatidiform mole and nonmolar abortion by assessment of proliferating cell nuclear antigen expression. *Placenta*, **15**, 551–6.
83. Brescia, R.J., Kurman, R. J., Main, C.S. *et al*. (1987) Immunocytochemical localization of chorionic gonadotropin, placental lactogen and placental alkaline phosphatase in the diagnosis of complete and partial moles. *International Journal of Gynecological Pathology*, **6**, 213–29.
84. Lage, J.M. (1991) Placentomegaly with massive hydrops of placental stem villi, diploid DNA content and fetal omphaloceles: possible association with Beckwith–Wiedeman syndrome. *Human Pathology*, **22**, 591–7.
85. McCowan, L.M.E. and Becroft, D.M.O. (1995) Beckwith–Wiedeman syndrome, placental abnormalities and gestational proteinuric hypertension. *Obstetrics and Gynecology*, **83**, 813–17.
86. Berkowitz, R.S., Goldstein, D.P. and Bernstein, M.R. (1985) Natural history of partial molar pregnancy. *Obstetrics and Gynecology*, **66**, 677–81.
87. Byrne, J., Blanc, W.A., Warburton, D. and Wigger, J. (1984) The significance of cystic hygroma in fetuses. *Human Pathology*, **15**, 61–7.
88. Suresh, U.R. Chawner, L., Buckley, C.H. and Fox, H. (1990) Do Agnor counts reflect cellular ploidy or cellular proliferation? A study of trophoblastic tissue. *Journal of Pathology*, **160**, 213–15.
89. Tommerup, N. and Vejerslev, L.O. (1985) Identification of triploidy by DA/DAPI staining of trophoblastic interphase nuclei. *Placenta*, **6**, 363–7.
90. Gaber, L.W., Redline, R.W., Mostoufi-Zadeh, M. and Driscoll, S.G. (1986) Invasive partial mole. *American Journal of Clinical Pathology*, **85**, 722–4.
91. Haines, M. (1955) Hydatidiform mole and vaginal nodules. *Journal of Obstetrics and Gynaecology of the British Empire*, **62**, 6–11.
92. Dinh-De, T. and Minh, H.N. (1961) Hydatidiform mole with recurrent vaginal metastases. *American Journal of Obstetrics and Gynecology*, **82**, 660–3.
93. Bagshawe, K.D. and Garnett, E.S. (1963) Radiological changes in the lungs of patients with trophoblastic tumours. *British Journal of Radiology*, **36**, 673–9.
94. Thiele, R.A. and de Alvarez, R.R. (1962) Metastasizing benign trophoblastic tumours. *American Journal of Obstetrics and Gynecology*, **84**, 1935–406.
95. Meyer, J.S. (1966) Benign pulmonary metastasis from hydatidiform mole: report of a case. *Obstetrics and Gynecology*, **28**, 826–9.
96. Jacobson, T.J. and Enzer, N. (1959) Hydatidiform mole with benign metastasis to lung: histologic evidence of regressing lesions in the lung. *American Journal of Obstetrics and Gynecology*, **78**, 868–75.
97. Ober, W.B., and Maier, R.C. (1981) Gestational choriocarcinoma of the fallopian tube. *Diagnostic Gynecology and Obstetrics*, **3**, 213–31.
98. Kika, K. and Matuda, I. (1957) Primary tubal hydatidiform mole: report of a case. *Obstetrics and Gynecology*, **9**, 224–7.
99. Muto, M.G., Lage, J.M., Berkowitz, R.S. *et al*. (1991) Gestational trophoblastic disease of the fallopian tube. *Journal of Reproductive Medicine*, **36**, 57–60.
100. Terada, S., Suzuki, N., Uchide, K. and Akasofu, K. (1993) Partial hydatidiform mole

in the fallopian tube. *Gynecological and Obstetric Investigation*, **35**, 240–2.

101. Fisher, R.A., Sheppard, D.M. and Lawler, S.D. (1982) Twin pregnancy with complete hydatidiform mole (46,XX) and fetus (46,XY): genetic origin proved by analysis of chromosome polymorphisms. *British Medical Journal*, **284**, 1218–20.
102. Vejerslev, L.O., Dueholm, M. and Hassing Nielsen, F. (1986) Hydatidiform mole: cytogenetic marker analysis in twin gestation. Report of two cases. *American Journal of Obstetrics and Gynecology*, **155**, 614–17.
103. Van de Kaa, C.A., Robben, J.C.M., Hopman, A.H.N. *et al.* (1995) Complete hydatidiform mole in twin pregnancy: differentiation from partial mole with interphase cytogenetic and DNA cytometric analysis on paraffin embedded tissue. *Histopathology*, **26**, 123–9.
104. Sauerbrei, E.E. Salem, S. and Fayle, B. (1980) Coexistent hydatidiform mole and live fetus in the second trimester. *Radiology*, **135**, 415–7.
105. Murray, J. and Dalrymple, C. (1992) Coexistent complete and partial hydatidiform moles in a twin pregnancy. *Abstracts of the VI World Congress on Gestational Trophoblastic Diseases*, Sydney, p. 7.
106. Honda, J., Ihara, S., Sato, A. *et al.* (1980) Hydatidiform mole concurrent with normal pregnancy (twins) following clomiphene therapy. *Acta Obstetrica Gynaecologica Japonica*, **32**, 2041–3.
107. Paradinas, F.J. Browne, P., Fisher, R.A. and Newlands, E.S. (1994) Diploid complete moles with coexistent embryonic tissues: incidence and prognosis. *Abstracts of the VII World Congress on Gestational Trophoblastic Diseases*, Hong Kong, p. 57.
108. Steller, M.A., Genest, D.R., Bernstein, M.R. *et al.* (1994) Natural history of twin pregnancy with complete hydatidiform mole and coexisting fetus. *Obstetrics and Gynecology*, **83**, 35–42.
109. Kato, M., Tanaka, K. and Takeuchi, S. (1982) The nature of trophoblastic disease initiated by transplantation into immunosuppressed animals. *American Journal of Obstetrics and Gynecology*, **142**, 497–505.
110. Fisher, R.A., Newlands, E.S., Jeffreys, A.J. *et al.* (1992) Gestational and nongestational trophoblastic tumors distinguished by DNA analysis. *Cancer*, **69**, 839–45.
111. Fisher, R.A., Soteriou, B.A., Meredith, L. *et al.* (1995) Previous hydatidiform mole identified as the causative pregnancy of choriocarcinoma following birth of normal twins. *International Journal of Gynecological Cancer*, **5**, 64–70.
112. Bagshawe, K.D., Dent, J. and Webb, J. (1986) Hydatidiform mole in England and Wales 1973–1983. *Lancet*, **ii**, 673–7.
113. Bagshawe, K.D., Wilson, H., Dublon, P. *et al.* (1973) Follow-up after hydatidiform mole: studies using radioimmunoassay for urinary human chorionic gonadotrophin (HCG). *Journal of Obstetrics and Gynaecology of the British Commonwealth*, **80**, 461–8.
114. Curry, S.L., Hammond, C.B., Tyrey, L. *et al.* (1975) Hydatidiform mole, diagnosis, management and long-term follow up of 347 patients. *Obstetrics and Gynecology*, **45**, 1–8.
115. Lurain, J.R., Brewer, J.I., Torok, E.E. and Halpern, B. (1983) Natural history of hydatidiform mole after primary evacuation. *American Journal of Obstetrics and Gynecology*, **145**, 591–5.
116. Davis, J.R., Surwit, E.A., Garay, J.P. and Fortier, K.J. (1994) Sex assignment in gestational trophoblastic neoplasia. *American Journal of Obstetrics and Gynecology*, **148**, 722–5.
117. Wake, N., Seki, T., Fujita, H. *et al.* (1984) Malignant potential of homozygous and heterozygous complete moles. *Cancer Research*, **44**, 1226–30.
118. Fisher, R.A. and Lawler, S.D. (1984) Heterozygous complete hydatidiform moles: do they have a worse prognosis than homozygous complete moles? *Lancet*, **ii**, 51.
119. Lage, J.M., Berkowitz, R.S., Rice, L.W. *et al.* (1991) Flow cytometric analysis of DNA content in partial hydatidiform moles with persistent gestational trophoblastic tumor. *Obstetrics and Gynecology*, **77**, 111–15.
120. Acosta-Sison, H. (1959) Ab initio choriocarcinoma: two unusual cases. *Obstetrics and Gynecolocy*, **13**, 350–2.
121. Chung, T.K.H., Cheung, T.H., Lam, S.K. and Chang, A.M.Z. (1995) Epidemiology and aetiology of trophoblastic disease. *Current Obstetrics and Gynaecology*, **5**, 2–5.

122. Elston, C.W. (1969) Cellular reaction to choriocarcinoma. *Journal of Pathology*, **97**, 261–8.
123. Deligdisch, L., Driscoll, S.G. and Goldstein, D.P. (1978) Gestational trophoblastic neoplasms: morphologic correlates of therapeutic response. *American Journal of Obstetrics and Gynecology*, **130**, 801–6.
124. Elston, C.W. (1987) Gestational trophoblastic disease, in *Haynes and Taylor Gynaecological Pathology*, Chapter 41 (ed. H. Fox), Churchill Livingstone, Edinburgh, pp. 1045–78.
125. Mazur, M.T. (1989) Metastatic gestational choriocarcinoma: unusual pathological variant following therapy. *Cancer*, **50**, 1370–7.
126. Paradinas, F.J. (1994) Value of histopathology in the diagnosis and prognosis of placental site trophoblastic tumour. *Abstracts of the VII World Congress on Gestational Trophoblastic Diseases*, Hong Kong, p. 49.
127. Bagshawe, K.D. and Noble, M.I.M. (1966) Cardio-respiratory aspects of trophoblastic tumours. *Quarterly Journal of Medicine*, **35**, 39–54.
128. Magrath, I.T., Golding, P.R and Bagshawe, K.D. (1971) Medical presentations of choriocarcinoma. *British Medical Journal*, **ii**, 633–7.
129. Knoop, C., Jacobovitz, D., Antoine, M. *et al.* (1994) Donor transmitted tumours in lung allograft recipients. *Transplantation*, **57**, 1679–80.
130. Emery, J.L. (1952) Chorionepithelioma in new-born male child with hyperplasia of interstitial cells of testis. *Journal of Pathology and Bacteriology*, **64**, 735–9.
131. Buckell, E.W.C. and Owen, T.K. (1954) Chorionepithelioma in mother and infant. *Journal of Obstetrics and Gynaecology of the British Empire*, **61**, 329–30.
132. Elston, C.W. and Bagshawe, K.D. (1972) The diagnosis of trophoblastic tumours from uterine curettings. *Journal of Clinical Pathology*, **25**, 111–18.
133. Flam, F., Lundstrom, V., Lindstedt, J. and Silfversward, C. (1989) Choriocarcinoma of the fallopian tube associated with induced superovulation in an IVF program: a case report. *European Journal of Obstetrics, Gynecology and Reproductive Biology*, **33**, 183–6.
134. Patton, G.W. and Goldstein, D.P. (1973) Gestational choriocarcinoma of the tube and ovary. *Surgery, Gynecology and Obstetrics*, **137**, 608–12.
135. Benjamin, F. and Rorat, E. (1978) Primary gestational choriocarcinoma of the ovary. *American Journal of Obstetrics and Gynecology*, **131**, 343–5.
136. Kuida, C.A., Braunstein, G.D., Shintaku, P. and Said, J.W. (1988) Human chorionic gonadotropin expression in lung, breast and renal carcinomas. *Archives of Pathology and Laboratory Medicine*, **112**, 282–5.
137. Azer, P.C., Braunstein, G.D., Van de Velde, R.L. *et al.* (1980) Ectopic production of pregnancy-specific beta 1-glycoprotein by a nontrophoblastic tumour *in vitro*. *Journal of Clinical Endocrinology and Metabolism*, **50**, 234–9.
138. Savage, J., Subby, W. and Okagaki, T. (1987) Adenocarcinoma of the endometrium with trophoblastic differentiation and metastases as choriocarcinoma: a case report. *Gynecological Oncolocy*, **26**, 257–62.
139. Fisher, R.A. and Newlands, E.S. (1993) Rapid diagnosis and classification of hydatidiform moles using polymerase chain reaction. *American Journal of Obstetrics and Gynecology*, **168**, 563–9.
140. Paradinas, F.J. and Fisher, R.A. (1995) Pathology and molecular genetics and trophoblastic disease. *Current Obstetrics and Gynaecology*, **5**, 6–12.
141. Tanimura, A., Natsuyama, H., Kawano, M., *et al.* (1985) Primary choriocarcinoma of the lung. *Human Pathology*, **16**, 1281–4.
142. Pushchak, M.J. and Farhi, D.C. (1987) Primary choriocarcinoma of the lung. *Archives of Pathology and Laboratory Medicine*, **111**, 447–9.
143. Saigo, P.E. and Rosen, P.P. (1981) Mammary carcinoma with choriocarcinomatous features. *American Journal of Surgical Pathology*, **5**, 773–8.
144. Green, D.M. (1990) Mucoid carcinoma of the breast with choriocarcinoma in its metastases. *Histopathology*, **16**, 504–6.
145. Kubosawa, H., Nagao, K., Kondo, Y. *et al.* (1984) Coexistence of adenocarcinoma and choriocarcinoma in the sigmoid colon. *Cancer*, **54**, 866–88.

146. Matthews, T.H., Heaton, G.E. and Christopherson, W.M. (1986) Primary duodenal choriocarcinoma. *Archives of Pathology and Laboratory Medicine*, **110**, 550–2.
147. Nakanuma, Y., Unoura, M., Noto, H. and Ohta, G. (1986) Human chorionic gonadotropin in primary liver carcinoma in adults: an immunohistochemical study. *Virchows Arch. Pathol. Anat. Histopathol.*, **409**, 365–73.
148. Watanabe, I., Yamaguchi, M. and Kasai, M. (1987) Histologic characteristics of gonadotropin-producing hepatoblastoma: a survey of seven cases from Japan. *Journal of Pediatric Surgery*, **22**, 406–11.
149. Maeyama, M., Furuki, Y., Munemura, M. *et al.* (1985) *In vivo* and *in vitro* studies on the production of placental proteins (human chorionic gonadotropin hCG, human placental lactogen and pregnancy specific beta 1-glycoprotein) in an adrenal choriocarcinoma. *Obstetrics and Gynecology*, **65**, 593–6.
150. Obe, J.A., Rosen, N. and Koss, L.G. (1983) Primary choriocarcinoma of the urinary bladder: report of a case with probable epithelial origin. *Cancer*, **52**, 1405–9.
151. Shah, V.M., Newman, J. Croker, J. *et al.* (1986) Ectopic beta-human chorionic gonadotropin production by bladder urothelial neoplasia. *Archives of Pathology and Laboratory Medicine*, **110**, 107–11.
152. Kurman, R.J., Scully, R.E. and Norris, H.J. (1976) Trophoblastic pseudotumour of the uterus: an exaggerated form of 'syncytial endometritis' simulating a malignant tumour. *Cancer*, **38**, 1214–26.
153. Gloor, E., Dialdas, J., Hartimann, J. *et al.* (1983) Placental site trophoblastic tumor (trophoblastic pseudotumor) of the uterus with metastases and fatal outcome: clinical and autopsy observations of a case. *American Journal of Surgical Pathology*, **7**, 483–7.
154. Young, R.H. and Scully, R.E. (1984) Placental-site trophoblastic tumor: current status. *Clinical Obstetrics and Gynecology*, **27**, 248–58.
155. Eckstein, R.P., Russell, P., Friedlander, M.L. *et al.* (1985) Metastasizing placental site trophoblastic tumour: a case study. *Human Pathology*, **16**, 632–6.
156. Fisher, R.A., Paradinas, F.J., Newlands, E.S. and Boxer, G.M. (1992) Genetic evidence that placental site trophoblastic tumours can originate from a hydatidiform mole or a normal conceptus. *British Journal of Cancer*, **65**, 355–8.
157. Bower, M., Paradinas, F.J., Fisher, R.A. *et al.* (1996) Placental site trophoblastic tumour: clinical experience and genetic origin. *Clinical Cancer Genetics* (in press).
158. Fukunaga, M. and Ushigome, S. (1993) Metastasizing placental site trophoblastic tumour. *American Journal of Surgical Pathology*, **17**, 1003–10.
159. How, J., Scurry, J., Grant, P. *et al.* (1995) Placental site trophoblastic tumour: report of three cases and review of the literature. *International Journal of Gynecological Cancer*, **5**, 241–9.
160. Young, R.H., Scully, R.E. and McCluskey, R.T. (1985) A distinctive glomerular lesion complicating placental site trophoblastic tumour: report of two cases. *Human Pathology*, **16**, 35–42.
161. Nagelberg, S.B. and Rosen, S.W. (1985) Clinical and laboratory investigation of a virilised woman with placental site trophoblastic tumour. *Obstetrics and Gynecology*, **65**, 527–34.
162. Paradinas, F.J. (1992) Pathology and classification of trophoblastic tumours, in *Gynecologic Oncology* (eds M. Coppleson, J.M. Monaghan, C.P. Morrow and M.H.N. Tattersall), Churchill Livingstone, Edinburgh. pp. 1013–26.
163. Collins, R.J., Ngan, H.Y.S. and Wong, L.C. (1990) Placental site trophoblastic tumour: with features between an exaggerated placental site reaction and a placental site trophoblastic tumour. *International Journal of Gynecological Pathology*, **9**, 170–7.
164. Sugimori, H., Kashimura, Y., Kashimura, M. *et al.* (1978) Nuclear DNA content of trophoblastic tumours. *Acta Cytologica (Baltimore)*, **22**, 542–5.
165. Fukunaga, M. and Ushigome, S. (1993) Malignant trophoblastic tumours: immunohistochemical and flow cytometric comparison of choriocarcinoma and placental site trophoblastic tumours. *Human Pathology*, **24**, 1098–106.
166. Gloor, E. and Hürlimann, J. (1981) Trophoblastic pseudotumour of the uterus:

Clinicopathologic report with immunohistochemical and ultrastructural studies. *American Journal of Surgical Pathology*, **5**, 5–13.

167. Dessau, R., Rustin, G., Dent, J. *et al*. (1990) Surgery and chemotherapy in the management of placental site tumour. *Gynecological Oncology*, **339**, 56–9.
168. Finkler, N., Berkowitz, R., Driscoll, S. *et al*. (1988) Clinical experience with placental site trophoblastic tumours at the New England Trophoblastic Disease Center. *Obstetrics and Gynecology*, **71**, 854–7.
169. Lee, K.C. and Chan, J.K. (1990) Placental site nodule. *Histopathology*, **16**, 193–5.
170. Shitabata, P.K. and Rutgers, J.L. (1994) The placental site nodule: an immunohistochemical study. *Human Pathology*, **25**, 1295–30.
171. Huettner, P.C. and Gersell, D.J. (1994) Placental site nodule: a clinicopathologic study of 38 cases. *International Journal of Gynecological Pathology*, **13**, 191–8.
172. Silva, E.G., Tornos, C., Lage, J. *et al*. (1993) Multiple nodules of intermediate trophoblast following hydatidiform moles. *International Journal of Gynecological Pathology*, **12**, 324–32.
173. Klein, J. (1963) Delayed appearance and rupture of lutein cysts with hydatidiform mole. *Obstetrics and Gynecology*, **21**, 30–2.

HUMAN CHORIONIC GONADOTROPIN ASSAY 5

Laurence A. Cole

5.1 INTRODUCTION

Human chorionic gonadotropin (hCG) is a single name, yet refers to multiple molecules, varying in their peptide or carbohydrate moieties. This heterogeneity, while apparent in normal pregnancy, is most evident in trophoblast disease. We describe this heterogeneity, particularly as it applies to trophoblast disease.

hCG is a large glycoprotein, with at least 11 distinct antibody sites. There are over 100 commercial assays available for measuring serum and urine levels of hCG. Each uses a slightly different combination of antibodies to these 11 hCG sites, and so detects slightly different things. This causes variability in hCG test results, particularly when testing trophoblast disease. We outline the types of antibodies used in hCG assays, some examples of commercial assays, inter-assay variability in trophoblast disease, and the optimal types of test for trophoblast disease applications.

Trophoblast disease, particularly invasive mole and choriocarcinoma, are marked by nicked or cleaved hCG molecules, carbohydrate-variant molecules, and by higher proportions of hCG free β-subunit in serum samples. We describe these tests and their potential use in the differential diagnosis of complete and partial hydatidiform mole, and benign and invasive disease.

It can be difficult to diagnose and treat patients with borderline hCG levels – those with levels persistently hovering around the detection limit of the assay, 2–10 U/l. We consider the possibility of measuring hCG free β-subunit or hCG β-core fragment, to help decipher whether residual trophoblast tissue is present.

5.2 THE HETEROGENEITY OF hCG

hCG is a glycoprotein hormone composed of two dissimilar subunits, α and β, joined non-covalently (Figure 5.1). The α-subunit of hCG is similar to that of the pituitary glycoprotein hormones; the β-subunit, however, is unique and distinguishes hCG from these other hormones. The hormone is produced by trophoblast tissue in pregnancy and trophoblast disease, and in small amounts by certain cancer tissues. The principal function of hCG is to promote progesterone production by the ovarian corpus luteum.

In addition to intact hCG, the hormone, a variety of broken-up or degraded hCG molecules are detected in serum and urine samples. All of these have little or no biological activity[1–7]. The following sections des-

Gestational Trophoblastic Disease.
Edited by B.W. Hancock, E.S. Newlands and R.S. Berkowitz.
ISBN 0 412 63100 8

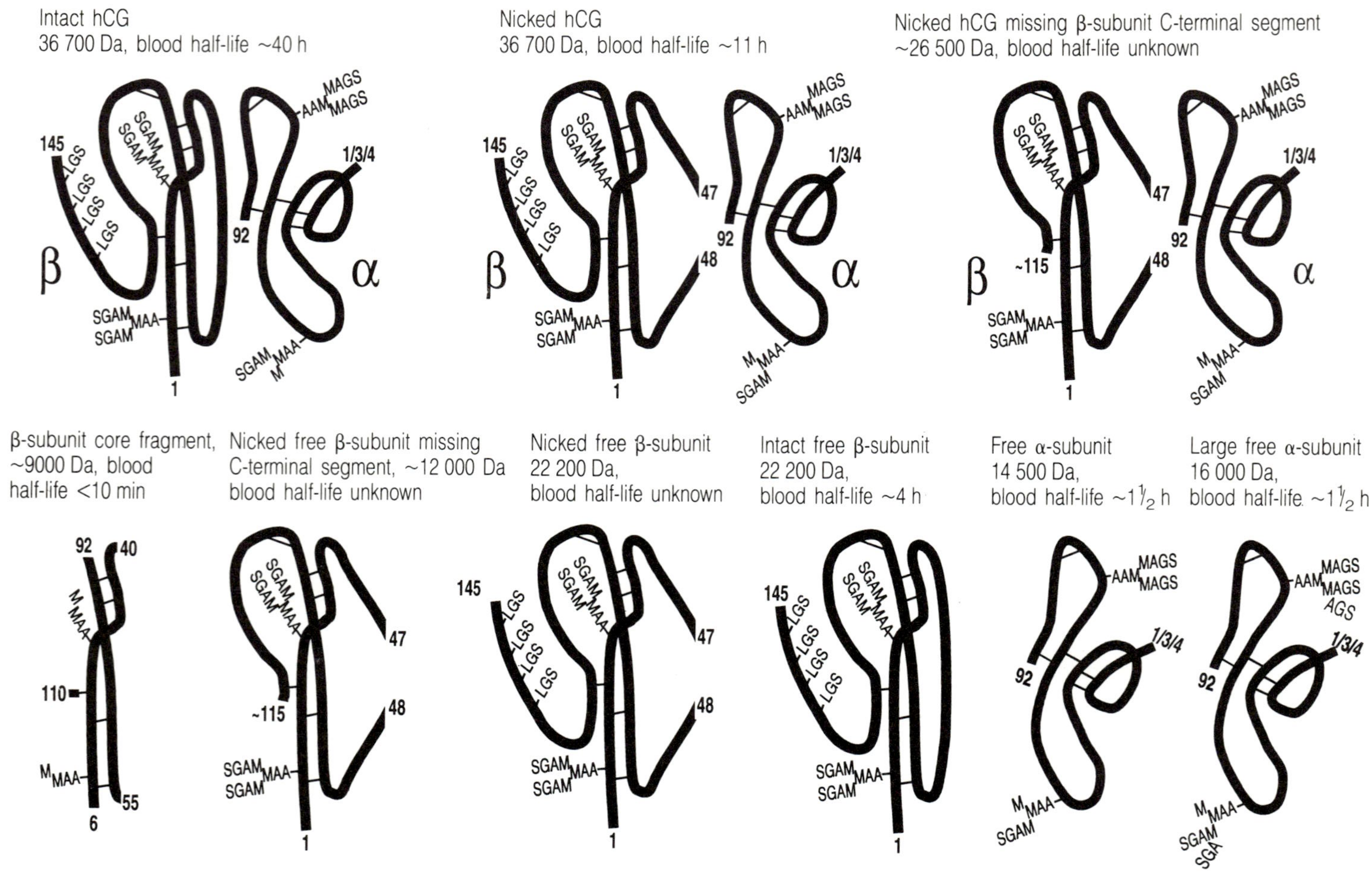

Figure 5.1 Outline structures of hCG and related molecules. Thick black lines represent the polypeptide chains. Numbers are the amino acid numbers in the chains. The thin lines represent disulfide linkages. Structures are folded according to the amino acid sequences of Morgan *et al.*[20], and to match the disulfide linkages of Lapthorn *et al.*[21]. Nicking site is that determined by Kardana *et al.*[5], and structure of β-core fragment that established by Birken *et al.*[4]. Approximate oligosaccharide structures are illustrated as chains of letters. A is *N*-acetylglucosamine, M is mannose, G is galactose, S is sialic acid and L is *N*-acetylgalactosamine. *N*-linked oligosaccharide structures were determined by Mizuochi *et al.*[23] and *O*-linked structure by Cole[24], and sugar structure on large free α-subunit by Blithe *et al.*[7]. Circulating half-lives are the slow components determined by Nisula and Wehmann[22]. Nicked hCG half-life is adjusted for dissociation half-time[3].

cribe these molecules and their occurrences in pregnancy and trophoblast disease serum and urine samples.

5.2.1 PEPTIDE HETEROGENEITY

The structure of intact hCG (the hormone) is outlined in Figure 5.1 (two-dimensional representation). It is composed of a 92 amino acid α-subunit, with two sugar side chains, associated with a 145 amino acid β-subunit with six sugar side chains. In addition to intact hCG, α-subunit *N*-terminal variations, nicked hCG, nicked hCG missing the β-subunit C-terminal segment, and free subunits and fragments can also be detected in serum or urine samples. A proportion of all hCG samples have degraded α-subunits, missing residues 1 and 2, or 1, 2 and 3[5]. A varying proportion is also cut or nicked between residues 43 and 44, between residues 44 and 45, or between 47 and 48 on the β-subunit[1,2,5]. While these different nicks do not remove any amino acids, they diminish the biological activity of hCG[3]. Nicked hCG can also be detected in serum samples missing the β-subunit C-terminal peptide (CTP) segment[3]. Nicked hCG is unstable, continuously splitting into nicked free β-subunit and free α-subunit (dissociation half-time 22 h versus >700 h for intact hCG[6]). Nicked free β-subunit and free α-subunit are also detected in serum samples. In addition, a large free α-subunit with abnormal sugar side chains and a regular free β-subunit are secreted by trophoblast tissue, and detected in serum samples[7]. Nicked free β-subunit may be continuously degraded to nicked free β-subunit missing the CTP and to β-core fragment[4–6]. β-Core fragment is a terminal degradation product, comprising β-subunit residues 6–40, 55–92 and 110, held together by disulfide bridges[4]. β-Subunit missing the β-subunit CTP and β-core fragment are most abundant in urine samples, in which they can account for as much as 90% of the hCG β-subunit-related molecules[3].

The β-subunit heteromers, nicked hCG, nicked hCG missing the β-subunit CTP, free β-subunit, nicked free β-subunit, nicked free β-subunit missing the β-subunit CTP and β-core fragment, and α-subunit N-terminal heterogeneity, are all much more abundant in trophoblast disease serum and urine than in pregnancy samples[2,3,5,8–19]. The abundance of nicked, dissociated and other broken-up molecules complicates the measurement of hCG in trophoblast disease. Firstly, its confounded by the uncertainty of what to measure, just intact hCG, intact and nicked hCG, or whether to measure all hCG-related molecules. Secondly, it is confused by the variability of what assays measure.

Nicked hCG missing the β-subunit CTP is unique to trophoblast disease patient serum and urine samples[5,8]. The proportion of free β-subunit molecules is much higher in trophoblast disease samples. In our experience, free β-subunit (nicked and non-nicked) accounts for $0.53 \pm 0.18\%$ of hCG levels in five- to eight-week pregnancies, $5.2 \pm 5.6\%$ in hydatidiform mole and $12 \pm 8.0\%$ in invasive mole and choriocarcinoma[10]. Similar levels have been reported by others[9–17]. Nicked hCG molecules account for $10 \pm 10\%$ of hCG molecules in 7–11-week pregnancies ($n = 40$), and $28 \pm 17\%$ of molecules in trophoblast disease[8]. Other reports also describe more extreme nicking or exclusive nicking in trophoblast disease[1,2,5,18]. The heterogeneity problem is not limited to initial pre-therapy samples; the proportions of nicked hCG molecules and free β-subunit can rise to as much as 100% of the hCG level during the clearance of hormone following evacuation of a hydatidiform mole, or during remission or recurrence of choriocarcinoma[19].

5.2.2 CARBOHYDRATE HETEROGENEITY

hCG α-subunit has two *N*-linked sugar units,

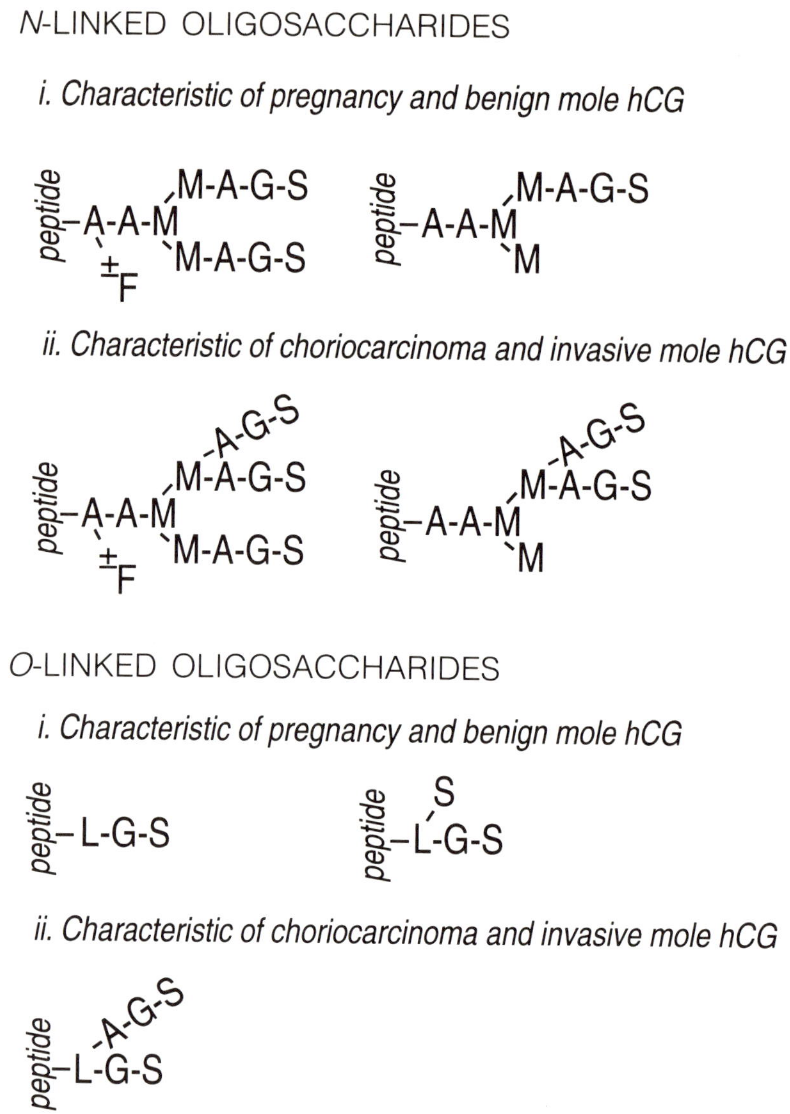

Figure 5.2 The oligosaccharide structure of hCG in normal pregnancy and benign mole, and in invasive mole plus choriocarcinoma. Approximate oligosaccharide structures are illustrated as chains of letters. A is *N*-acetylglucosamine, M is mannose, G is galactose, S is sialic acid and L is *N*-acetylgalactosamine. *N*-Linked oligosaccharide structures were determined by Mizuochi *et al.*[23] and *O*-linked structure by Cole[24].

linked to amino acid residues 52 and 78 (Figure 5.1). hCG β-subunit also has two, at residues 13 and 30. Carbohydrate variants of hCG have been detected in samples from invasive mole and choriocarcinoma. Pregnancy hCG has an *N*-linked sugar unit with mainly one or two antenna sequences (-M-A-G-S sequence, Figure 5.2). Invasive mole and choriocarcinoma molecules have an additional antenna sequence (-A-G-S, Figure 5.2), or two or three antennae[23]. The β-subunit of hCG also has 4 *O*-linked sugar units at serine residues 121, 127, 132 and 138 (Figure 5.1)[24,25]. Simple trisaccharide and tetrasaccharide structures are found in normal pregnancy hCG, and a hexasaccharide structure with an additional antenna sequence (-A-G-S, Figure 5.2), on invasive mole and choriocarcinoma molecules[24,25]. While pregnancy hCG molecules have a conservative 10–14 sialic acid residues on the *N*- and *O*-linked oligosaccharides, choriocarcinoma molecules have anywhere from zero to 19 sialic acid residues. This causes charge heterogeneity[23,24]. This may affect the affinity of antibodies for hCG. Sialic acid-deficient molecules can give exaggerated results, and molecules with additional sialic acid residues can give reduced responses in competitive hCG immunoassays[26,27].

5.3 hCG ASSAY

In the 1940s and 1950s a rodent uterine weight test was used to measure hCG and lutropin. This was replaced in 1960 by the competitive radioimmunoassay. This used anti-hCG antisera and detected hCG and lutropin. In 1972 Vaitukaitis and colleagues developed the βhCG radioimmunoassay using antisera to hCG β-subunit[28]. This assay, also called the βhCG test, was the first to distinguish hCG and luteinizing hormone. The βhCG assay was the test of choice in the 1970s and early 1980s, and is still used by some laboratories today. Physicians ordered a βhCG test, rather than just an hCG test, to make sure they were getting the new test that does not detect lutropin. With time, the word βhCG became synonymous with hCG. The term βhCG is still, erroneously, used today, even though we use very different types of hCG immunoassay.

The arrival of monoclonal antibodies led to more sophisticated immunoassays. Multiple-site sandwich assays were developed, which are generally more sensitive and more specific than the βhCG test. With short incubations and automated instruments, such as the Abbott Labs. IMX, the Baxter Diagnostics Stratus, and the Ciba-Corning Magic Light, these new sandwich assays have become much more rapid also. Today hCG levels are measured by many different combinations of sandwich assay or less often by the βhCG radioimmunoassay, in any of over 100 different commercial kits.

The βhCG radioimmunoassay detected all forms of hCG and its free β-subunit, and urine β-core fragment (Figure 5.1)[8]. Most of the new sandwich assays, however, are more specific, and do not detect all broken-up hCG molecules. Broken-up molecules are more prevalent in trophoblast disease blood samples. As such, some sandwich assays give lower hCG values or even false negative results with trophoblast disease samples. The instruction sheets in most hCG kits claim that the assay is only approved for or only tested for normal pregnancy applications. Care must be taken in choosing hCG kits for detecting and monitoring trophoblast disease samples.

5.3.1 PRINCIPLE OF IMMUNOASSAY

To understand hCG assays, and the problems that arise in trophoblast disease, one must first understand how the assays work. There are two basic types of immunoassay: the non-competitive or sandwich assay, and the competitive test, like the βhCG radioimmunoassay. The principles of both types of test are outlined in Figure 5.3. In non-competitive (sandwich) assays, tubes, wells or beads are coated with a capture antibody. The sample is added, and hCG slowly binds to the capture antibody. The labeled antibody is added. This is raised against a distant site on hCG (to capture antibody), and is labeled with a dye, with an enzyme that can catalyze the formation of a

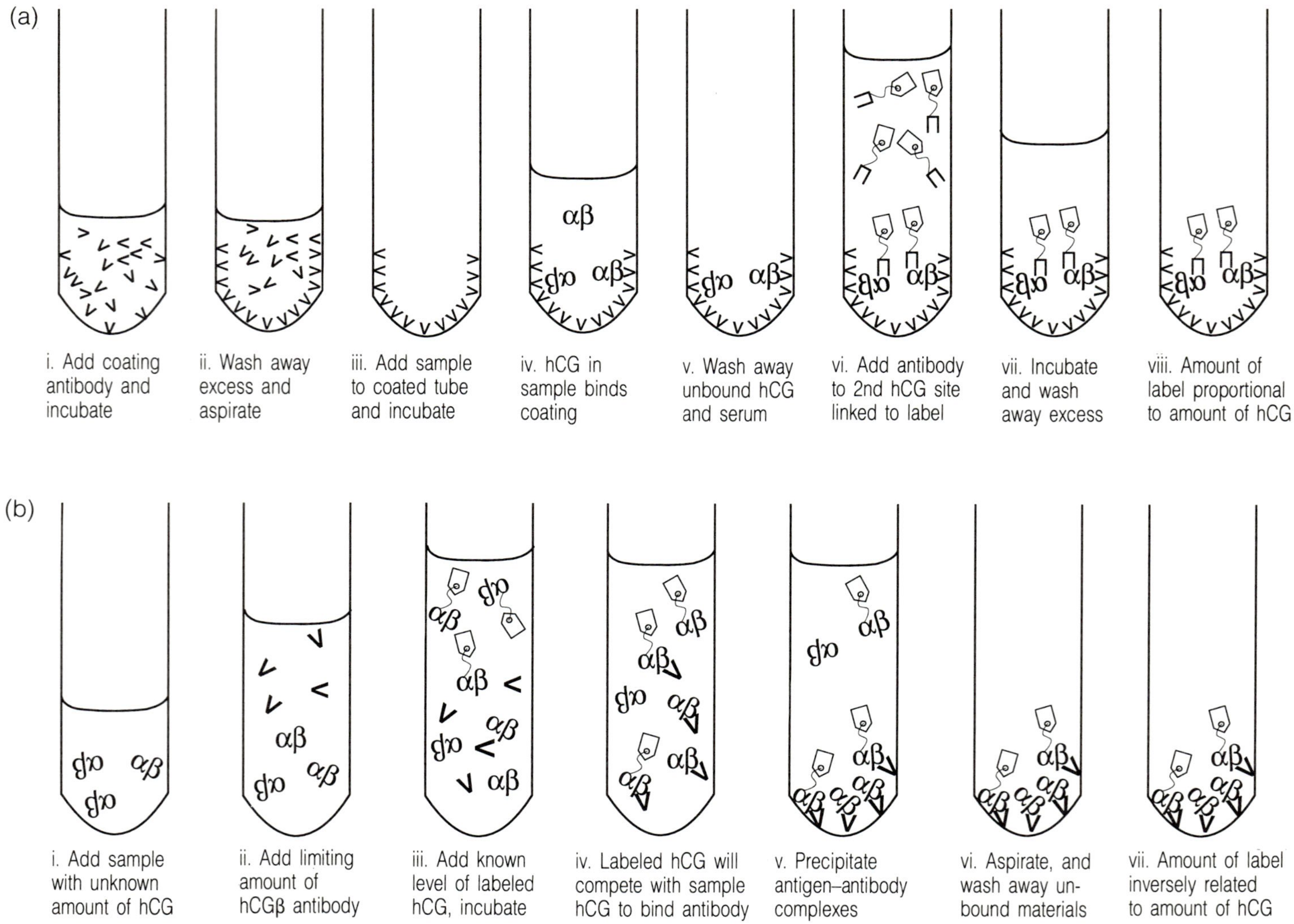

Figure 5.3 Competitive and non-competitive hCG assay methods. Arrow heads indicate antibody; $\alpha\beta$ is hCG; parcel tag represents an enzyme, radioactive or chemical label, which may be attached to an antibody or antigen. (a) Non-competitive assay method; (b) competitive assay method.

colored product, or with radioactive iodine. A sandwich forms, capture antibody: hCG-labeled antibody. The excess labeled antibody is washed away, and the amount of label determined by spectrometry, gamma counting or other methods. The amount of label is proportional to the amount of hCG.

In the competitive assay method, a known amount of dye, enzyme or radioactive labeled hCG, competes with a sample hCG to bind a limited amount of βhCG antibody. The greater the unknown amount of hCG the smaller the proportion of labeled hCG binding the antibody. The antigen–antibody complexes are precipitated, separated, and the amount of label determined. The amount of label in the precipitate is inversely proportional to the level of sample hCG.

5.3.2 COMMERCIAL hCG ASSAYS

The specificity of a sandwich-type hCG assay is controlled by the combination of antibodies employed. We know of 11 general types of hCG antibody (Table 5.1). Anti-β1 is the βhCG antibody described by Vaitukaitis[28]. This antibody binds a site common to all forms of hCG, free β-subunit and β-core fragment. This is used in the competitive βhCG radioimmunoassay, which may equally detect all of these molecules. Examples of commercial assays using anti-β1 and the competitive protocol are listed in Table 5.2.

Combinations of the 11 general types of hCG antibody are used in commercial sandwich-type assays. A common combination is anti-hCG coating antibody with labeled anti-β1. This combination detects only intact (non-nicked) hCG molecules. If anti-free β1 is added as a second coating antibody, intact hCG and free β-subunit are detected. Another common arrangement is an anti-α coating antibody with labeled anti-β1. This type of assay binds all forms of hCG, nicked, intact or missing the β-subunit CTP. If the anti-α coating is supplemented with a β-subunit antibody, anti-β2 or anti-free β, then all forms of hCG and free β-subunit are detected. Another common combination uses two β-subunit antibodies, anti-β1 and anti-β2. This type of assay may detect all forms of hCG, free β-subunit and urine β-core fragment. Some assays use antibodies to the β-subunit CTP (anti-βCTP), in combination with anti-α or anti-β1. These combinations, while detecting intact and nicked hCG, do not detect molecules missing the β-subunit CTP, present in some trophoblast disease samples. Table 5.2 gives 27 examples of commercial hCG sandwich-type immunoassays, using eight different combinations of antibodies. Manufacturers, kit names, probable methods, antibody combinations and specificities are presented.

5.3.3 INTER-ASSAY VARIABILITY

Fifteen pregnancy serum samples, and 15 from different patients with trophoblast disease, were each tested in seven different commercial hCG assays. The assays included two competitive βhCG radioimmunoassays (Amersham Amerlex M and Diagnostic Products HCG), two anti-β1, anti-β2 type sandwich assays (Abbott 15/15 and Biomerica hCG), one anti-βCTP : anti-β1 type sandwich assay (Organon NML), one anti-α : anti-β1 type sandwich assay (Hybritech Tandem-R) and one anti hCG plus anti-free β1 : anti-β1 type sandwich assay (Serono MAIAclone). The greatest assay-to-assay variation was 46% in 15 pregnancy serum samples (Figure 5.4a). This was found in sample 3. In this sample, the Diagnostic Products HCG assay result was 5940 μg/l, and the Organon NML assay value was 11 020 μg/l. The coefficient of variation was 9.9% for 105 pregnancy determinations with seven assays. Bigger assay-to-assay variation was found with the trophoblast disease samples. Sample 1 was 201 600 μg/l in the Amersham Amerlex M and

Table 5.1 Antibody sites on hCG, hCG subunits and β-core fragment

	Site	*Antibody specificity*
Anti-hCG	Interface of α-β-subunit dimer including nick site	Intact (non-nicked) hCG only
Anti-α	Region of α-subunit common to hCG and free α-subunit	All forms of hCG, and free α-subunit
Anti-free α	Region unique to the folding of free α-subunit	Free α-subunit
Anti-β1	Region on β-subunit common to all β-subunit-related molecules	All forms of hCG and free β-subunit, plus β-core fragment
Anti-β2	Region on β-subunit close to CTP	All forms of hCG and free β-subunit, plus β-core fragment
Anti-β3	Region unique to the folding of nicked β-subunit	Nicked hCG and nicked free β-subunit
Anti-βCTP	Region in βCTP (β-subunit residues 110–145)	Intact and nicked hCG, and intact and nicked free β-subunit
Anti-free β1	Region unique to folding of free β-unit, close to CTP	All forms of free β-subunit
Anti-free β2	Region unique to folding of free β-subunit, including nick site	Intact (non-nicked) free β-subunit only
Anti-β core 1	Region unique to folding of free β-subunit, not including nick site	β-Core fragment and all forms of free β-subunit
Anti-β core 2	Region unique to folding of β-core fragment	β-Core fragment

was 3990 μg/l in the Organon NML assay (Figure 5.4,b). This was a 51-fold difference. Differences of two-fold or more in assays values were found in four of the 15 trophoblast disease samples (samples 1, 9, 11 and 12). The coefficient of variation was 17% for 105 determinations with seven assays.

Two types of assay gave particularly low or variable results with trophoblast disease serum samples. The Serono MAIAclone anti-hCG plus anti-free β1 : anti-β1 sandwich assay, detects intact hCG and not nicked molecules. It gave consistently low results with trophoblast disease samples (Figure 5.4b). Results for the 15 trophoblast disease samples averaged 75% of the mean values of the seven assays. The range was 51–91% of mean values. Similar low results have been found with other anti-hCG plus anti-free β1 : anti-β and anti-hCG : anti-β1 sandwich-type assays[19]. The Organon NML anti-βCTP : anti-β1 sandwich assay, which detects

Table 5.2 Examples of quantitative serum pregnancy test kits

Distributor	*Kit*	*How detected*[a] *Labeled antibody conjugate (method)*	*Antibody types*[ab] *captured antibody : labeled antibody*	*Specificity*[a]
Medix Biotech	HCG ELISA	Enzyme–antibody (spectrometric)	Anti-hCG : anti-β1	Intact hCG (non-nicked hCG only)
Tosoh Medics	HCG	Enzyme–antibody (spectrometric)	Anti-hCG : anti-β1	
BioMerieux Vitek	HCG	Enzyme–antibody (spectrometric)	Anti-hCG : anti-β1	
Baxter Diagnostics	Stratus HCG	Enzyme–antibody (spectrometric)	Anti-hCG : anti-β1	
Sunita Chemicals	HCG	^{125}I-labeled antibody (radioactivity)	Anti-hCG : anti-β1	
Bioclone Australia	HCG IRMA	^{125}I-labeled antibody (radioactivity)	Anti-hCG : anti-β1	
Bioclone Australia	βHCG ELISA	Enzyme–antibody (spectrometric)	Anti-hCG + anti-free β1 : anti-β1	Intact hCG + free β
Serono Diagnostics	MAIAclone	^{125}I-labeled antibody (radioactivity)	Anti-hCG + anti-free β1 : anti-β1	
Miles	Immuno-1	Enzyme–antibody (spectrometric)	Anti-hCG + anti-free β1 : anti-β1	
Wallac	Delfia HCG	Lanthanide–antibody (fluorescent)	Anti-α : anti-β1	Total hCG (intact + nicked)
PB Diagnostics	Opus HCG	Enzyme–antibody (spectrometric)	Anti-α : anti-β1	
Dupont	ACA HCG	Enzyme–antibody (spectrometric)	Anti-α : anti-β1	
Hybritech	Tandem-R	^{125}I-labeled antibody (radioactivity)	Anti-α : anti-β1	
Hybritech	Tandem-E	Enzyme–antibody (spectrometric)	Anti-α : anti-β1	
Binax	HCG	^{125}I-labeled antibody (radioactivity)	Anti-α : anti-β1	
V-Tech	Target hCG	Enzyme–antibody (spectrometric)	Anti-α : anti-β1	
Guildhay	HCG ELISA	Enzyme–antibody (spectrometric)	Anti-α : anti-β1	
Abbott Laboratories	IMX HCG	Enzyme–antibody (fluorescent)	Anti-α : anti-β CTP[c]	
Hybritech	Tandem-R total	^{125}I-labeled antibody (radioactivity)	Anti-α + anti-free β2 : anti-β1	Total hCG + free β
Ciba Corning	Magic Light	Antibody–acridinium (luminescence)	Anti-α + anti-β2 : anti-β1	
Ciba Corning	ACS 180	Antibody–acridinium (luminescence)	Anti-α + anti-β2 : anti-β1	
Tosoh Medics	βHCG	Enzyme–antibody (spectrometric)	Anti-β2 : anti-β1	
Sanofi Diagnostic	Access system	Enzyme–antibody (spectrometric)	Anti-β2 : anti-β1	
Baxter Diagnostics	Stratus βHCG	Enzyme–antibody (spectrometric)	Anti-β2 : anti-β1	
Abbott Laboratories	β-HCG 15/15	Enzyme–antibody (spectrometric)	Anti-β2 : anti-β1	
Immunonuclear	Gammadab	^{125}I-labeled antigen, competitive (radioactivity)	Anti-β1	Total hCG + free β
Binax	βHCG RIA	^{125}I-labeled antigen, competitive (radioactivity)	Anti-β1	
ICN Biomedicals	HCGβ RIA	^{125}I-labeled antigen, competitive (radioactivity)	Anti-β1	
Amersham	Amerlex-M	^{125}I-labeled antigen, competitive (radioactivity)	Anti-β1	
Diagnostic Products	HCG	^{125}I-labeled antigen, competitive (radioactivity)	Anti-β1	
Organon Teknika	NML	^{125}I-labeled antibody (radioactivity)	Anti-βCTP : anti-β1[c]	Total hCG[c] + free β
Abbott Laboratories	IMX βHCG	Enzyme–antibody (fluorescent)	Anti-βCTP : anti-β1[c]	

[a]As indicated in instruction booklets, by telephone technical support services, or in published reports.
[b]Antibody sites are those listed in Table 5.1.
[c]Does not detect hCG missing C-terminal peptide segment.

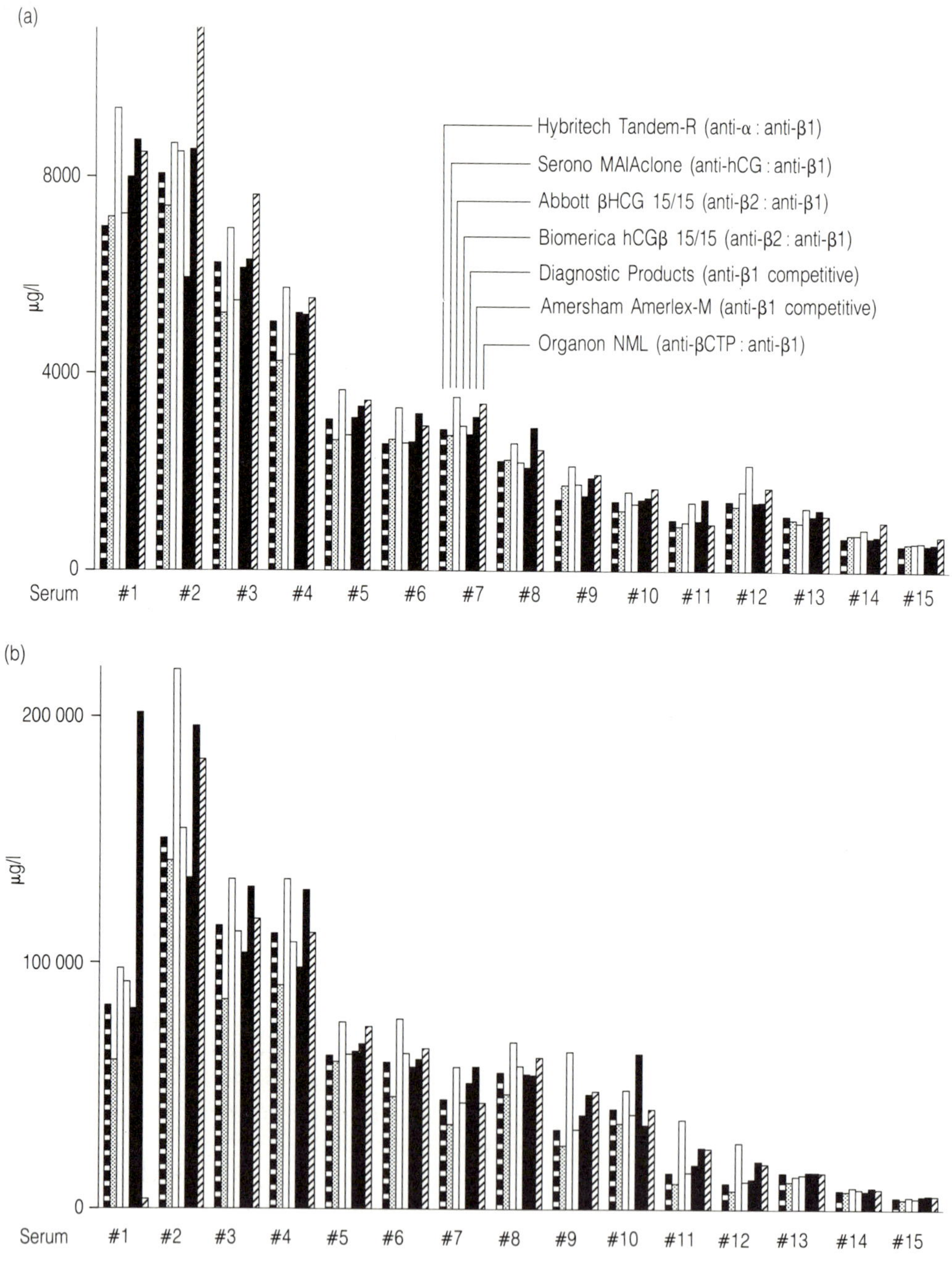

Figure 5.4 Inter-assay discordance in hCG determinations. Fifteen serum samples from first-trimester pregnancy (a) and 15 from trophoblast disease (b), were each tested with seven different commercial hCG immunoassays. From left to right the bars are Hybritech Tandem-R kit (checkerboard bar), Serono MAIAclone kit (poker-dot bar), Abbott hCGβ 15/15 and Biomerica hCGβ kits (white bars), Diagnostic Products hCG and Amersham Amerlex M kits (black bars), and Organon NML kit (striped bar). The types of assay and antibodies used are listed in Tables 5.1 and 5.2.

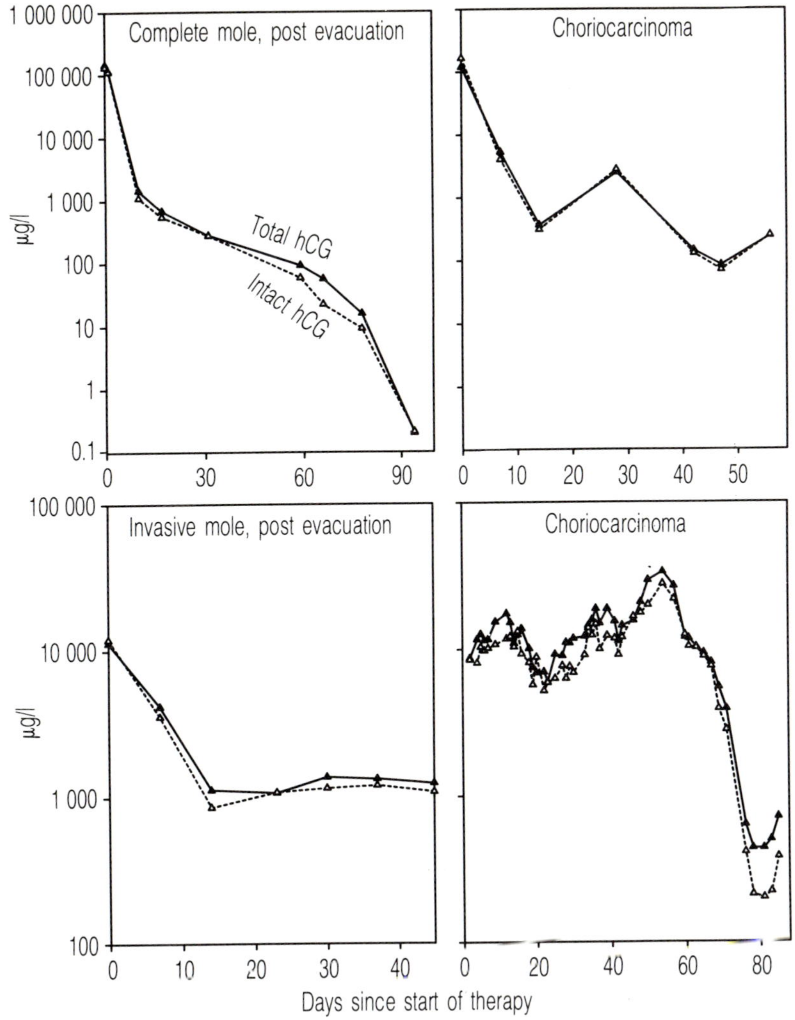

Figure 5.5 Intact hCG and total hCG (intact plus nicked hCG) levels in serum samples from four patients undergoing therapy for trophoblast disease. Intact hCG was determined by an anti-hCG : anti-β1-type immunoassay, and total hCG by an anti-α : anti-β test[19].

molecules containing the βCTP, gave sporadic results; in one case giving values 5.0% of the mean concentration. Similar results have been found with other anti-βCTP : anti-β1 sandwich assays[19]. Both of these types of assay gave good results with pregnancy serum, 82–96%, and 86–130% of mean values. We infer that anti-hCG plus anti-free β1 : anti-β1, anti-hCG : anti-β1, and anti-βCTP : anti-β1 sandwich assays, while appropriate for detecting pregnancy, may not be the best for detecting hCG in patients with trophoblast disease.

We compared total and intact hCG assay values in serial serum samples following the evacuation of hydatidiform mole and chemotherapy for choriocarcinoma. We

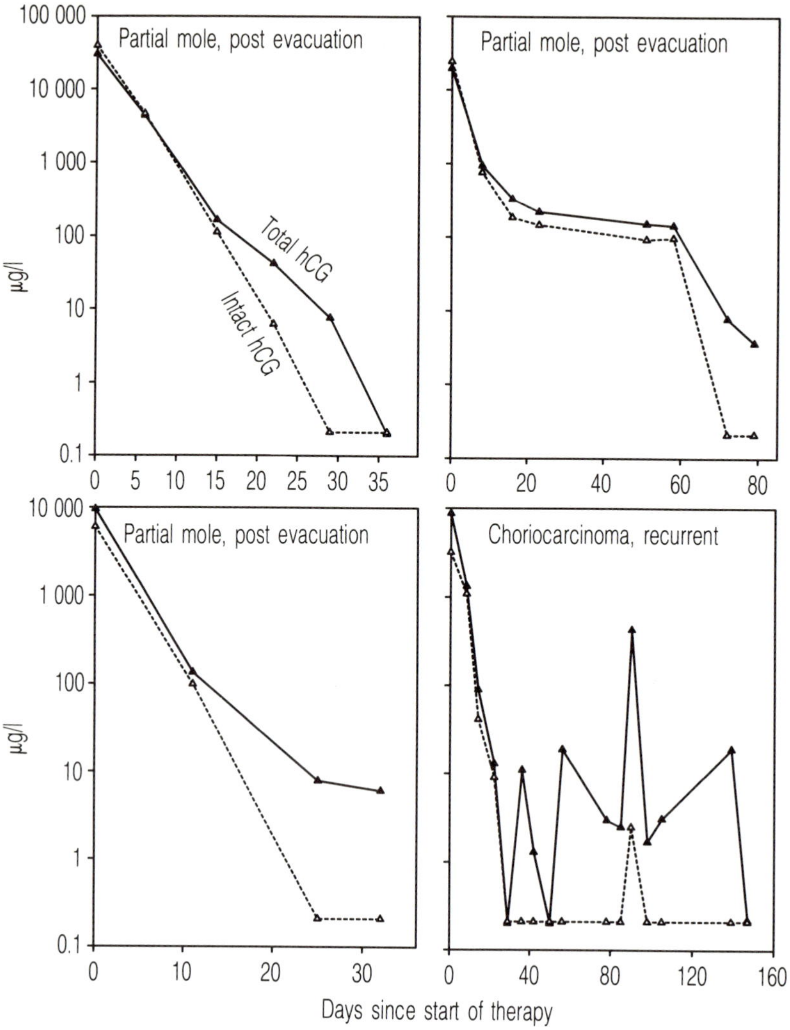

Figure 5.6 Intact hCG and total hCG (intact plus nicked hCG) levels in serum samples from four additional patients undergoing therapy for trophoblast disease. Intact hCG was determined by an anti-hCG : anti-β1-type immunoassay, and total hCG by an anti-α:anti-β test[19].

measured total hCG using an anti-α : anti-β1 sandwich assay and intact hCG using an anti-hCG : anti-β1 assay[19]. In five of eight cases, the intact hCG and total hCG profiles diverged (Figures 5.5 and 5.6). In three cases following evacuation of partial mole, intact hCG levels declined more rapidly than total hCG, becoming undetectable (<0.2 μg/l or <2 U/l eight more days before total hCG measurements. In a fourth case (Figure 5.5, lower right panel) – a patient with triple therapy-resistant choriocarcinoma – intact hCG levels were consistently 20–50% lower than the total hCG concentration. In the fifth case (Figure 5.6, lower right panel) – recurrent choriocarcinoma – intact hCG levels failed to rise during three of four recurrences of disease. We again infer that

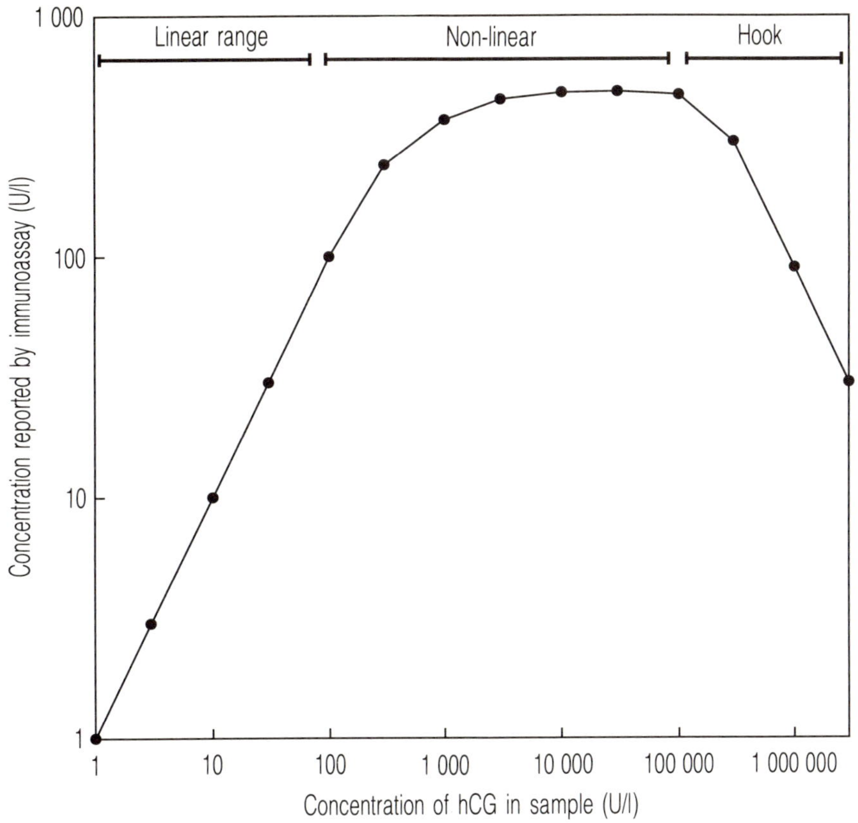

Figure 5.7 The hook effect on hCG immunoassay results. The horizontal axis is the actual concentration of hCG (logarithmic) in the serum sample, and the vertical axis (logarithmic) is the concentration reported by sandwich type immunoassays. Dose–response curve is marked 'linear range' for the area that yields accurate results, 'non-linear' for the area giving meaningless results, and 'hook' for the part relating to erroneous hook effect results.

anti-hCG : anti-β type sandwich assays may not be appropriate for detecting hCG in patients with trophoblast disease.

5.3.4 HOOK EFFECT

The range of hCG levels in trophoblast disease patient serum samples is very wide, from 1 to 1 500 000 U/l. They can reach 10 times the concentration of pregnancy hCG. For normal pregnancy, serum samples are diluted one- to 1000-fold for hCG assay; this covers the range 1–100 000 U/l. If a trophoblast disease serum sample contains 500 000 U/l hCG, it would need to be diluted 10 000-fold or greater to be in the range of the assay. This is not normally done. If it is tested in a sandwich assay, using a pregnancy test protocol (no dilution), it can erroneously give a result in the assay range (Figure 5.7).

In sandwich assays, beads, tubes or plates are coated with a large excess of antibody. An excess of labeled antibody is also used. When a vast 10 000-fold excess of hCG is present it may occupy almost all immobilized antibody sites and nearly all labeled antibody sites, limiting sandwich formation. As such, an undiluted sample, containing a very high concentration of hCG, can give the same low result (leaves few antibody sites to form a sandwich) as that 10 000-fold diluted (few antibody–hCG–antibody sandwiches) (Figure 5.7). The hook effect only occurs when vast, >5000-fold, errors in dilution are made. It can be prevented by making multiple 10-fold dilutions of a sample, and by showing that only one is within the assay range, and that others are above or below that range.

If a laboratory tests a sample, does not know that it is from trophoblast disease, and makes no or minimal dilutions, it may report an erroneous hook effect result. This may be as much as 50 000-fold below the true hCG concentration. The hook effect is one of the biggest causes of erroneous results with trophoblast disease samples. It can be avoided by marking laboratory request slips for hCG assay as being for trophoblast disease. Confusion can also be avoided by requesting multiple dilutions on the request slip.

5.3.5 CHOICE OF ASSAY FOR MONITORING TROPHOBLAST DISEASE

Care must be taken in choosing hCG assays, or external testing laboratories for trophoblast disease samples. Anti-hCG : anti-β1 type assays, and anti-hCG + anti-free anti-β1 : anti-β1 type sandwich assays, the Serono MAIAclone and many others detect intact or biologically active hCG. This makes them particularly good for pregnancy hormone determinations. The data presented here, and previously published data[19], indicate that this type of assay is not appropriate for trophoblast disease applications. Anti-βCTP : anti-β1 type sandwich assays, like the Organon NML, are also good for pregnancy testing. Again, based on the data presented here, and on previously published data[19], these assays are not ideal for trophoblast disease hCG determinations. For patients with trophoblast disease, total hCG plus free β assays, anti-α + anti-β2 : anti-β1 sandwich type assays, competitive βhCG radioimmunoassays or anti-β1 : anti-β2 sandwich type assays are suggested for serum samples. Assays measuring all forms of hCG, total hCG (anti-α : anti-β sandwich assay) may also be suitable, except that they do not detect free β-subunit, the principal antigen in some choriocarcinoma samples[12,14]. Laboratories might want to consider using one of these assays for all serum determinations or using an intact hCG assay for measuring hormone in pregnancy, and a separate assay for monitoring the various forms of hCG in patients with trophoblast disease.

5.4 hCG-RELATED MOLECULES IN THE DIAGNOSIS OF TROPHOBLAST DISEASE

Measurements of free β-subunit, carbohydrate-variant hCG and nicked hCG may be useful in screening for trophoblast disease, or in the differential diagnosis of mole and invasive disease. Trophoblast disease is rare in the USA, affecting less than one in 1500 pregnancies. If it were more common, as it is in Southeast Asia and in certain African nations, these screening and differential diagnosis methods would be used routinely, like the triple screen tests for Down's syndrome pregnancy.

5.4.1 FREE β-SUBUNIT

Free β-subunit measurements have proven useful in the diagnosis of trophoblast disease. In 1983 we used immunoassays to demonstrate elevated levels of free β-subunit in trophoblast disease serum samples[11]. Since then, many other reports have expanded upon these findings[9,10,12–17]. In our experience, none of 12 women with first-trimester pregnancy and 17 of 18 with trophoblast disease had free β levels in excess of 1.0% of the hCG concentration. Free

β-subunit levels averaged $0.53 \pm 0.18\%$ (standard deviation) of hCG in the pregnancy, and $7.3 \pm 6.3\%$ in the trophoblast disease samples (Student's t test, $p < 0.0003$). These data suggested 97% efficiency in screening for trophoblast disease[9]. Similar results and testing efficiency have been reported by others [13,14,16,17]. The free β-subunit test may be useful in screening pregnant women for trophoblast disease[9].

Ozturk and colleagues used free β-subunit measurement in the differential diagnosis of pregnancy ($0.40 \pm 0.26\%$ of hCG level) and complete mole ($1.8 \pm 1.0\%$ of hCG level; in Student's t test, $p < 10^{-8}$), and of complete mole and choriocarcinoma ($9.2 \pm 4.8\%$ of hCG level; in Student's t test, $p < 10^{-8}$)[17]. Particularly high free β-subunit levels were detected by Ozturk and colleagues prior to and during recurrences of choriocarcinoma[17]. This indicated an application for free β-subunit measurements in predicting recurrence of choriocarcinoma. Berkowitz and colleagues used the free β-subunit test to differentiate those with partial (1.0% of hCG level) and complete moles (2.4% of hCG level; in Student's t test, $p < 0.005$)[13]. This indicated a further discriminatory application for the free β-subunit test.

These and other publications clearly show how free β measurements may aid the physician in the diagnosis of trophoblast disease, in differentiation of moles and possibly in following the therapy of choriocarcinoma. Commercial free β-subunit assays are sold by Diagnostic Products Corp., Bioclone Inc. CIS, and other companies.

5.4.2 hCG CARBOHYDRATE VARIANTS

As shown in Figure 5.2, markedly different *N*-linked and *O*-linked sugar structures are attached to invasive disease hCG[23–25]. Two alterations mark invasive disease hCG. The first is the number of antennae, and the second is the quantity of terminal sialic acid residues on invasive disease hCG. Both of these differences can be detected in serum samples using carbohydrate-specific antibodies or lectin–antibody sandwich assays. In 1987, Imamura and colleagues developed a peanut lectin–anti-β1 sandwich assay. Peanut lectin binds *O*-linked sugar units with a terminal galactose residue (missing sialic acid)[29]. They used the assay to detect sialic acid-deficient hCG. Using this test they could distinguish choriocarcinoma from benign mole or normal pregnancy serum samples. Similar results were reported by Birken and colleagues using a competitive radioimmunoassay with antisera developed against sialic acid-free hCG βCTP[30]. In 1988, Endo and colleagues used *Datura stramonium* lectin to identify hCG molecules with *N*-linked sugar unit having three antennae[31]. The method distinguished invasive mole and choriocarcinoma from benign mole and normal pregnancy samples. All of these procedures may potentially be useful in the diagnosis of invasive trophoblast disease.

5.4.3 NICKED hCG

hCG molecules are more extensively nicked in trophoblast disease serum samples[1–3,8,18,19]. Nicked hCG measurements are another credible method for diagnosing trophoblast disease. In our experience, nicked molecules account for 6% of hCG molecules in pregnancy serum samples (7–13 weeks, $n = 41$), and 17% of those in trophoblast disease samples ($n = 20$) (Figure 5.8). Greater than 10% nicking was detected in 14 of 41 (34%) normal pregnancy, and 18 of 20 (90%) trophoblast disease samples.

5.5 NEGATIVE, BORDERLINE OR AMBIGUOUS hCG LEVELS

Once or twice a month we receive calls from gynecologists treating trophoblast disease, or clinical laboratories running immunoassays,

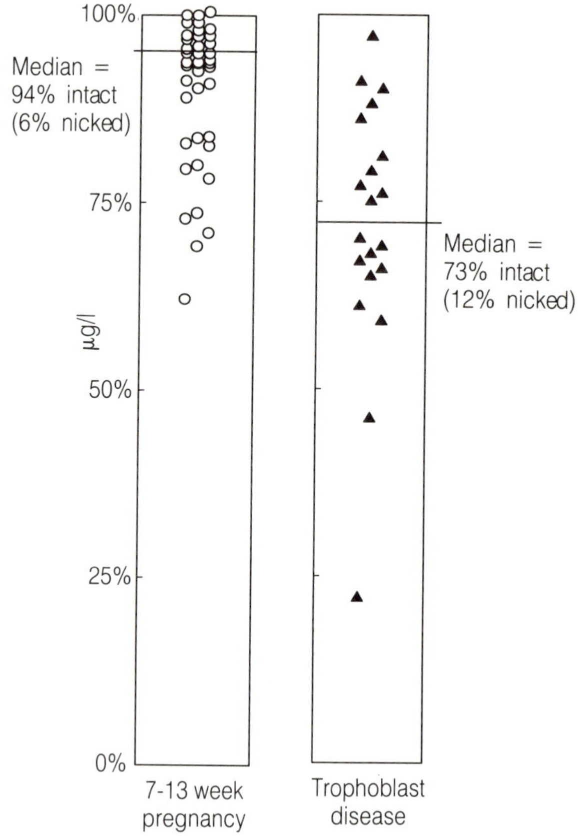

Figure 5.8 Proportions of intact and nicked hCG molecules in pregnancy and trophoblast disease patient serum samples. Intact hCG was determined by an anti-hCG : anti-β1-type immunoassay, and total hCG (intact plus nicked) by an anti-α : anti-β test[19]. Nicked hCG was estimated as the difference between the two immunoassay results[6].

who have puzzling hCG results. The problem is always the same: 'cannot detect hCG'. We hear about consistent borderline positive hCG levels (1–10 U/l) or occasional positive or ambiguous hCG levels, detected in the months following the evacuation of a hydatidiform mole. We have used a free β-subunit test to analyze supplied samples. In some samples we detected significant free β-subunit levels. These have helped the gynecologist decide whether to implement chemotherapy. In some cases in which free β-subunit was detected with a specific free β-subunit assay, hCG plus free β-subunit or βhCG type assays failed to detect the free β-subunit. These hCG assays may not detect all forms of free β-subunit.

We are familiar with two cases of trophoblast disease with negative serum hCG, and highly elevated urine assay values. Tests in our laboratory identified β-core fragment in the urine samples. This is the terminal degradation product of hCG. In these patients, the hCG was probably rapidly degraded, becoming most evident as β-core fragment in urine samples. The most common hCG problems we encounter with outside laboratories are hook effect errors, assay-to-assay discordance, or use of inappropriate assays. These problems are discussed in the preceding sections.

REFERENCES

1. Bidart, J.-M., Puisieux, A., Troalen, F. *et al.* (1988) Characterization of the cleavage product in the human choriogonadotropin β-subunit. *Biochemical and Biophysical Research Communications*, **154**, 626–32.
2. Nishimura, R., Ide, K., Utsunomiya, T. *et al.* (1988) Fragmentation of the β-subunit of human chorionic gonadotropin produced by choriocarcinoma. *Endocrinology*, **123**, 420–5.
3. Cole, L.A., Kardana, A., Andrade-Gordon, P. *et al.* (1991) The heterogeneity of hCG: II. The occurrence, biological and immunological activities of nicked hCG. *Endocrinology*, **129**, 1559–68.
4. Birken, S., Armstrong, E.G., Kolks, M.A.G. *et al.* (1988) Structure of human chorionic gonadotropin β-subunit core fragment from pregnancy urine. *Endocrinology*, **123**, 572–80.
5. Kardana, A., Elliott, M.E., Gawinowicz, M.A. *et al.* (1991) The heterogeneity of hCG: I. Characterization of peptide variations in 13 individual preparations of hCG. *Endocrinology*, **129**, 1541–9.
6. Cole, L.A., Kardana, A., Park, S-Y. and Braunstein, G.D. (1993) The deactivation of hCG by nicking and dissociation. *Journal of Clinical Endocrinology and Metabolism*, **76**, 704–13.
7. Blithe, D.L. and Nisula, B.C. (1985) Variations in the oligosaccharides on free and combined α-subunits of human choriogonadotropin in pregnancy. *Endocrinology*, **117**, 2218–28.
8. Cole, L.A. and Kardana, A. (1992) Discordant results in human chorionic gonadotropin assays. *Clinical Chemistry*, **38**, 263–9.
9. Kardana, A. and Cole, L.A. (1992) Polypeptide nicks cause erroneous results in human chorionic gonadotropin free β-subunit assays. *Clinical Chemistry*, **38**, 26–31.
10. Cole, L.A., Kroll, T.D. and Ruddon, R.W. (1984) Differential occurrence of free α and free β subunits of human chorionic gonadotropin (hCG) from pregnancy sera. *Journal of Clinical Endocrinology and Metabolism*, **50**, 1200–2.
11. Cole, L.A., Hartle, R.J., Laferla, J.J. and Ruddon, R.W. (1983) Detection of the free beta subunit of human chorionic gonadotropin (hCG) in cultures of normal and malignant trophoblast cells, pregnancy sera, and sera of patients with choriocarcinoma, *Endocrinology*, **113**, 1176–8.
12. Ozturk, M., Bellet, D., Manil, L. *et al.* (1987) Physiological studies of human chorionic gonadotropin (hCG), αhCG, and βhCG as measured by specific monoclonal immunoradiometric assays. *Endocrinology*, **120**, 549–57.
13. Berkowitz, R., Ozturk, M., Goldstein, D. *et al.* (1989) Human chorionic gonadotropin and free subunits' serum levels in patients with partial and complete hydatidiform moles. *Obstetrics and Gynecoloy*, **74**, 212–16.
14. Fan, C., Goto, S., Furuhashi, Y. and Tomoda, Y. (1987) Radioimmunoassay of the serum free beta-subunit of human chorionic gonadotropin in trophoblastic disease. *Journal of Clinical Endocrinology and Metabolism*, **64**, 313–18.
15. Khazaeli, M.B., Hedayat, M.M., Hatch, K.D. *et al.* (1986) Radioimmunoassay of free beta subunit of human chorionic gonadotropin as a prognostic test for persistent trophoblastic disease in molar pregnancy. *American Journal of Obstetrics and Gynecology*, **155**, 320–5.
16. Khazaeli, M. B., Buchina, E. S., Pattillo, R. A. *et al.* (1989) Radioimmunoassay of free beta subunit of human chorionic gonadotropin in diagnosis of high-risk and low-risk gestational trophoblastic disease. *American Journal of Obstetrics and Gynecology*, **160**, 444–9.
17. Ozturk, M., Berkowitz, R., Goldstein, D. *et al.* (1988) Differential production of human chorionic gonadotropin and free subunits in gestational trophoblast disease. *American Journal of Obstetrics and Gynecology*, **158**, 193–9.
18. Puisieux, A., Bellet, D., Troalen, F. *et al.* (1990) Occurrence of fragmentation of free and combined forms of the β-subunit of human chorionic gonadotropin. *Endocrinology*, **126**, 687–94.
19. Cole, L.A. (1994) New perspectives in measuring human chorionic gonadotropin levels for measuring and monitoring trophoblast disease. *Journal of Reproductive Medicine*, **39**, 193–200.

20. Morgan, F.J., Birken, S. and Canfield, R.E. (1975) The amino acid sequence of human chorionic gonadotropin: the α-subunit and β-subunit. *Journal of Biological Chemistry*, **225**, 5247–57.
21. Lapthorn, A.J., Harris, D.C., Littlejohn, A. *et al.* (1994) Crystal structure of human chorionic gonadotropin, *Nature*, **369**, 455–60.
22. Nisula, B.C. and Wehmann, R.E. (1980) Distribution, metabolism, and excretion of human chorionic gonadotropin and its subunits in man, in *Chorionic Gonadotropin* (ed. S.J. Segal), Plenum Press, New York, pp. 199–212.
23. Mizuochi, T., Nishimura, R., Derappe, C. *et al.* (1983) Structures of the asparagine-linked sugar chains of human chorionic gonadotropin produced in choriocarcinoma: appearance of triantennary sugar chains and unique biantennary sugar chains. *Journal of Biological Chemistry*, **225**, 14126–9.
24. Cole, L.A. (1987) The *O*-linked oligosaccharides are strikingly different on pregnancy and choriocarcinoma hCG. *Journal of Clinical Endocrinology and Metabolism*, **65**, 811–13.
25. Amano, J., Nishimura, R., Mochizuki, M. and Kobata, A. (1988) Comparative study of the mucin-type sugar chains of human chorionic gonadotropin present in the urine of patients with trophoblastic diseases and healthy pregnant women. *Journal of Biological Chemistry*, **263**, 1157–65.
26. Birken, S. and Canfield, R.E. (1980) Chemistry and immunochemistry of human chorionic gonadotropin, in *Chorionic Gonadotropin* (ed. S.J. Segal), Plenum Press, New York, pp. 65–88.
27. Schwartz, S., Krude, H., Kleiber, R. *et al.* (1991) Number and topography of epitopes of human chorionic gonadotropin (hCG) are shared by desialylated and deglycosylated hCG. *Molecular and Cellular Endocrinology*, **80**, 33–40.
28. Vaitukaitis, J.L., Braunstein, G.D. and Ross, G.T. (1972) A radioimmunoassay which specifically measures human chorionic gonadotropin in the presence of human luteinizing hormone. *American Journal of Obstetrics and Gynecology*, **113**, 751–60.
29. Imamura, S., Armstrong, G.A., Birken, S. *et al.* (1987) Highly specific and sensitive measurements of desialylated forms of human chorionic gonadotropin with lectin immunoradiometric assays. *Clinica Chimica Acta*, **163**, 339–49.
30. Birken, S., Agosto, G., Amr, S. *et al.* (1988) Characterization of antisera distinguishing carbohydrate structures in the β carboxyl-terminal region of human chorionic gonadotropin. *Endocrinology*, **122**, 2054–63.
31. Endo, T., Iino, K., Nozawa, S. *et al.* (1988) Immobilized *Datura stramonium* agglutinin column chromatography, a novel method to discriminate the urinary hCGs of patients with invasive mole and choriocarcinoma from those of normal pregnant women and patients with hydatidiform mole. *Japanese Journal of Cancer Research*, **79**, 160–4.

STAGING AND CLASSIFICATION SYSTEMS 6

Ho-Kei Ma, Ling-Chui Wong and Hextan Ngan

6.1 INTRODUCTION

Although it is universally recognized that an accurate and precise staging and classification system for gestational trophoblastic diseases (GTD) is needed to enable clinicians to assess the prognosis or risk of patients, to individualize and to optimize their treatment, to date there is still a variety of staging and classification systems used by centers treating GTD. This makes meaningful comparison of treatment results and evaluation of new treatment protocols impossible, and hampers improvement in the management of the disease.

During the 1991 Fédération Internationale de Gynécologie et d'Obstétrique (FIGO) Oncology Committee meeting held in Singapore, a revised staging system was proposed and the details of the revised FIGO staging (Table 6.1) were published in 1992[1]. This new system is simple and user friendly. In this chapter, we shall review the historical background leading to the formulation of the 1992 FIGO staging and we shall try to compare its effectiveness in prognostic prediction with that of the World Health Organization (WHO) scoring system. The prognosis and treatment results of the patients of different stages of the new FIGO system will be reported and discussed.

Table 6.1 1992 Revised FIGO staging system for GTD

Stage	
I.	Disease confined to the uterus
II.	Disease extends outside of the uterus but is limited to the genital structures (adnexa, vagina, broad ligament)
III.	Disease extends to lungs with or without known genital tract involvement
IV.	Disease at other metastatic sites
Substage	
A.	No risk factor
B.	One risk factor
C.	Two risk factors
Risk factors	
1.	hCG higher than 100 000 U/l
2.	Duration from termination of antecedent pregnancy to diagnosis more than 6 months

6.2 HISTORICAL REVIEW

6.2.1 MORPHOLOGICAL/HISTOLOGICAL CLASSIFICATION

For many centuries, morphological/histological classification was the only class-

Gestational Trophoblastic Disease.
Edited by B.W. Hancock, E.S. Newlands and R.S. Berkowitz.
ISBN 0 412 63100 8

Table 6.2 Sänger's classification for GTD

1. Decidual sarcoma with participation of chorionic elements: a. Diffuse, ulcerated type b. Nodular, non-ulcerated type c. Mixed nodular–ulcerative type
2. Decidual sarcoma with participation of chorionic elements, following hydatidiform mole
3. Interstitial, destructive hydatidiform mole

ification. In 1276, it was first recorded that the Countess of Henneberg delivered 365 'children'. From the description of the 'children', the pregnancy was clearly a hydatidiform mole. In 1840, Wilton[2] published a report on a patient with chorioadenoma destruens who had a fatal intraperitoneal hemorrhage from the tumor, which had perforated the uterus. In 1877, the first case of choriocarcinoma was described by Chiari[3]. Sixteen years later, Sänger[4] proposed the first morphological classification (Table 6.2). Two years later, Marchand[5] proposed to call this group of diseases chorionepithelioma malignum and he classified the diseases into typical and atypical forms and related the different forms to the prognosis of the patients.

It was Ewing[6] in 1910 who classified the diseases into groups called syncytial endometritis, chorioadenoma destruens (invasive mole) and choriocarcinoma. Ewing's classification is the basis of classifications used by many centers today. Since then, many workers, notably Novak, Ishizuka, Hertz, Park and Driscoll, reported their findings on the morphology and histology of the different groups and their variants. The prognosis and the course of the disease of the different groups of GTD were studied by many. The prognostic significance of the different groups of GTD and the diagnostic problems were the subjects of many publications. In 1967, the International Union Against Cancer (UICC) compiled a clinical and morphological classification[7] (Table 6.3). It becomes clear that GTD consists of a group of related conditions which develop following any type of pregnancy and these conditions range from the benign to the most malignant form. The different morphological groups generally differ in their prognosis.

However, in recent years, surgery was seldom done for GTD patients. Therefore in many patients it was impossible to establish a morphological or histological diagnosis at the onset of the disease. Patients could only be classified retrospectively based on their clinical course. This type of classification could not be used prospectively to guide clinicians in the choice of treatment. It was obvious that a different classification was needed. However, a morphological classification was adopted by the GTD Registration Committee of the Japan Society of Obstetrics and Gynecology for reporting of their GTD data[8] (Table 6.4) but many centers outside of Japan had adopted a clinical classification or had used clinical classification in addition to a morphological one. It was also known that histological grade of the lesion, i.e. the degree of differentiation and proliferation of the trophoblasts, did not correlate well with the behavior of the tumor and hence histological grading could not be used to predict patient outcome.

6.2.2 ANATOMICAL STAGING SYSTEM

Clinicians are used to staging gynecological malignant diseases based on anatomical criteria. An anatomical staging system for GTD would be a popular and logical one. The disease can be staged at the time of diagnosis. In 1982, the FIGO Oncology Committee proposed an anatomical staging system (Table 6.5) and promoted its use universally for reporting of GTD data. How-

Table 6.3 UICC 1967 classification for GTD

A. Gestational
B. Non-gestational
I. CLINICAL DIAGNOSIS

1. Non-metastatic

2. Metastatic
   a. Local (pelvic)
   b. Extrapelvic (specify location)

3. Other required information
   a. Evidence
      i. Morphological
      ii. Non-morphological

   b. Antecedent pregnancy. Specify duration
      i. Normal
      ii. Aborted
      iii. Molar
   c. Previous treatment
      i. Untreated
      ii. Treated. Specify

II. MORPHOLOGICAL DIAGNOSIS

1. Hydatidiform mole
   a. Non-invasive
   b. Invasive

2. Choriocarcinoma

3. Uncertain[a]

4. Other required information
   a. Diagnostic basis. Specify
      i. C = Curettage
      ii. U = Excised uterus
      iii. N = Necropsy
      iv. O = Other
   b. Date of diagnosis (with respect to date of onset of treatment)
   c. Subsequent change in morphological diagnosis. Specify diagnostic basis as in II.4a

[a]'Syncytial endometritis' is not considered neoplasia.

ever, it was soon found that the prognosis of patients in the same stage varied greatly. For some years, it was known that there were a number of clinical features besides the anatomical extent of the disease that affected the prognosis of the patients. The FIGO anatomical staging was not universally adopted as was hoped.

Table 6.4 Registration Committee, Japan Society of Obstetrics and Gynecology Classification for GTD

1. Total (or complete) hydatidiform mole
2. Partial hydatidiform mole
3. Invasive (or destructive) hydatidiform mole
4. Choriocarcinoma
5. Persistent trophoblastic disease
   a. Post-molar persistent hCG
   b. Clinical invasive (or destructive) mole
   c. Clinical choriocarcinoma

Table 6.5 1982 FIGO anatomical staging system for GTD

Stage	
I.	Confined to the uterus corpus
II.	Metastases to pelvis and vagina
III.	Metastases to lung
IV.	Distant metastases

In China, Song[9] independently formulated a classification based on his own data (Table 6.6) which was very similar to that of the FIGO anatomical staging. Since 1962, Song's classification has been used by all Chinese centers.

6.2.3 CLINICAL CLASSIFICATION

For a long time, it was well known that GTD patients with metastases had a worse prognosis than those without metastasis. The early methods for detection of metastasis were physical examination, chest X-rays, electroencephalogram, arteriogram and the detection of an increased level of human chorionic gonadotropin (hCG) in the cerebrospinal fluid. These methods would detect metastasis late and only when the size of metastasis was large (>2 cm in diameter). Therefore, the large volume of the tumor rather than the site of the metastasis might be the poor prognostic factor. In addition to a morphological classification, delegates at the 1965 UICC Conference held in the Philippines agreed to adopt a clinical classification (Table 6.3) which divided the patients into non-metastatic and metastatic groups. In the same year, Ross and his co-workers[10] identified clinical features that were associated with poor prognosis; these features were high hCG level, duration of disease longer than four months, and the presence of brain and/or liver metastasis. In

Table 6.6 Song's classification for GTD

Stage		
I.		Disease confined to the uterus
II.	A	Disease extends to adnexa and parametria
	B	Disease extends to vagina
III.	A	Disease extends to lung and metastases less than 3 cm in diameter or mottling in less than half of one lung
	B	Disease extends to lung and metastases bigger than 3 cm in diameter or mottling in more than half of one lung
IV.		Disease extends to other organs, e.g. brain, liver, kidney and bowel

Reproduced with permission from Song *et al*, Trophoblastic tumours: diagnosis and treatment; published by People Health, Beijing.

Table 6.7 Hammond's Southeastern Trophoblastic Disease Center Clinical Classification for GTD

I. Non-metastatic GTD

II. Metastatic GTD
  A. Good prognosis
    1. Urinary hCG < 100 000 IU/24 h urine or <40 000 IU/l serum
    2. Symptoms present for less than 4 months
    3. No brain or liver metastases
    4. No prior chemotherapy
    5. Pregnancy event is not term delivery (i.e. mole, ectopic or spontaneous abortion)

  B. Poor prognosis
    1. Urinary hCG > 100 000 IU/24 h urine or >40 000 IU/l
    2. Symptoms present for more than 4 months
    3. Brain or liver metastases
    4. Prior chemotherapeutic failure
    5. Antecedent term pregnancy

1973 Hammond *et al.*[11] reported the treatment results of their patients based on a clinical classification that divided patients into non-metastatic and metastatic, with the metastatic GTD patients divided into good and poor prognostic groups (Table 6.7). In addition to the prognostic factors identified by Ross, Hammond added antecedent term pregnancy and previous chemotherapy failure as poor prognostic indicators. Since then, the majority of US centers have used a clinical classification similar to Hammond's.

In The Netherlands, since 1983 centers have used a clinical classification proposed by the Dutch Working Group for Trophoblastic Tumors (Table 6.8) to guide the choice of chemotherapy for an individual patient[12]. The Dutch classification is very similar to Hammond's classification except it also included the number of organ sites of metastasis outside of the uterus as a prognostic factor.

History has shown that these clinical classifications are largely accurate in predicting prognosis. They can be used prospectively to guide the choice of chemotherapeutic regimen, i.e. single or multiple agents for a patient. However, the relative importance of each factor is not taken into account.

6.2.4 PROGNOSTIC SCORING SYSTEM

In 1976, Bagshawe[13] suggested a prognostic scoring system which gave different weighting to different prognostic factors and based on the score, patients were divided into high-, medium- and low-risk groups. In addition to factors used by Hammond, age, parity, ABO blood group, number of metastases, diameter of the largest tumor mass, lymphocytic infiltration and immune status were included in the scoring system (Table 6.9). Bagshawe's prognostic score could not be calculated for patients in developing countries because of incomplete investigations. Some of the tests were not available in developing countries where GTD was prevalent. In 1983, a WHO Working Group[14] proposed a modification of the Bagshawe system (Table 6.10). The WHO scoring system is widely used by centers in developing countries. It is easy to use and reflects the prognosis of the patients.

Table 6.8 Classification by the Dutch Working Group for GTN

Low-risk GTN
Demands all of the following conditions:

1. Antecedent pregnancy: hydatidiform mole, abortion
2. No metastases or metastases in both of the following conditions:
   a. One organ site
   b. Site in the small pelvis, vagina or lung
3. No previous chemotherapy.
4. Interval between evacuation and start of chemotherapy less than 12 months

High-risk GTN
Demands one or more of the following conditions:

1. Failure of previous chemotherapy
2. Metastases in one or more of the following organs:
   a. Brain
   b. Liver
   c. Spleen
   d. Kidney
   e. Gastrointestinal tract
3. Metastases in more than one site (outside the uterus)
4. Antecedent pregnancy: term
5. Interval between end of antecedent pregnancy and start of chemotherapy more than 12 months

6.3 REVISED FIGO STAGING SYSTEM

6.3.1 REVISED FIGO STAGING SYSTEM

Clinical classifications, WHO prognostic score and the FIGO staging have now been used for many years. It is assumed that the score, or stage of classified groups of GTD indicates the prognosis of the patients. However, there is no agreement on the best system or classification and none has been shown to be clearly superior to the others. The relative importance of the prognostic factors is being debated. Evaluation of these published systems[12,15–20] showed that some of the prognostic factors might not significantly affect the patient's prognosis or treatment outcome. Unfortunately, different evaluation criteria were used in these studies. The chemotherapeutic regimen used besides classification, stage and prognostic score also influenced the prognosis and treatment outcome. The WHO score was generally found to be more predictive of prognosis than

Table 6.9 Bagshawe's prognostic scoring system for GTD (1976)

Score	*0*	*10*	*20*	*40*
Age (years)	<39	>39		
Parity	1, 2, >4	3 or 4		
Antecedent pregnancy	Mole	Abortion	Term	
Histological diagnosis (AP)	Invasive mole	Not known	Choriocarcinoma	
Interval (AP to start of chemotherapy) in months	<4	4–7	7–12	>12
HCG (plasma IU/l or urine IU/day)	10^3–10^4	$<10^3$	10^4–10^5	$>10^5$
ABO groups (patient × husband)	A × A O or A × B O or A × AB	O × O A × O O × A B × B AN × B	B × O or A AB × O or A	
No. of metastases seen	None	1–4	4–8	>8
Site of metastases	Not detected Lungs Vagina	Spleen Kidney	Gastrointestinal tract Liver	Brain
Largest tumor mass diameter	3 cm	3–5 cm	5 cm	
Lymphocytic infiltration of tumor	Marked	Moderate or unknown	Slight	
Immune status	Reactive	Unknown	Unreactive	
Relapse after previous chemotherapy			Yes	

Modified 1983; see Table 11.1.

the FIGO anatomical staging[17–20]. Our own study of 55 patients with metastatic disease[19] treated by the same multiple-agent chemotherapy, i.e. Bagshawe's CHAMOCA (see Chapter 11), showed that of the eight prognostic factors identified only the interval from the antecedent pregnancy to diagnosis of GTD, the level of hCG, and possibly the number of metastatic organ sites were significantly associated with fatal outcome. hCG is clearly a very good tumor marker and a more superior indicator of

Table 6.10 WHO prognostic scoring system for GTD

	0	*1*	*2*	*4*
Age	<39	>39		
Antecedent pregnancy	Mole	Abortion	Term pregnancy	
Interval	4	4–6	7–12	>12
Pretreatment hCG (log)	<3	<4	<5	>5
ABO group (female × male)		O × A	B	
		A × O	AB	
Largest tumor (cm)		3–5	5	
Site of metastasis		Spleen, kidney	Gastrointestinal tract, liver	Brain
Number of metastases identified		1–4	4–8	>8
Previous chemotherapy failed			Single drug	2 or more

< 4, low risk; 5–7, medium risk; >7, high risk.
Reproduced, by permission of WHO, from: *Gestational trophoblastic diseases. Report of a WHO Scientific Group*. Geneva, World Health Organisation, 1983 (Technical Report Series, No. 692)

tumor volume than the number or size of metastases. If our findings are correct, it is possible to combine an anatomical staging and a prognostic clinical classification. The number of prognostic factors can be greatly reduced. The FIGO Oncology Committee met in Singapore during the XIIIth World Congress of Obstetrics and Gynaecology and reviewed the recent data. The Committee decided to add substages to its anatomical staging. The new FIGO staging fulfills some of the criteria of a good classification because it is simple, easy for clinicians to remember and use, and the risk factors can be assessed by the patient's history and by the estimation of the hCG, which should be available in any center. As it is new, it has not been evaluated.

6.3.2 EVALUATION OF THE 1992 REVISED FIGO STAGING SYSTEM

We recognize the limitations of our publication[19], which concluded that five of the eight prognostic factors were unimportant and could be discarded, and we decided to compare the effectiveness of the new FIGO staging with that of the WHO scoring system. 'Drug resistance', which is defined as the necessity of change of chemotherapeutic regimen because of poor response, relapse and death, is regarded as an indicator of poor prognosis or outcome. Poor response to chemotherapy was defined as less than one log fall of the hCG level after one course of chemotherapy. From 1983 to 1993, 207 GTD patients were treated in the Department of

Table 6.11 Comparison of WHO score and FIGO revised staging

FIGO stage		*WHO low risk Score ≤4*		*WHO medium risk Score 5–7*		*WHO high risk Score >7*	
		No.	*%*[a]	*No.*	*%*[a]	*No.*	*%*[a]
I.	a	87	78.4	6	11.3	0	0
	b	1	0.9	4	7.6	3	7.0
	c	0	0	1	1.9	0	0
II.	a	2	1.8	2	3.8	1	2.3
	b	0	0	0	0	1	2.3
	c	0	0	0	0	1	2.3
III.	a	12	10.8	14	26.4	0	0
	b	1	0.9	2	3.8	12	27.9
	c	0	0	0	0	1	2.3
IV.	a	8	7.2	23	43.3	12	28.0
	b	0	0	1	1.9	8	18.6
	c	0	0	0	0	4	9.3

[a]Percentage of same WHO risk group.

Obstetrics and Gynecology of the University of Hong Kong in Queen Mary Hospital. Patients were scored according to the WHO system and were also staged according to the new FIGO system.

Table 6.11 shows the risk grouping according to the WHO score and the new FIGO stage of the patients. Stage Ia patients constituted the majority of the low-risk patients (78.4%). All the low-risk patients except two would be in substage a; 55.9% of the WHO high-risk patients would be in stage IV; 75.4% of medium-risk patients would be stages III and IV. However, 69.7% of the medium-risk patients would be stages IIIa and IVa. This means that the substaging is essential for prediction of patient risk within a stage. The close correlation between the substages and the WHO risk score is shown in Figures 6.1 and 6.2. The new FIGO staging correlated well with the WHO risk score in these 207 patients.

Table 6.12 shows the treatment results of

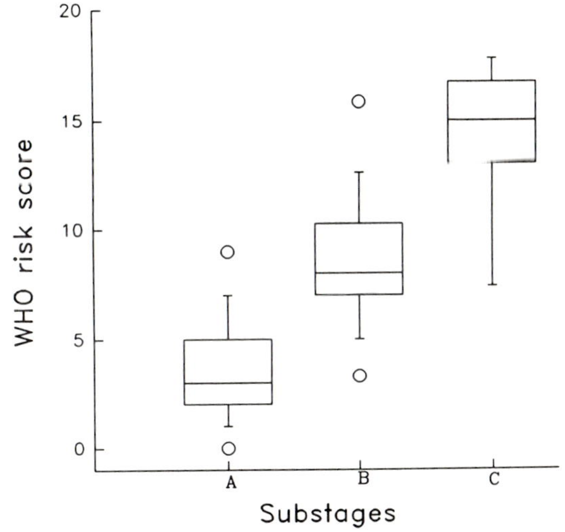

Figure 6.1 WHO risk score and FIGO substages. Upper and lower borders of the box show 75th and 25th percentiles, middle line shows 50th percentile, the upper and lower whiskers show 90th and 10th percentiles, and the two circles show 95th and 5th percentiles.

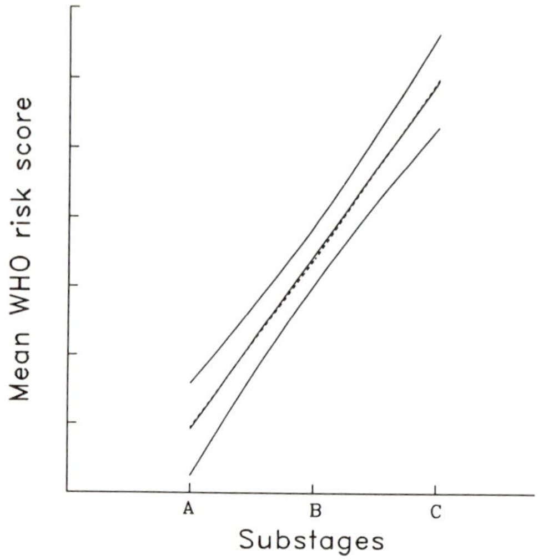

Figure 6.2 Regression line between mean WHO risk score and FIGO substages. The middle line represents the regression of mean WHO risk score and FIGO substages. The upper and lower solid lines show 5th and 95th confidence intervals on the regression.

the 207 patients in the WHO risk groups. The percentage of patients who developed drug resistance, relapsed and died increased with increased risk. One hundred of the 111 low-risk patients (90.0%) were treated by single drug and the rest by a multiple-agent regimen. The single drug administered was either methotrexate or etoposide; the multiple-agent regimens most frequently used were methotrexate and actinomycin, and CHAMOCA. Twenty of the 53 medium-risk patients (37.7%) and six of the 43 high-risk patients (14.0%) were treated by single drug. Table 6.13 shows that there were more patients who developed drug resistance, relapsed and died in the group treated by multiple agents.

The treatment outcome of the different FIGO stages is shown in Table 6.14. There was only one patient in stages Ic, IIb, IIc and IIIc, and fewer than 10 patients in stages Ib, IIa, IVb and IVc. Report on treatment results of such small numbers of patients is not meaningful. Therefore, these stage groups are not shown in Table 6.14. Patients who have tumor only in the uterus or pelvis usually do not have a long history, and hCG level is generally low. With modern sophisticated diagnostic aids, early detection of distant metastasis is expected and if confirmed it is not surprising to have many stage IIIa and IVa patients. Therefore, 26 of the 42 stage III (61.9%) and 43 of the 56 stage IV patients (76.8%) were in substage a, i.e. without any

Table 6.12 Treatment results of WHO risk groups

WHO risk group	*Total no.*	*Drug resistance*[a]		*Relapse*[b]		*Death*	
		No.	*%*[c]	*No.*	*%*[c]	*No.*	*%*[c]
Low (score ≤ 4)	111	1	0.9	4	3.6	0	0
Medium (score 5–7)	53	5	9.4	2	3.8	3	5.7
High (score >7)	43	17	39.5	7	16.3	10	23.3

[a]Drug resistance versus WHO risk group; $\chi^2 = 47.0$, $p < 0.0001$.
[b]Relapse versus WHO risk group; $\chi^2 = 9.2$, $p < 0.01$.
[c]Percentage in the same WHO risk group.

Table 6.13 Results of single and multiple drug treatment

Regimen	*Total no.*	*Drug resistance*		*Relapse*		*Death*	
		No.	*%*[a]	*No.*	*%*[a]	*No.*	*%*[a]
Single	126	11	8.7	6	4.8	5	4.0
Multiple	81	12	14.8	7	8.6	8	9.9

[a]Percentage of the same treatment group.

Table 6.14 Treatment results of FIGO stages

FIGO stage	*Substage*	*Patient no.*	*Drug resistance*		*Relapse*		*Death*	
			No.	*%*[a]	*No.*	*%*[a]	*No.*	*%*[a]
I.		102	4	3.9	3	2.9	0	0
	a	93	1	1.1	2	2.2	0	0
III.		42	8	19.1	8	19.1	8	19.1
	a	26	2	7.7	2	7.7	2	7.7
	b	15	5	33.3	6	40.0	5	33.3
IV.		56	11	19.6	2	3.6	5	8.9
	a	43	6	14.0	2	4.7	1	2.3

[a]Percentage in same stage or substage.

risk factor. The treatment results of these patients, although with advanced disease, were good and they had relatively low risk. This again proved that substaging is essential to discriminate the low-, medium- and high-risk patients. However, occasionally there would be patients with localized disease but large tumor volume or long history and these patients must be regarded as medium or high risk.

6.3.3 RECOMMENDATIONS ON RISK GROUPING OF THE REVISED FIGO STAGES

Figure 6.3 shows the risk score of the FIGO stages which seem to divide themselves into low-, medium- and high-risk groups. After studying the treatment results, we recommend that stage Ia patients should be considered as low risk and be treated by single drug; stage Ib, c, IIa, IIIa and IVa patients should be considered medium risk and all other stages high risk. We suggest that high-risk patients should be treated with multiple drugs. Medium-risk patients in many centers, including ours, would be treated by multiple drugs; if a single drug is used, the response must be monitored closely with prompt change of regimen if the response is unsatisfactory. An indication of the likely treatment results of our suggested grouping and treatment scheme is shown in Table 6.15. Our data showed that a stage Ia patient has only a 1.1% chance of not responding to a single drug. It is unnecessary to subject the patient to the risk and toxicity of multiple

Table 6.15 Treatment results of different FIGO risk groups

FIGO stage (risk group)		No. of patients	Drug resistance[a] No.	Drug resistance[a] %[a]	Relapse[b] No.	Relapse[b] %[a]	Death No.	Death %[a]
Stage Ia (low risk)		93	1	1.1	2	2.2	0	0
	Single	91	1	1.1	2	2.2	0	0
	Multiple	2	0	0	0	0	0	0
Stage Ib, c, IIa, IIIa, IVa (medium risk)		83	11	13.3	5	6.0	3	3.6
	Single	29	6	20.7	3	10.3	2	6.9
	Multiple	54	5	9.3	2	3.7	1	1.9
Stage IIb, c, IIIb, c, IVb, c, (high risk)		31	11	35.5	6	19.4	10	32.3
	Single	6	4	66.7	1	16.7	3	50.0
	Multiple	25	7	28.0	5	20.0	7	28.0

[a]Drug resistance versus the FIGO risk groups; $\chi^2 = 28.5$, $p < 0.0001$.
[b]Relapse versus FIGO risk groups; $\chi^2 = 11.7$, $p < 0.003$.
Single, patients treated by single-drug chemotherapy.
Multiple, patients treated by multiple-drug chemotherapy.

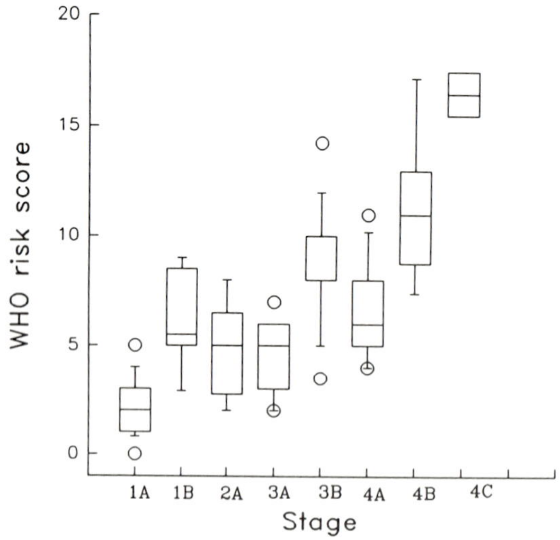

Figure 6.3 WHO risk score of the 8 FIGO stages (explanation: see Figure 6.1).

drugs. The treatment results of using multiple drugs to treat a medium- or high-risk patient are probably significantly better than a single drug.

6.3.4 USE OF COMPUTED TOMOGRAPHY OF LUNG IN STAGING

We wondered whether the use of computed tomography (CT) scanning of the lungs would increase the number of stage IIIa patients and decrease the discriminating effect of the system. In 51 of the 207 patients in the present series, CT scanning of the lungs was performed and metastasis which was not detected on chest X-ray was seen in seven of the stage Ia and one of the stage IIa patients. In none of the substage b or c patients had chest X-ray missed the lung metastasis. Therefore, if CT scanning of the lungs was used for pretreatment evaluation to detect lung metastasis in our series of patients there would be eight more stage IIIa patients. These patients might have been overtreated, because all these eight patients were treated with a single drug with good response and went into sustained complete remission. There is no doubt that CT scanning of the lungs can detect small lung metastasis. The prognosis of these patients with very small tumor volume is good. The use of CT scanning of the lungs as routine pretreatment evaluation will not improve the effectiveness of the new FIGO staging and may result in overtreatment of some patients. It is also expensive and exposes the patient to additional radiation.

6.4 SUMMARY AND CONCLUSION

A historical review of staging and classification systems for GTD was presented. An attempt was made to evaluate the 1992 revised FIGO staging system. Our analysis of 207 GTD patients treated from 1983 to 1993 has shown that the new FIGO staging with the new substages is useful. Further evaluation is needed. If our findings are substantiated, the staging should be adopted for reporting by all centers treating GTD so that treatment results and experience can be collated and compared meaningfully.

REFERENCES

1. FIGO Oncology Committee Report (1992) *Int. J. Gynecol. Obstet.*, **39**, 149–50.
2. Wilton W. (1840) Hydatids, terminating fatally, by haemorrhage. *Lancet*, **i**, 691–3.
3. Chiari, H. (1877) Über drei Fälle von primärem Karcinom in Fundus und Corpus des Uterus. *Med. Jahrb.*, **7**, 364–8.
4. Sänger, M. (1893) Über Sarcoma uteri deciduocellulare und andere deciduale Geschwülste. *Arch. Gynäk.*, **44**, 89–148.
5. Marchand, F. (1895) Über die sogenannten 'decidualen Geschwülste' im Anschluss an normale Geburten, Abort, Blasenmol and Extrauterin-Schwangerschaft. *Monastschr. Geburtshilfe Gynaekol.*, **1**, 417–18, and 531–62.
6. Ewing, J. (1910) Chorioma: a clinical and pathological study. *Surg. Gynecol. Obstet.*, **10**, 366–92.
7. Ishizuka N., Brewer, J.W., Hreshchyshyn, M.M. *et al.* (1967) Choriocarcinoma, in *UICC Monograph Series*, Vol. 3 (eds J.F. Holland and M.M. Hreshchyshyn), Springer, Berlin, Appendix 1.
8. Registration Committee for Trophoblastic Disease of the Japan Society of Obstetrics and Gynecology (1982) Report of the Registration Committee for Trophoblastic Disease. *Acta Obstet. Gynecol. Jpn.*, **34**, 1805–12.
9. Song, H.C., Wu, P.C., Tong, M.Y. and Wang, Y.O. (1981) *Trophoblastic Tumours Diagnosis and Treatment*. People Health, Beijing, pp. 128–9.
10. Ross, G.T., Goldstein, D.P., Hertz, R. *et al.* (1965) Sequential use of methotrexate and actinomycin D in the treatment of metastatic choriocarcinoma and related trophoblastic diseases in women. *Am. J. Obstet. Gynecol.*, **93** 223–9.
11. Hammond, C.B., Borchert, L.G., Tyrey L. *et al.* (1973) Treatment of metastatic disease: good and poor prognosis. *Am. J. Obstet. Gynecol.*, **115**, 451–7.
12. Dijkema, H.E., Aalders J.G., De Bruiju, H.W.A. and Laurini, R.N. (1986) Risk factors in gestational trophoblastic disease, and consequences for primary treatment. *Eur. J. Obstet. Gynecol. Reprod. Biol.*, **22**, 145–52.
13. Bagshawe, K.D. (1976) Risk and prognostic factors in trophoblastic neoplasia. *Cancer*, **38** 1373–85.
14. World Health Organization (1983) *Gestational Trophoblastic Disease*. *WHO Tech. Rep. Ser.* 692.
15. DuBeshter, B. (1991) High-risk factors in metastatic gestational trophoblastic neoplasia. *J. Reprod. Med.*, **36**, 9–13.
16. Azab, M.B., Pejovic, M.H., Theodore C. *et al.* (1988) Prognostic factors in gestational trophoblastic tumors: A multivariate analysis. *Cancer*, **62**, 585–92.
17. Lurain, J.R., Casanova, L.A., Miller, D.S. and Rademaker, A.W. (1991) Prognostic factors in gestational trophoblastic tumours: a proposed

new scoring system based on multivariate analysis. *Am. J. Obstet. Gynecol.*, **164**, 611–16.

18. Mortakis, A.E. and Braga, C.A. (1990) 'Poor prognosis' metastatic gestational trophoblastic disease: the prognostic significance of the scoring system in predicting chemotherapy failures. *Obstet. Gynecol.*, **76**, 272–7.
19. Ngan, H.Y.S., Lopes, A.D.B., Lauder, I.J. *et al.* (1994) An evaluation of the prognostic factors in metastatic gestational trophoblastic disease. *Int. J. Gynecol. Cancer*, **4**, 36–42.
20. Dubc-Lissoir, J., Sweizig, S., Schlaerth, J.B. and Morrow, C.P. (1992) Metastatic gestational trophoblastic disease: a comparison of prognostic classification systems. *Gynecol. Oncol.*, **45**, 40–5.

CLINICAL FEATURES OF MOLAR PREGNANCIES AND GESTATIONAL TROPHOBLASTIC TUMORS

7

A.C. Evans Jr, John T. Soper and Charles B. Hammond

7.1 INTRODUCTION

Successful management and cure of gestational trophoblastic disease (GTD) depends upon prompt, accurate diagnosis and institution of individualized therapeutic modalities. Because GTD encompasses a multitude of clinical entities, each with myriad presentations, clinicians must remain alert to identify patients exhibiting signs and symptoms consistent with GTD[1,2]. Armed with a high index of suspicion, physicians may target such individuals and launch the appropriate diagnostic barrage, leading to triage for treatment early in the course of disease.

The focus of this chapter is the diverse manifestations of GTD. We will review common presenting features as well as unusual but instructive cases. Standard and newer diagnostic procedures for making the clinical diagnosis of GTD will also be presented.

7.2 SPECTRUM OF DISEASE

GTD arises as a neoplastic derivative of the fetal allograft which escapes immunological surveillance and has the potential to invade its maternal host[3]. Pathogenic and histological features of GTD in its various rubrics are detailed elsewhere in this volume and will not be reiterated here. For the purposes of this chapter, terminology of GTD states will be as follows: molar pregnancies will be considered to comprise complete and partial hydatidiform moles, and gestational trophoblastic tumor (GTT) will refer to invasive mole, choriocarcinoma, and persistent GTD after completion of pregnancy (whether of molar or non-molar type).

Complete hydatidiform moles (CHM) and partial hydatidiform moles (PHM) differ in their invasive potential and propensity for malignant transformation. Approximately 8–20% of patients with CHM may be expected to develop persistent trophoblastic disease following uterine evacuation[4–7]. Prospective study has demonstrated no difference in requirement for chemotherapy between patients with homozygous CHM (those derived from duplication of male haploid genome) and those with heterozygous CHM (those resulting from dispermic fertilization[6]. PHM gives rise to persistent trophoblastic disease in less than 3% of cases[5–7].

Invasive mole (IM) is a histologically benign condition resulting from invasion of abnormal trophoblasts into myometrium and/or embolization of molar tissue through pelvic venous plexi. Fifteen per cent of patients with IM have metastases; these most commonly lodge in the vagina and lungs[8].

Gestational Trophoblastic Disease.
Edited by B.W. Hancock, E.S. Newlands and R.S. Berkowitz.
ISBN 0 412 63100 8

Gestational choriocarcinoma (CC) is a malignancy which arises from trophoblastic tissue of term pregnancies, ectopic gestations, spontaneous/induced abortions or molar elements[9–16]. CC invades and metastasizes early and is often widespread at the time of diagnosis. Lung metastases are present in almost all patients with extrauterine disease; other sites often involved include brain, liver, vagina, kidney and intestines[17]. Fifty per cent of cases arise from molar gestations (2% of all CHM), one-quarter develop from aborted pregnancies and the remaining cases follow term deliveries[8].

Placental site trophoblastic tumor (PSTT) is a rare manifestation of GTT which develops at placental implantation site and may complicate any type of pregnancy[18–21]. PSTT is resistant to chemotherapy but responds well to surgery if the disease is localized[22].

Because many cases of GTT are identified by clinical criteria and no pathological diagnosis exists, treatment of this tumor is based upon clinical parameters. Thus, there is little distinction between IM and CC in terms of the way that treatment strategy is planned. More important than the type of GTT is the accurate and rapid diagnosis so that treatment may be administered promptly.

7.3 EPIDEMIOLOGAL CHARACTERISTICS

In the USA approximately 3000 cases of hydatidiform mole and 500 to 750 cases of malignant GTT are diagnosed each year[2]. The incidence of CHM is between 50 and 150 per 100 000 pregnancies[23–26]. Incidence data relating to PHM has been more difficult to quantify given the lack of reliable histopathological diagnosis.

Asian populations have at least a two-fold higher incidence of CHM, which does not seem to be related to differences in environmental or dietary factors[24,26]. Molar gestations are increased in older and very young women of reproductive age[26]. When compared to women between the ages of 25 and 29, gravid females below age 20 have a 1.3-fold higher incidence of molar gestation; those over age 45 possess a 19-fold increased risk. Women over 50 have as much as a 200- to 400-fold elevated risk of hydatidiform mole[27,28]. Risk remains relatively constant between the ages of 20 and 39[26]. Advanced paternal age may yield a higher risk of CHM[23,29,30]. Neither maternal nor paternal age has been linked to elevated risk of PHM[30].

History of previous molar gestation increases risk of a subsequent occurrence by a factor of 10[31]. Type, number and nature of previous pregnancies do not otherwise seem to influence risk for development of molar gestation[32]. Conflicting evidence exists regarding dietary contribution to formation of hydatidiform mole, with deficiency of vitamin A derivatives and protein being most commonly implicated[26].

CC occurs in approximately 2.2 per 100 000 pregnancies in the USA[26]. Risk of developing CC is increased 1000–2000 times for women with hydatidiform moles[33]. Therefore, it seems reasonable that epidemiological risk modifiers for CHM would correspondingly alter risk for the one-half of CC cases that follow molar pregnancies. It has been much more difficult to determine risk factors for gestations for which CC arises from apparently normal placental tissue.

It is well established that an increased incidence of CC occurs at the upper and lower extremes of the reproductive years[34, 35]. It has been suggested that non-white populations are at increased risk[34]. Certain parental ABO blood groups are linked to increased risk of CC development[36,37] but do not affect risk for hydatidiform mole[36]. No human leukocyte antigen (HLA) locus antigens have been found to be associated with development of GTT[26]. No other epidemiological variables have been consis-

Table 7.1 Clinical features of molar pregnancy

Finding	*Percentage of patients*	
	SERTDC[a]	*NERTDC*[b]
Vaginal bleeding	89	97
Anemia	n.d.	54
Excessive uterine enlargement	46	51
Ovarian enlargement	14[c]	50[d]
Pre-eclampsia	12	27
Hyperemesis gravidarum	14	26
Pain	10	n.d.
Hyperthyroidism	2	7

[a]Southeastern Regional Trophoblastic Disease Center.
[b]New England Trophoblastic Disease Center.
[c]Greater than 8 cm.
[d]Greater than 6 cm.
n.d., not determined.
Modified from references 4 and 38.

tently linked with CC, probably owing to the rarity of the disease.

7.4 CLINICAL MANIFESTATIONS

Clinical features of GTD in all of its manifestations range from common symptoms such as vaginal bleeding to more unusual presentations such as sudden death from hemorrhagic involvement of vital organs. Classic presentations of trophoblastic disease will be outlined here; rare and bizarre manifestations will be considered in a later section.

Vaginal bleeding is the most common presenting symptom of CHM; it is experienced by 89–97% of patients and may result in symptomatic anemia[4,38–40]. The majority of patients present prior to 20 weeks gestation[4]. Liquefaction of intrauterine clots may lead to leakage of fluid with the color and consistency of prune juice. Some patients pass molar vesicles. Table 7.1 lists some of the most common symptoms found in association with molar gestation.

Approximately 40–50% of women with CHM experience uterine enlargement in excess of four weeks greater than of that expected based on last menstrual period[4,38,39]. Increased uterine size results from trophoblastic hyperplasia with expansion and hemorrhage within the uterine cavity. Although uterine size greater than dates is regarded as a classic manifestation of molar pregnancy, about 15–40% of patients have a 'small-for-dates' uterus[4,38,39].

Hyperemesis gravidarum complicates about 15–25% of cases of CHM and is usually associated with uterine enlargement and markedly elevated human chorionic gonadotropin (hCG) levels[4,38,39]. Pre-eclampsia is associated with 12–27% of CHM[4,38] but is rare if molar pregnancy is diagnosed prior to 10–12 weeks[39]. Curry *et al.* noted that, of 347 patients treated at the Southeastern Regional Trophoblastic Disease Center, 81% of those with pre-eclampsia had an excessively enlarged uterus[4]. Development of the syndrome of hypertension, proteinuria and edema in early pregnancy should raise suspicion of a molar gestation.

Clinically evident hyperthyroidism is a feature of CHM in 2–7% of patients[4,38]. Presenting symptoms include thyroid enlargement, tachycardia, fever and tremor; occasional women present with thyroid storm. Conflicting evidence exists with respect to whether hCG is the thyrotropic factor responsible for stimulating thyrotoxicosis[41,42].

Pulmonary insufficiency is associated with about 2% of cases of CHM[43,44]. In these cases, acute respiratory distress occurs after molar evacuation and is almost invariably associated with marked uterine enlargement. Although acute respiratory distress syndrome has been presumed to arise because of trophoblastic embolization, this notion has been challenged[45]. Other conditions associated with CHM can lead to respiratory distress. These include high-output congestive heart failure secondary to anemia or hyperthyroidism, pre-eclampsia or fluid overload[43]. Symptoms and signs of acute respiratory distress syndrome include dyspnea, tachycardia and tachypnea. Examination usually reveals extensive rales. Intensive care unit support and assisted ventilation may be required. With appropriate attention, respiratory distress usually abates in two to three days.

Theca lutein cysts of the ovary are commonly associated with CHM. Almost 50% of patients in one series had ovarian cysts greater than 6 cm in diameter[38]. Ovarian enlargement of 8 cm or more was found in 14% of patients treated at the Southeastern Regional Trophoblastic Disease Center[4]. Another study found that 26% of women with CHM had some adnexal enlargement; mean cyst size was 7 cm with a range of 3–20 cm[46]. These cysts have been assumed to arise as a result of extremely high hCG levels[38]; however, Montz *et al.* demonstrated that growth and regression of cysts are often unrelated to hCG levels[46]. Cyst fluid may consist of serous or serosanguinous liquor. In the University of Southern California (USC) study cited[46], three of 102 patients (2.9%) experienced symptoms related to cysts (torsion, hemoperitoneum, ascites). Laparoscopy has been employed to relieve unbearable pelvic pressure or torsion[38]. In general, intervention is unnecessary and the cysts resolve within 12 weeks[46].

Fever or evidence of a bleeding diathesis should be investigated if present because uterine infection and disseminated intravascular coagulation are variably associated with molar pregnancy. Fetal heart tones are invariably absent in patients with CHM. Sometimes CHM is diagnosed on the basis of histopathological examination of uterine curettings following pregnancy termination. This highlights the importance of routinely submitting for pathological review any tissue obtained from uterine evacuation or curettage.

PHMs are rarely diagnosed prior to uterine evacuation. Most patients present with signs and symptoms suggesting incomplete or missed abortion[47,48]. Any of the clinical manifestations of CHM may be associated with PHM, but they tend to be more subdued. Excessive uterine enlargement, pre-eclampsia and hCG values greater than 100 000 U/l are found in less than 10% of patients[47]. Hyperthyroidism, hyperemesis and theca lutein cysts are exceedingly rare. Fetal heart tones may be present in twin pregnancy of mole and fetus.

The most common symptom of invasive mole is irregular uterine bleeding following evacuation of a molar gestation. If metastasis has occurred, bleeding from vaginal or pulmonary sources may be present if these sites are affected. Diagnosis of persistent GTD after molar evacuation is usually made by observation of persistently elevated or rising hCG levels[49].

Presenting signs and symptoms of gestational CC are highly variable. The invasive nature of this tumor often leads to early metastasis. Additionally, some tumors are diagnosed long after the antecedent gestation and are widely disseminated. About two-thirds of the patients treated for GTT at the Brewer Trophoblastic Disease Center had metastases when diagnosed[12]. Vaginal bleeding is the most common symptom.

Symptoms and signs associated with metastatic sites of CC are often present owing to extensive tissue invasion with secondary necrosis and hemorrhage. Vaginal metastases may bleed extensively, especially when biopsied. Uterine enlargement and irregularity may be noted. Metastases to the lung are present in over 80% of women with metastatic GTT[50]. Pulmonary involvement may cause cough, dyspnea, hemoptysis and/or pleuritic chest pain due to pulmonary infarction or pleural space invasion. Patients may experience abdominal pain if visceral involvement or hemoperitoneum is present. Neurological manifestations may include headaches, seizures, loss of consciousness and paralysis. Profound anemia may be another feature of metastatic CC.

Clinicians should be alert to the possibility of malignant GTT in any reproductive age woman with bizarre central nervous system symptoms, postpartum cerebrovascular accidents or radiographic evidence of metastatic tumor of unknown primary origin[1]. In these instances, a simple hCG determination may be life-saving.

Almost all patients with placental site trophoblastic tumors present with irregular vaginal bleeding; most others complain of amenorrhea[19–21,51]. Rarely, these tumors may cause virilization or nephrotic syndrome. Patients of all ages are affected. No association with gravidity or type of prior pregnancy has been identified[21]. Time from antecedent gestation to diagnosis varies from one week to 14 years[20,21].

7.5 PERSISTENT GTD FOLLOWING MOLAR EVACUATION

About 20% of patients with CHM develop malignant sequelae[4,8,40]. Eighty-five per cent of these individuals have disease localized to the uterus. Fewer than 4% of women with PHM contract persistent GTD[5,7,47,48]. Postmolar GTT arising from PHM is almost always invasive mole (as opposed to CC), tends not to metastasize and readily responds to chemotherapy[7,52].

Clinical features suggesting persistent GTD include plateauing or rising hCG levels, elevated hCG at four months post evacuation (greater than 20 000 U/l), hemorrhage from uterine or other metastatic foci, demonstrable metastases and histological verification of CC or PSTT. In the USA the hCG criteria often employed for defining post-molar GTT are rising levels over any two-week period with weekly determinations or no significant decline (less than 10%) over three weeks during surveillance[31,53]. Often no histological diagnosis exists and treatment is initiated based on hCG criteria; therefore, most investigators refer to categories of invasive and metastatic disease generically as 'GTT'. However, some researchers have advocated clinicopathological diagnosis of invasive mole or CC based on type of antecedent pregnancy and histological criteria[12]. Such classification has been demonstrated to affect prognosis for cure[12].

Several clinical findings are associated with increased risk for development of post-molar GTT[4,35,50,52–54]. About half of women with uterine size greater than 20 weeks or with theca lutein cysts develop persistent GTD after molar pregnancy. Thirty-five to forty per cent of women with a second molar gestation have progressive disease. Post-molar GTT ensues in one-quarter to one-third of patients with uterine size greater than dates or over age 40. Post-evacuation hemorrhage, trophoblastic embolization to lungs, and eclampsia have also been identified as high-risk factors[40,44,54,55]. The pattern of hCG regression[56] and ratio of free hCG β-subunit to total β-subunit[57] has been reported to predict persistent disease. Early studies suggested that extent of trophoblastic proliferation and degree of anaplasia were associated with increased risk of post-molar GTT[58], but this has not been confirmed[4,59]. About 35% of patients with molar pregnancies have one or more of the cited 'high-risk' factors; therefore, vigilant follow-up is warranted since those individuals destined to require further therapy for post-molar GTT cannot be predicted with certainty.

Women who develop post-molar GTT tend to be diagnosed earlier than women with malignant GTD arising from an aborted or term pregnancy. Surveillance of hCG levels affords relatively early diagnosis in the former condition. Diagnosis is often delayed beyond four months among women with antecedent normal or aborted gestations[13]. Furthermore, women with persistent GTD diagnosed by hCG surveillance often have non-metastatic disease and very few symptoms. Abnormal uterine bleeding that regularly accompanies invasive disease may sometimes be masked by oral contraceptive therapy.

7.6 METASTATIC GTT

GTT metastases have been reported in almost all conceivable sites. Organs most commonly involved are lung, vagina, central nervous system, liver, kidneys and gastrointestinal tract (Table 7.2). Symptoms and physical findings reflect the degree of involvement of the affected organ(s) and whether hemorrhage or necrosis is the prominent feature.

The most common extragenital site of involvement of GTT is the lung. Pulmonary involvement rarely causes symptoms. One series of 97 women with pulmonary involvement (88% had multiple lung nodules) revealed that only four patients had symptoms[60]. These symptoms comprised hemoptysis and/or chronic cough. None of the women had breathlessness.

A recent study at our center revealed that 15 of 17 (88%) patients with GTT involving a high-risk metastatic site had symptoms of extrapulmonary disease[61]. All 17 of these patients had lung metastases but none had pulmonary symptoms. Table 7.3 gives a sum-

Table 7.2 Distribution of metastases[a]

Site	*% Involvement*
Lung	78–93
CNS[b]	7–9
Vagina	5–16
Pelvis	4–7
Liver	1–4
Abdomen	2–4
Kidney	1
Bone	1
Breast	1
Adrenal	1

[a]Patients may have metastases affecting more than one site.
[b]Central nervous system.
Data modified from references 12, 43 and 61.

Table 7.3 Presenting symptoms of patients with extrapulmonary metastases

Site (no. of patients)	*Presentation (no. of patients)*
Central nervous system (11)	Seizure (6)
	Visual field cuts (1)
	Dysphasia (1)
	Abnormal neurological examination (1)
	None (2)
Liver (4)	None (4)
Gastrointestinal (3)	Gastrointestinal hemorrhage (3)
Kidneys (8)	Retroperitoneal hemorrhage (2)
	Pain/hematuria/mass (2)
	None (4)
Bone (2)	Bone pain (2)
Breast (1)	Mass lesion (1)

Data modified from references 61 and 123.

mary of presenting symptoms of women with high-risk GTT.

Researchers at the Brewer Trophoblastic Disease Center have studied causes of death among patients with metastatic GTT[50]. Hemorrhage from metastatic foci was the most common cause of death (42%). Sites involved (in descending order) were lungs, liver, gastrointestinal tract and peritoneal cavity. Intra-abdominal bleeds were more prevalent among patients with advanced disease who had not received a full course of therapy. Pulmonary insufficiency secondary to alveolar destruction, tumor burden and hemorrhage caused the demise of 31% of their non-survivors. Death was attributed to chemotherapeutic toxicity in 10% of cases, but toxicity was a complicating factor in several others. Less common causes of death (about 2%) included sepsis, uremia secondary to obstructive uropathy, acute tubular necrosis and pulmonary embolism. Eight per cent of patients (all with extensive metastases) died away from the hospital and their fatal events could not be assessed.

7.7 DIAGNOSTIC AIDS

Several laboratory and radiological tools are available to secure the clinical diagnosis of GTT and determine extent of disease. Standard and newer techniques are described here. Work-up, staging and prognostic indicators of GTT are addressed elsewhere in this volume.

Accurate, dependable assays of hCG are essential for reliable diagnosis and are the foundation upon which individualized therapeutic decisions are built[62]. In general, hCG levels correspond to tumor burden. Radioimmunoassay, fluoroimmunoassay and enzyme immunoassay are sensitive to below 5 U/l and provide reproducible results. These assays are based on antibody recognition of the hCG β-subunit, and typically measure both free β-subunit and intact hCG. Chromatographic separation is necessary if measurement of isolated α or β is required; this is not routinely done in clinical laboratories. Several reports exist suggesting measurement of free α- or β-subunit may have clinical relevance, but these findings have not been consistently demonstrated[57,62–64]. Despite the sensitivity and accuracy of most assays, the 'sandwich' assay which employs two distinct monoclonal antibodies directed against different epitopes of the intact hCG molecule may suggest a falsely low level of hCG when extremely high levels are present[65]. Thus, it is important for clinicians to understand the methodology employed for hCG quantification in the laboratory where their patients' sera are analyzed.

Investigators at the Charing Cross Hospital have advocated measurement of hCG in cerebrospinal fluid as an aid in diagnosing brain metastases and for monitoring therapeutic response in those with proven central nervous system involvement[66,67]. Detection of hCG in symptomatic older, postmenopausal women strongly suggests the diagnosis of latent GTT[35,68,69]. Serial hCG monitoring of women with disease in prolonged remission (greater than one year) often provides early evidence of recurrence[70]. GTT may rarely be associated with undetectable levels of hCG[71]. Significant amounts of hCG may be liberated by a number of tumors other than GTT; this should be borne in mind when working up any woman with elevated hCG levels who is suspected of harboring a malignancy.

α-Fetoprotein is not usually elevated except in cases of partial mole with significant fetal development or in cases of coexisting GTD and normal pregnancy[72]. Human placental lactogen (hPL) may help distinguish between CC and PSTT[22,51]. Low hCG levels in association with a relatively large tumor should raise suspicion of PSTT[21]. Immunohistochemical studies often reveal extensive staining for hPL and a trace presence of hCG[22,51]. Neither hCG nor hPL levels in tumor or serum are predictive of clinical behavior of PSTT[20–22,73]. CA-125 may be elevated in some cases of PSTT[74] or persistent GTD[75].

A hematocrit should be obtained in all women with GTD to assess for anemia. The presence of hyperemesis, pre-eclampsia, hyperthyroid symptoms, excessive hemorrhage, infection, hematuria, oliguria, melena or dyspnea may suggest the need for further studies such as blood count, platelets, electrolytes, blood urea nitrogen (BUN), creatinine, liver enzymes, thyroid profile, coagulation studies, urinalysis, stool guaiac, blood cultures or arterial blood gases[53,76]. Central hemodynamic monitoring may be required to watch cardiopulmonary status in unstable patients.

Radiological evaluation is often helpful for diagnosing molar gestation and in assessing patients for metastases of GTT. A chest X-ray is useful in evaluating women experiencing respiratory distress with suspected pulmonary edema, adult respiratory distress syndrome or extensive lung metastases. Chest roentgenology has utility as a screening tool for trophoblastic emboli in women with CHM. Excellent reviews of chest X-ray findings in women with pulmonary metastases of GTT are available[77,78]. Early findings include generalized increased lung markings often associated with small sacculations or dilated regions resembling a 'string of beads'. As lesions progress, patchy infiltrates and small nodules or miliary shadows are seen. More advanced disease results in medium (3–5 cm) to large (greater than 5 cm), round, low-density shadows with hazy or well-defined margins. Atelectasis, pneumothorax and effusion (usually hemothorax) are seen in many patients. Extensive pulmonary disease leads in some cases to cardiac enlargement and prominent pulmonary conus as a result of acute cor pulmonale[78].

Angiography was used heavily for diagnosing metastatic lesions in the liver, spleen and brain until the advent of computed tomography (CT) scans[79] and continues to be of use in selected cases for detecting small lesions or for determining the extent of vascular compromise by tumor[80,81]. Intravenous urography lacks the sensitivity and specificity necessary to screen for renal involvement[82].

Ultrasound is a useful non-invasive imaging method[83], especially when combined with hCG data[84]. CHM has the appearance of a vesicular mass in association with uterine enlargement and focal areas of hemorrhage. Theca–lutein cysts may be demonstrated. Location and size of invasive mole or CC lesions can be determined. Transvaginal sonography is especially helpful for diagnosing and subsequently following GTT lesions during chemotherapy[85–88]. Color flow Doppler can define regions of increased vascularity representative of invasive disease[89] and enhanced uterine perfusion distinct from that seen in conditions related to pregnancy or abortion[85]. Ultrasound and color Doppler imaging of extrauterine disease may demonstrate tumor vascularity and blood flow patterns and can be employed to target lesions for percutaneous sampling[90].

CT scan is an effective means of screening for central nervous system and abdominopelvic metastases[61]. Chest CT is more sensitive than chest X-ray for detecting pulmonary metastases; about 40% of patients with presumed non-metastatic GTT have pulmonary lesions when screened with CT scan[91]. In our experience, these women lack pulmonary symptoms. Magnetic resonance imaging has been shown to accurately define the degree of uterine invasion by GTT and is useful for monitoring tumor responsiveness to therapy[92–94].

Traditional histopathological review of biopsy material reliably provides a diagnosis of GTT when present, but categorization of the lesions varies among pathologists[95–97]. Molar ploidy analysis by flow cytometry is useful in distinguishing PHM from CHM[98]. More sophisticated genetic techniques including polymerase chain reaction and restriction fragment length polymorphism analysis are accurate and sensitive means for tumor classification[6,99–101]. Oncogene involvement in the evolution of GTD is under investigation and may provide prognostic data and therapeutic strategies in the future[102]. Cytological study of pulmonary artery aspirates may help in the differential diagnosis of pulmonary lesions or may provide tissue diagnosis of GTT when biopsies of other sites are negative or unavailable[103–105].

7.8 UNUSUAL PRESENTATIONS

Patients with GTT often present with non-gynecological complaints; alternatively, gynecological symptoms are sometimes ignored, attributed to normal peripartum or postabortal state, or are not appreciated by non-gynecologists. Clinicians of all disciplines who care for women in the reproductive age range must be aware of the possibility of GTT and, where applicable, should rule the diagnosis in or out. In preceding sections we have outlined common features of GTD; here we focus on non-classic manifestations.

Catastrophic hemorrhagic events may provide the initial presentation of GTD. A number of reports exist describing women suffering massive hemoperitoneum secondary to rupture of hepatic splenic or pelvic foci of GTT[1,106–108]. Severe hemorrhage has also occurred following liver biopsy of nodules that were not suspected of being CC[109]. The presentation may mimic that of ruptured eccyesis[14,15,110]. Gastrointestinal bleeding also occurs. Esophageal, gastric and small bowel metastases have caused hematemesis and severe melena[1,108,111–114]. Acute intracranial hemorrhage is another rare presentation of metastatic GTT leading to sudden collapse and loss of consciousness. Such events may occur within days of delivery[115,116] or molar evacuation[117], or at times remote from these events[108,118,119]. Aneurysms occasionally develop at sites of metastasis[108,117,120]. Intrathoracic hemorrhage sometimes leads to hemoptysis, dyspnea, chest pain, bloody effusion and hypovolemia[1,106,114,121]. Kidney involvement may cause massive retroperitoneal hemorrhage[122,123].

Mass effect, tissue invasion and paraneoplastic syndromes may lead to bizarre presentations. Intussusception caused by CC has been described[124]. Intestinal obstruction[125] and colonic pseudo-obstruction have been reported[126]. Renal metastases may cause abdominal pain, hematuria or oliguria[1,122,127] but sometimes are found as mass lesions during radiological screening for metastases[123,128]. Neurological manifestations may include hemiparesis[106], paresthesias[1], seizures[1] or Jacksonian epilepsy[129]. Pulmonary hypertension secondary to tumor emboli can mimic pulmonary thromboembolus or right-sided heart failure[130,131]. Fatal ischemic heart disease from coronary artery embolism of CC has been reported[132]. CC has also presented as an intracavitary tumor of the left atrium with classic symptoms and findings of left atrial myxoma[133]. Herpes gestationis has been described associated with GTD[134]. Thyrotoxicosis is sometimes the initial finding in GTD patients[135,136]. Recurrent bacteremia has led to the diagnosis of GTD[137].

Metastases of GTT may occur almost anywhere in the body. Unusual sites such as bone[106], breast[138] and others must be diagnosed since their presence may affect therapeutic decisions and prognosis. Rare instances of metastases to the fetus have been documented[139,140].

Rarely, 'twin' gestations comprising molar pregnancies in concert with a fetus occur[141–145]. These patients tend to be diagnosed with molar gestation at a later stage than those with single molar pregnancies. They also have been shown to have higher pre-evacuation hCG levels and an elevated risk of developing persistent trophoblastic disease[142]. Ultrasound diagnosis can be achieved in about two-thirds of cases. Chromosomal studies can also be helpful if there is a triploid (partial) mole and a diploid fetus. No fetal anomalies have been described in association with this condition; the fetal survival is about 25%. Despite the later diagnosis and higher rates of GTT among these patients, all reported patients with dual normal–molar pregnancies have survived. Little data are available to assist in the counselling of women with this diagnosis. Decisions regarding continuation of the gestation should be based on whether or not concomitant problems such as pre-eclampsia, hemorrhage or respiratory distress are present and on the desires of the patient. These women should be informed of the elevated risk of malignant sequelae associated with coexisting molar and normal pregnancies.

Several reports of CC in association with intrauterine pregnancy exist[106,146]. Fetal compromise is often found in such cases. Grossly, CC in a term placenta may be misinterpreted as a placental infarct[147]. Sometimes pathological examination of the placenta yields the first sign of CC and has led to the diagnosis of metastases in otherwise asymptomatic patients[148].

Many other unusual situations have been documented that provide diagnostic challenges. Postmenopausal women may harbor latent GTT[68,69,106,149]. Serum hCG levels may be undetectable in some patients[71]. Factitious cases of GTD have been reported in women who feigned symptoms and surreptitiously exchanged blood samples so that they might receive medical attention and unwarranted surgery[150]. CC rarely may arise from totipotent cells in extragonadal sites and may be misdiagnosed as GTD[151].

7.9 POST TREATMENT

The diagnosis of mole or malignant neoplasia in a woman anticipating routine pregnancy has obvious psychological consequences. GTD patients have been shown to have clinically significant fatigue, anger, anxiety, confusion and sexual dysfunction[152]. These concerns should be addressed and psychiatric referral obtained if indicated.

Current chemotherapeutic regimens allow preservation of fertility in most GTD patients. Normal reproductive outcome should be anticipated in women with prior molar gestations; there is no increased risk of stillbirth, abortion, preterm delivery or congenital anomalies[153,154]. The risk of recurrent mole is about 2%[154]. Similarly, patients with post-molar GTT and CC cured by chemotherapy can expect therapeutic outcomes no different from that of the general population[154].

Patients should employ reliable contraception to prevent confusion caused by intercurrent pregnancy and the attendant rise in hCG. Hormonal contraception has been proven to be safe and very effective[155].

Serial serum hCG levels should be determined for at least one year after remission is accomplished. Patients should also be queried on each visit regarding any symptoms suspicious for recurrence (especially irregular vaginal bleeding). Most recurrences of GTT occur within one year of achieving remission[156]. However, late recurrences have been reported years after primary remission[70]; the incidence of such cases is less than 1%.

7.10 SUMMARY

GTD may present in an unlimited number of ways. Astute clinicians should be able to secure the diagnosis if it is considered and appropriate history, examination, laboratory, radiological and pathological techniques are employed.

REFERENCES

1. Hammond, C.B., Hertz, R., Ross, G.T. *et al.* (1967) Diagnostic problems of choriocarcinoma and related trophoblastic neoplasms. *Obstetrics and Gynecology*, **29**, 224–9.
2. Hammond, C.B. and Parker, R.T. (1970) Diagnosis and treatment of trophoblastic disease: a report from the Southeastern Regional Center. *Obstetrics and Gynecology*, **35**, 132–43.
3. Lawler, S.D. and Fisher, R.A. (1987) Immunological aspects, in *Gestational Trophoblastic Disease*, (eds A.E. Szulman and H.J. Buchsbaum), Springer-Verlag, New York, pp. 77–87.
4. Curry, S.L., Hammond, C.B., Tyrey, L. *et al.* (1975) Hydatidiform mole: diagnosis, management, and long-term followup of 347 patients. *Obstetrics and Gynecology*, **45**, 1–8.
5. Bagshawe, K.D., Lawler, S.D., Paradinas, F.J. *et al.* (1990) Gestational trophoblastic tumours following initial diagnosis of partial hydatidiform mole. *Lancet*, **335**, 1074–6.
6. Lawler, S.D., Fisher, R.A. and Dent, J. (1991) A prospective genetic study of complete and partial hydatidiform moles. *American Journal of Obstetrics and Gynecology*, **164**, 1270–7.
7. Goto, S., Yamada, A., Ishizuka, T. *et al.* (1993) Development of postmolar trophoblastic disease after partial molar pregnancy. *Gynecologic Oncology*, **48**, 165–70.
8. Lurain, J.R. (1990) Gestational trophoblastic tumors. *Seminars in Surgical Oncology*, **6**, 347–53.
9. Miller, J.M., Jr, Surwit, E.A. and Hammond, C.B. (1979) Choriocarcinoma following term pregnancy. *Obstetrics and Gynecology*, **53**, 207–12.
10. Berkowitz, R.S., Goldstein, D.P. and Bernstein, M.R. (1984) Choriocarcinoma following term gestation. *Gynecologic Oncology*, **17**, 52–7.
11. Hammond, C.B., Borchert, L.G., Tyrey, L. *et al.* (1973) Treatment of metastatic trophoblastic disease: good and poor prognosis, *American Journal of Obstetrics and Gynecology*, **115**, 451–7.
12. Lurain, J.R., Brewer, J.I., Torok, E.E. *et al.* (1982) Gestational trophoblastic disease: treatment results at the Brewer Trophoblastic Disease Center. *Obstetrics and Gynecology*, **60**, 354–60.
13. Soper, J.T., Clarke-Pearson, D. and Hammond, C.B. (1988) Metastatic gestational trophoblastic disease: prognostic factors in previously untreated patients. *Obstetrics and Gynecology*, **71**, 338–43.
14. Lurain, J.R., Sand, P.K. and Brewer, J.I. (1986) Choriocarcinoma associated with ectopic pregnancy. *Obstetrics and Gynecology*, **68**, 286–7.
15. Kucukozkan, T., Savan, K., Aydin, E. *et al.* (1992) Choriocarcinoma associated with ectopic pregnancy after tubal sterilisation. *Acta Obstetricia et Gynecologica Scandinavica*, **71**, 636–8.
16. Lurain, J.R., Casanova, L.A., Miller, D.S. *et al.* (1991) Prognostic factors in gestational trophoblastic tumors: a proposed new scoring system based on multivariate analysis. *American Journal of Obstetrics and Gynecology*, **164**, 611–16.
17. Mazur, M.T. and Kurman, R.J. (1987) Choriocarcinoma and placental site trophoblastic tumor, in *Gestational Trophoblastic Disease* (eds A.E. Szulman and H.J. Buchsbaum), Springer-Verlag, New York, pp. 45–68.
18. Rosenshein, N.B., Wijnen, H. and Woodruff, J.D. (1980) Clinical importance of the diagnosis of trophoblastic pseudotumors. *American Journal of Obstetrics and Gynecology*, **136**, 635–8.
19. Finkler, N.J., Berkowitz, R.S., Driscoll, S.G. *et al.* (1988) Clinical experience with placental site trophoblastic tumors at the New England Trophoblastic Disease Center. *Obstetrics and Gynecology*, **71**, 854–7.
20. Lathrop, J.C., Lauchlan, S., Nayak, R. *et al.* (1988) Clinical characteristics of placental site trophoblastic tumor (PSTT). *Gynecologic Oncology*, **31**, 32–42.
21. Finkler, N.J. (1991) Placental site trophoblastic tumor: diagnosis, clinical behavior and treatment. *Journal of Reproductive Medicine*, **36**, 27–30.

22. Dessau, R., Rustin, G.J., Dent, J. *et al.* (1990) Surgery and chemotherapy in the management of placental site tumor. *Gynecologic Oncology*, **39**, 56–9.
23. Yes, S. and MacMahon, B. (1968) Epidemiologic features of trophoblastic disease. *American Journal of Obstetrics and Gynecology*, **101**, 126–32.
24. McCorriston, C.C. (1968) Racial incidence of hydatidiform mole: a study in a contained polyracial community. *American Journal of Obstetrics and Gynecology*, **101**, 377–82.
25. Hayashi, K., Bracken, M.B., Freeman, D.H., Jr *et al.* (1982) Hydatidiform mole in the United States (1970–1977): a statistical and theoretical analysis. *American Journal of Epidemiology*, **115**, 67–77.
26. Buckley, J. (1987) Epidemiology of gestational trophoblastic diseases, in *Gestational Trophoblastic Disease* (eds A.E. Szulman and H.J. Buchsbaum), Springer-Verlag, New York, pp. 8–26.
27. Nakano, R., Sasaki, K., Yamoto, M. *et al.* (1980) Trophoblastic disease: analysis of 342 patients. *Gynecologic and Obstetric Investigation*, **11**, 237–42.
28. Bagshawe, K.D., Dent, J. and Webb, J. (1986) Hydatidiform mole in England and Wales 1973–83, *Lancet*, **ii**, 673–7.
29. La Vecchia, C., Parazzini, F., Decarli, A. *et al.* (1984) Age of parents and risk of gestational trophoblastic disease. *Journal of the National Cancer Institute*, **73**, 639–42.
30. Parazzini, F., La Vecchia, C. and Pampallona, S. (1986) Parental age and risk of complete and partial hydatidiform mole. *British Journal of Obstetrics and Gynaecology*, **93**, 582–5.
31. Soper, J.T., Hammond, C.B. and Lewis, J.L., Jr (1992) Gestational trophoblastic disease, in *Principles and Practice of Gynecologic Oncology* (eds W.J. Hoskins, C.A. Perez and R.C. Young), Lippincott, Philadelphia, pp. 795–825.
32. Atrash, H.K., Hogue, C.J. and Grimes, D.A. (1986) Epidemiology of hydatidiform mole during early gestation. *American Journal of Obstetrics and Gynecology*, **154**, 906–9.
33. Park, W.W. and Lees, J.C. (1950) Choriocarcinoma: a general review, with analysis of 516 cases. *Archives of Pathology*, **49**, 73–104.
34. Brinton, L.A., Bracken, M.B. and Connelly, R.R. (1986) Choriocarcinoma incidence in the United States. *American Journal of Epidemiology*, **123**, 1094–100.
35. Bandy, L.C., Clarke-Pearson, D.L. and Hammond, C.B. (1984) Malignant potential of gestational trophoblastic disease at the extreme ages of reproductive life. *Obstetrics and Gynecology*, **64**, 395–9.
36. Dawood, M.Y., Teoh, E.S. and Ratnam, S.S. (1971) ABO blood group in trophoblastic disease. *Journal of Obstetrics and Gynaecology of the British Commonwealth*, **78**, 918–23.
37. Bagshawe, K.D., Rawlins, G., Pike, M.C. *et al.* (1971) ABO blood-groups in trophoblastic neoplasia. *Lancet*, **i**, 553–6.
38. Golstein, D.P and Berkowitz, R.S. (1982) *Gestational Trophoblastic Neoplasms: clinical principles of diagnosis and management*. W.B. Saunders, Philadelphia, pp. 1–301.
39. Kohorn, E.I. (1984) Molar pregnancy: presentation and diagnosis. *Clinical Obstetrics and Gynecology*, **27**, 181–91.
40. Morrow, C.P., Kletzky, O.A., Di Saia, P.J. *et al.* (1977) Clinical and laboratory correlates of molar pregnancy and trophoblastic disease. *American Journal of Obstetrics and Gynecology*, **128**, 424–30.
41. Amir, S.M., Osathonondh, R., Berkowitz, R.S. *et al.* (1984) Human chorionic gonadotropin and thyroid function in patients with hydatidiform mole. *American Journal of Obstetrics and Gynecology*, **150**, 723–8.
42. Nisula, B.C. and Taliadouros, G.S. (1980) Thyroid function in gestational trophoblastic neoplasia: evidence that the thyrotropic activity of human chorionic gonadotropin mediates the thyrotoxicosis of choriocarcinoma. *American Journal of Obstetrics and Gynecology*, **138**, 77–85.
43. Twiggs, L.B., Morrow, C.P. and Schlaerth, J.B. (1979) Acute pulmonary complications of molar pregnancy. *American Journal of Obstetrics and Gynecology*, **135**, 189–94.
44. Kohorn, E.I. (1987) Clinical management and the neoplastic sequelae of trophoblastic embolization associated with hydatidiform mole. *Obstetrical and Gynecological Survey*, **42**, 484–8.
45. Hankins, G., Wendel, G.D., Snyder, R.R. *et*

al. (1987) Trophoblastic embolization during molar evacuation: central hemodynamic observations. *Obstetrics and Gynecology*, **69**, 368–72.

46. Montz, F.J., Schlaerth, J.B. and Morrow, C.P. (1988) The natural history of theca lutein cysts. *Obstetrics and Gynecology*, **72**, 247–51.
47. Berkowitz, R.S., Goldstein, D.P. and Bernstein, M.R. (1985) Natural history of partial molar pregnancy. *Obstetrics and Gynecology*, **66**, 677–81.
48. Szulman, A.E. (1987) Clinicopathologic features of partial hydatidiform mole. *Journal of Reproductive Medicine*, **32**, 640–3.
49. Lurain, J.R. and Brewer, J.I. (1982) Invasive mole. *Seminars in Oncology*, **9**, 174–80.
50. Lurain, J.R. (1987) Natural history, in *Gestational Trophoblastic Disease* (eds A.E. Szulman and H.J. Buchsbaum), Springer-Verlag, New York, pp. 69–76.
51. Yamamoto, Y., Otsuka, H., Numoto, S. *et al.* (1987) Placental-site trophoblastic tumor of the uterus: clinicopathological and immunohistochemical observations of a case. *Acta Pathologica Japonica*, **37**, 1979–86.
52. Goldstein, D.P. (1991) Gestational trophoblastic neoplasia in the 1990s. *Yale Journal of Biology and Medicine*, **64**, 639–51.
53. Morrow, C.P. (1984) Postmolar trophoblastic disease: diagnosis, management, and prognosis. *Clinical Obstetrics and Gynecology*, **27**, 211–20.
54. Parazzini, F., Mangili, G., Belloni, C. *et al.* (1988) The problem of identification of prognostic factors for persistent trophoblastic disease. *Gynecologic Oncology*, **30**, 57–62.
55. Newman, R.B. and Eddy, G.L. (1989) Eclampsia as a possible risk factor for persistent trophoblastic disease. *Gynecologic Oncology*, **34**, 212–15.
56. Schlaerth, J.B., Morrow, C.P., Kletzky, O.A. *et al.* (1981) Prognostic characteristics of serum human chorionic gonadotropin titer regression following molar pregnancy. *Obstetrics and Gynecology*, **58**, 478–82.
57. Khazaeli, M.B., Buchina, E.S., Patillo, R.A. *et al.* (1989) Radioimmunoassay of free beta-subunit of human chorionic gonadotropin in diagnosis of high-risk and low-risk gestational trophoblastic disease. *American Journal of Obstetrics and Gynecology*, **160**, 444–9.
58. Hertig, A.T. and Sheldon, W.H. (1947) Hydatidiform mole: a pathologico-clinical correlation of 200 cases. *American Journal of Obstetrics and Gynecology*, **53**, 1–32.
59. Rice, L.W., Genest, D.R., Berkowitz, R.S. *et al.* (1991) Pathologic features of sharp curettings in complete hydatidiform mole: predictors of persistent gestational trophoblastic disease. *Journal of Reproductive Medicine*, **36**, 17–20.
60. Kumar, J., Ilancheran, A. and Ratnam, S.S. (1988) Pulmonary metastases in gestational trophoblastic disease: a review of 97 cases. *British Journal of Obstetrics and Gynaecology*, **95**, 70–4.
61. Hunter, V., Raymond, E., Christensen, C. *et al.* (1990) Efficacy of the metastatic survey in the staging of gestational trophoblastic disease. *Cancer*, **65**, 1647–50.
62. Tyrey, L. (1988) Human chorionic gonadotropin assays and their uses. *Obstetrics and Gynecology Clinics of North America*, **15**, 457–75.
63. Quigley, M.M., Tyrey, L. and Hammond, C.B. (1980) Alpha-subunit in sera of choriocarcinoma patients in remission. *Journal of Clinical Endocrinology and Metabolism*, **50**, 98–102.
64. Quigley, M.M., Tyrey, L. and Hammond, C.B. (1980) Utility of assay of alpha subunit of human chorionic gonadotropin in management of gestational, trophoblastic malignancies. *American Journal of Obstetrics and Gynecology*, **138**, 545–9.
65. Levavi, H., Neri, A., Bar, J. *et al.* (1993) 'Hook effect' in complete hydatidiform molar pregnancy: a falsley low level of beta-HCG. *Obstetrics and Gynecology*, **82**, 720–1.
66. Bagshawe, K.D. and Harland, S. (1976) Immunodiagnosis and monitoring of gonadotrophin-producing metastases in the central nervous system. *Cancer*, **38**, 112–18.
67. Soma, H., Takayama, M., Tokoro, K. *et al.* (1980) Radioimmunoassay of hCG as an early diagnosis of cerebral metastases in choriocarcinoma patients. *Acta Obstetricia et Gynecologica Scandinavica*, **59**, 445–8.
68. Sonobe, H., Taguchi, K., Ogawa, K. *et al.* (1976) Latent vaginal choriocarcinoma in a postmenopausal woman. *Acta Pathologica Japonica*, **26**, 611–18.

69. Tsukamoto, N., Iwasaka, T., Kashimura, Y. *et al.* (1985) Gestational trophoblastic disease in women aged 50 or more. *Gynecologic Oncology*, **20**, 53–61.
70. Vaughn, T.C., Surwit, E.A. and Hammond, C.B. (1980) Late recurrences of gestational trophoblastic neoplasia. *American Journal of Obstetrics and Gynecology*, **138**, 73–6.
71. Lemonnier, M.C., Glezerman, M., Vauclair, R. *et al.* (1986) Choriocarcinoma associated with undetectable levels of human chorionic gonadotropin. *Gynecologic Oncology*, **25**, 48–52.
72. Ollendorff, D.A., Goldberg, J.M., Abu-Jawdeh, G.M. *et al.* (1990) Markedly elevated maternal serum alpha-fetoprotein associated with a normal fetus and choriocarcinoma of the placenta. *Obstetrics and Gynecology*, **76**, 494–7.
73. Fukunaga, M. and Ushigome, S. (1993) Metastasizing placental site trophoblastic tumor: an immunohistochemical and flow cytometric study of two cases. *American Journal of Surgical Pathology*, **17**, 1003–10.
74. Hopkins, M.P., Drescher, C.W., McQuillan, A. *et al.* (1992) Malignant placental site trophoblastic tumor associated with placental abruption, fetal distress, and elevated CA-125. *Gynecologic Oncology*, **47**, 267–71.
75. Koonings, P.P. and Schlaerth, J.B. (1993) CA-125: a marker for persistent gestational trophoblastic disease? *Gynecologic Oncology*, **49**, 240–2.
76. Twiggs, L.B. (1984) Nonneoplastic complications of molar pregnancy. *Clinical Obstetrics and Gynecology*, **27**, 199–210.
77. Libshitz, H.I., Baber, C.E. and Hammond, C.B. (1977) The pulmonary metastases of choriocarcinoma. *Obstetrics and Gynecology*, **49**, 412–16.
78. Sung, H.C., Wu, P.C., Hu, M.H. *et al.* (1982) Roentgenologic manifestations of pulmonary metastases in choriocarcinoma and invasive mole. *American Journal of Obstetrics and Gynecology*, **142**, 89–97.
79. Maroulis, G.B., Hammond, C.B., Johnsrude, I.S. *et al.* (1975) Arteriography and infusional chemotherapy in localized trophoblastic disease. *Obstetrics and Gynecology*, **45**, 397–406.
80. Watanabe, A.S. and Smoker, W.R. (1989) Computed tomography and angiographic findings in metastatic choriocarcinoma. *Journal of Computer Assisted Tomography*, **13**, 319–22.
81. Hillard, A.E., Allen, R.W. and Beale, G. (1993) Metastatic choriocarcinoma: correlation of MRI, CT, and angiography. *Southern Medical Journal*, **86**, 1299–302.
82. Smith, E.B., Dunnick, N.R., Nelson, P. *et al.* (1985) Renal metastases of malignant gestational trophoblastic disease: the use of intravenous urography in staging. *Gynecologic Oncology*, **20**, 317–24.
83. Munyer, T.P., Callen, P.W., Filly, R.A. *et al.* (1981) Further observations on the sonographic spectrum of gestational trophoblastic disease. *Journal of Clinical Ultrasound*, **9**, 349–58.
84. Romero, R., Horgan, J.G., Kohorn, E.I. *et al.* (1985) New criteria for the diagnosis of gestational trophoblastic disease. *Obstetrics and Gynecology*, **66**, 553–8.
85. Taylor, K.J., Schwartz, P.E. and Kohorn, E.I. (1987) Gestational trophoblastic neoplasia: diagnosis with Doppler US. *Radiology*, **165**, 445–8.
86. Schneider, D.F., Bukovsky, I., Weinraub, Z. *et al.* (1990) Transvaginal ultrasound diagnosis and treatment follow-up of invasive gestational trophoblastic disease. *Journal of Clinical Ultrasound*, **18**, 110–13.
87. Ansbacher, R., Hopkins, M.P., Roberts, J.A. *et al.* (1990) Localization of trophoblastic disease with vaginal ultrasonography: a report of two cases. *Journal of Reproductive Medicine*, **35**, 835–8.
88. Mangili, G., Spagnolo, D., Valsecchi, L. *et al.* (1993) Transvaginal ultrasonography in persistent trophoblastic tumor. *American Journal of Obstetrics and Gynecology*, **169**, 1218–23.
89. Desai, R.K. and Desberg, A.L. (1991) Diagnosis of gestational trophoblastic disease: value of endovaginal color flow Doppler sonography. *American Journal of Roentgenology*, **157**, 787–8.
90. Liaw, Y.S., Yang, P.C., Yuan, A. *et al.* (1993) Ultrasonography and color Doppler imaging of metastatic pulmonary choriocarcinoma. *Chest*, **104**, 1600–1.
91. Mutch, D.G., Soper, J.T., Baker, M.E. *et al.* (1986) Role of computed axial tomography of the chest in staging patients with non-

metastatic gestational trophoblastic disease. *Obstetrics and Gynecology*, **68**, 348–52.

92. Powell, M.C., Buckley, J., Worthington, B.S. *et al.* (1986) Magnetic resonance imaging and hydatidiform mole. *British Journal of Radiology*, **59**, 561–4.
93. Hricak, H., Demas, B.E., Braga, C.A. *et al.* (1986) Gestational trophoblastic neoplasm of the uterus: MR assessment. *Radiology*, **161**, 11–16.
94. Kohorn, E.I. (1993) Evaluation of the criteria used to make the diagnosis of nonmetastatic gestational trophoblastic neoplasia. *Gynecologic Oncology*, **48**, 139–47.
95. Messerli, M.L., Parmley, T., Woodruff, J.D. *et al.* (1987) Inter- and intra-pathologist variability in the diagnosis of gestational trophoblastic neoplasia. *Obstetrics and Gynecology*, **69**, 622–6.
96. Driscoll, S.G. (1987) Problems and pitfalls in the histopathologic diagnosis of gestational trophoblastic lesions. *Journal of Reproductive Medicine*, **32**, 623–8.
97. Howat, A.J., Beck, S., Fox, H. *et al.* (1993) Can histopathologists reliably diagnose molar pregnancy? *Journal of Clinical Pathology*, **46**, 599–602.
98. Bocklage, T.J., Smith, H.O. and Bartow, S.A. (1994) Distinctive flow histogram pattern in molar pregnancies with elevated maternal serum human chorionic gonadotropin levels. *Cancer*, **73**, 2782–90.
99. Fukuyama, R., Takata, M., Kudoh, J. *et al.* (1991) DNA diagnosis of hydatidiform mole using the polymerase chain reaction. *Human Genetics*, **87**, 216–18.
100. Fisher, R.A. and Newlands, E.S. (1993) Rapid diagnosis and classification of hydatidiform moles with polymerase chain reaction. *American Journal of Obstetrics and Gynecology*, **168**, 563–9.
101. Fisher, R.A., Newlands, E.S., Jeffreys, A.J. *et al.* (1992) Gestational and nongestational trophoblastic tumors distinguished by DNA analysis. *Cancer*, **69**, 839–45.
102. Surti, U. (1987) Genetic concepts and techniques, in *Gestational Trophoblastic Disease* (eds A.E. Szulman and H.J. Buchsbaum), Springer-Verlag, New York, pp. 111–21.
103. Twiggs, L.B. and Phillips, G.L. (1986) Documentation of subclinical trophoblastic embolization with invasive cardiac monitoring in a woman with a molar pregnancy: a case report. *Journal of Reproductive Medicine*, **31**, 277–9.
104. Bhuvaneswaran, J.S., Venkitachalam, C.G. and Sandhyamani, S. (1993) Pulmonary wedge aspiration cytology in the diagnosis of recurrent tumour embolism causing pulmonary arterial hypertension. *International Journal of Cardiology*, **39**, 209–12.
105. Abati, A., Landucci, D., Danner, R.L. *et al.* (1994) Diagnosis of pulmonary microvascular metastases by cytologic evaluation of pulmonary artery catheter-derived blood specimens. *Human Pathology*, **25**, 257–62.
106. Kim, S.J. (1982) Difficult cases of trophoblastic disease and its classification and management. *Seminars in Oncology*, **9**, 234–8.
107. Erb, R.E. and Gibler, W.B. (1989) Massive hemoperitoneum following rupture of hepatic metastases from unsuspected choriocarcinoma. *American Journal of Emergency Medicine*, **7**, 196–8.
108. Giannakopoulos, G., Nair, S., Snider, C. *et al.* (1992) Implications for the pathogenesis of aneurysm formation: metastatic choriocarcinoma with spontaneous splenic rupture. Case report and a review. *Surgical Neurology*, **38**, 236–40.
109. Alveyn, C.G. and Loehry, C.A. (1988) Hepatic metastases due to choriocarcinoma. *Postgraduate Medical Journal*, **64**, 941–2.
110. Muto, M.G., Lage, J.M., Berkowitz, R.S. *et al.* (1991) Gestational trophoblastic disease of the fallopian tube. *Journal of Reproductive Medicine*, **36**, 57–60.
111. Villet, W.T., Du Toit, D.F. and Conroy, C. (1979) Unusual presentation of choriocarcinoma: a case report. *South African Medical Journal*, **55**, 96–8.
112. Trillo, A.A., Accettullo, L.M. and Yeiter, T.L. (1979) Choriocarcinoma of the esophagus: histologic and cytologic findings. A case report. *Acta Cytologica*, **23**, 69–74.
113. Suski, E., Pavlides, C. and Matsumoto, T. (1979) Massive lower gastrointestinal bleeding: unusual presentation of metastatic choriocarcinoma. *International Surgery*, **64**, 53–5.
114. Deligdisch, L. and Waxman, J. (1984) Metastatic gestational trophoblastic neoplasm. A

study of two cases in unusual clinical settings and review of the literature. *Gynecologic Oncology*, **19**, 323–8.

115. Gurwitt, L.J., Long, J.M. and Clark, R.E. (1975) Cerebral metastatic choriocarcinoma: a postpartum cause of 'stroke'. *Obstetrics and Gynecology*, **45**, 583–8.
116. Pihl, K., Malmstrom, H. and Simonsen, E. (1990) Choriocarcinoma presenting with cerebral metastases after full-term pregnancy. *Acta Obstetricia et Gynecologica Scandinavica*, **69**, 433–5.
117. Pullar, M., Blumbergs, P.C., Phillips, G.E. *et al.* (1985) Neoplastic cerebral aneurysm from metastatic gestational choriocarcinoma: case report. *Journal of Neurosurgery*, **63**, 644–7.
118. Dagi, T.F. and Maccabe, J.J. (1980) Metastatic trophoblastic disease presenting as a subarachnoid hemorrhage: report of two cases and review of the literature. *Surgical Neurology*, **14**, 175–84.
119. Ilancheran, A., Ratnam, S.S. and Baratham, G. (1988) Metastatic cerebral choriocarcinoma with primary neurological presentation. *Gynecologic Oncology*, **29**, 361–4.
120. Noterman, J., Verhest, A., Baleriaux, D. *et al.* (1989) A ruptured cerebral aneurysm from choriocarcinomatous origin: a case report and a review. *Neurosurgical Review*, **12**, 71–4.
121. McLeod, D.T. (1988) Gestational choriocarcinoma presenting as endobronchial carcinoma. *Thorax*, **43**, 410–11.
122. Newman, L.B., Morgan, T.E., Bucy, J.G. *et al.* (1975) Choriocarcinoma and bilateral renal metastases. *Urology*, **5**, 658–61.
123. Soper, J.T., Mutch, D.G., Chin, N. *et al.* (1988) Renal metastases of gestational trophoblastic disease: a report of eight cases. *Obstetrics and Gynecology*, **72**, 796–8.
124. Nkanza, N.K. and King, C.S. (1989) Choriocarcinoma presenting as an intussusception: a case report. *Central Afrian Journal of Medicine*, **35**, 389–92.
125. Kristoffersson, A., Emdin, S. and Jarhult, J. (1985) Acute intestinal obstruction and splenic hemorrhage due to metastatic choriocarcinoma. A case report. *Acta Chirurgica Scandinavica*, **151**, 381–4.
126. Bandy, L.C., Clarke-Pearson, D.L. and Hammond, C.B. (1985) Pseudoobstruction of the colon complicating choriocarcinoma. *Gynecologic Oncology*, **20**, 402–7.
127. Devasia, A., Nath, V., Abraham, B. *et al.* (1994) Hematuria, renal mass and amenorrhea: indicators of a rare diagnosis. *Journal of Urology*, **151**, 409–10.
128. Mack, R.B., Katz, S.M. and Amenta, P.S. (1992) Choriocarcinoma of the kidney. *Journal of the American Osteopathic Association*, **92**, 799–802.
129. Jacobson, R.J., Morley, J.E., Shires, R. *et al.* (1976) Choriocarcinoma presenting as Jacksonian epilepsy. *South African Medical Journal*, **50**, 131–4.
130. Gangadharan, V.P., Chitrathara, K., Sivaramakrishnan, R. *et al.* (1993) Pulmonary hypertension: a rare presentation of choriocarcinoma. *Acta Oncologica*, **32**, 461–2.
131. Yutani, C., Imakita, M., Ishibashi-Ueda, H. *et al.* (1993) Pulmonary hypertension due to tumor emboli: a report of three autopsy cases with morphological correlations to radiological findings. *Acta Pathologica Japonica*, **43**, 135–41.
132. Vasiljevic, J.D. and Abdulla, A.K. (1990) Coronary embolism by metastatic choriocarcinoma of the uterus: an unusual cause of ischemic heart disease. *Gynecologic Oncology*, **38**, 289–92.
133. Kishore, A.G., Desai, N. and Nayak, G. (1992) Choriocarcinoma presenting as intracavitary tumor in the left atrium. *International Journal of Cardiology*, **35**, 405–7.
134. Slazinski, L. and Degefu, S. (1982) Herpes gestationis associated with choriocarcinoma. *Archives of Dermatology*, **118**, 425–8.
135. Krige, L.P. and di Bisceglie, A. (1984) Pitfalls in the diagnosis of gestational choriocarcinoma: a case report. *South African Medical Journal*, **65**, 26–7.
136. O'Reilly, S., Lyons, D.J., Harrison, M. *et al.* (1993) Thyrotoxicosis induced by choriocarcinoma: a report of two cases. *Irish Medical Journal*, **86**, 124–7.
137. Holt, P. and Nicholas, R. (1981) Recurrent bacteraemia: an unusual presentation of choriocarcinoma. *British Medical Journal (Clinical Research)*, **282**, 1835–6.
138. Kumar, P.V., Esfahani, F.N. and Salimi, A. (1991) Choriocarcinoma metastatic to the breast diagnosed by fine needle aspiration.

Acta Cytologica, **35**, 239–42.

139. Avril, M.F., Mathieu, A., Kalifa, C. *et al.* (1986) Infantile choriocarcinoma with cutaneous tumors: an additional case and review of the literature. *Journal of the American Academy of Dermatology*, **14**, 918–27.
140. Belchis, D.A., Mowry, J. and Davis, J.H. (1993) Infantile choriocarcinoma: re-examination of a potentially curable entity. *Cancer*, **72**, 2028–42.
141. Steller, M.A., Genest, D.R., Bernstein, M.R. *et al.* (1994) Natural history of twin pregnancy with complete hydatidiform mole and coexisting fetus. *Obstrectics and Gynecology*, **83**, 35–42.
142. Steller, M.A., Genest, D.R., Bernstein, M.R. *et al.* (1994) Clinical features of multiple conception with partial or complete molar pregnancy and coexisting fetuses. *Journal of Reproductive Medicine*, **39**, 147–54.
143. Khoo, S.K., Monks, P.L. and Davies, N.T. (1986) Hydatidiform mole coexisting with a live fetus: a dilemma of management. A recent review (1965–1986) and report of 2 new cases. *Australian and New Zealand Journal of Obstetrics and Gynaecology*, **26**, 129–35.
144. Kuhn, R.J., Long, A.R. and Fortune, D.W. (1980) Choriocarcinoma coexistent with intrauterine pregnancy. *Australian and New Zealand Journal of Obstetrics and Gynaecology*, **20**, 94 8.
145. Jones, W.B. and Lauersen, N.H. (1975) Hydatidiform mole with coexistent fetus. *American Journal of Obstetrics and Gynecology*, **122**, 267–72.
146. Hallam, L.A., McLaren, K.M., el-Jabbour, J.N. *et al.* (1990) Intraplacental choriocarcinoma: a case report. *Placenta*, **11**, 247–51.
147. Surwit, E.A. and Hammond, C.B. (1980) Treatment of metastatic trophoblastic disease with poor prognosis. *Obstetrics and Gynecology*, **55**, 565–70.
148. Lage, J.M. and Roberts, D.J. (1993) Choriocarcinoma in a term placenta: pathologic diagnosis of tumor in an asymptomatic patient with metatastatic disease. *International Journal of Gynecological Pathology*, **12**, 80–5.
149. McLellan, R., Buscema, J., Currie, J.L. *et al.* (1991) Placental site trophoblastic tumor in a postmenopausal woman. *American Journal of Clinical Pathology*, **95**, 670–5.
150. Board, J.A. and Hammond, C.B. (1980) Factitious trophoblastic disease: Munchausen's mole. *Southern Medical Journal*, **73**, 831–2.
151. Van Nostrand, K.M., Lucci, J.A., 3rd, Liao, S.Y. *et al.* (1994) Primary lung choriocarcinoma masquerading as a metastatic gestational neoplasm. *Gynecologic Oncology*, **53**, 361–5.
152. Wenzel, L., Berkowitz, R.S., Robinson, S. *et al.* (1992) The psychological, social, and sexual consequences of gestational trophoblastic disease. *Gynecologic Oncology*, **46**, 74–81.
153. Goldstein, D.P., Berkowitz, R.S. and Bernstein, M.R. (1984) Reproductive performance after molar pregnancy and gestational trophoblastic tumors. *Clinical Obstetrics and Gynecology*, **27**, 221–7.
154. Berkowitz, R.S., Goldstein, D.P., Bernstein, M.R. *et al.* (1987) Subsequent pregnancy outcome in patients with molar pregnancy and gestational trophoblastic tumors. *Journal of Reproductive Medicine*, **32**, 680–4.
155. Curry, S.L., Schlaerth, J.B., Kohorn, E.I. *et al.* (1989) Hormonal contraception and trophoblastic sequelae after hydatidiform mole (a Gynecologic Oncology Group Study). *American Journal of Obstetrics and Gynecology*, **160**, 805–9.
156. Surwit, E.A. and Hammond, C.B. (1981) Recurrent gestational trophoblastic disease. *Gynecologic Oncology*, **12**, 177–85.

PRESENTATION AND MANAGEMENT OF MOLAR PREGNANCY 8

Ross S. Berkowitz and Donald P. Goldstein

Our understanding of the cytogenetics, epidemiology, pathology and clinical management of hydatidiform mole has advanced considerably over the past 40 years. It is now well recognized that molar pregnancy comprises two distinct entities, complete and partial, which differ on the basis of chromosomal pattern, gross and microscopic histopathology and clinical presentation. Other chapters in this text by Drs Fisher, Kim and Paradinas review the current status of the cytogenetics, epidemiology and pathology of molar disease. In this chapter, our focus will be on the presentation, diagnosis and principles of management of patients with complete and partial hydatidiform mole.

8.1 PRESENTATION OF COMPLETE MOLAR PREGNANCY AND MANAGEMENT OF COMPLICATIONS

The following description of the clinical presentation of complete mole is partially based upon our experience with 308 patients between 1965 and 1975 at the New England Trophoblastic Disease Center (NETDC)[1]. The experience from our center is consistent with the published observations of other investigators. However, partial mole was initially distinguished from complete mole by Vassilakos *et al.* in 1977 and Szulman and Surti in 1978 on the basis of karyotype and histopathology[2–4]. It is therefore important to note that all studies concerning molar pregnancy which include patients before 1980 may have included some patients with partial mole. However, the vast majority of patients with molar pregnancy in studies before 1980 most likely involved cases of classic complete hydatidiform mole, since most cases of partial mole were interpreted as being non-molar abortions.

8.1.1 VAGINAL BLEEDING

Vaginal bleeding is the most common presenting symptom in patients with complete mole, occurring in 97% of our cases. Curry *et al.* and Kohorn also noted a high incidence of vaginal bleeding in 312 (89%) of 347 and in 188 (94%) of 200 patients with molar pregnancy, respectively.[5,6]. Molar chorionic villi may disrupt maternal vessels by separating from the decidua and the endometrial cavity may be distended by large volumes of retained blood. Retained blood may undergo oxidation and 'prune juice-like' fluid may leak from the uterine cavity. Because bleeding may be prolonged, considerable and occult, 54% of our patients

Gestational Trophoblastic Disease.
Edited by B.W. Hancock, E.S. Newlands and R.S. Berkowitz.
ISBN 0 412 63100 8

were anemic at presentation (hemoglobin <10 g/100 ml).

8.1.2 EXCESSIVE UTERINE ENLARGEMENT

The uterine size was palpably larger than gestational age in 51% of our patients with complete mole. Uterine size was larger than dates by four weeks in 46% and 38% of patients with complete mole in the studies by Curry *et al.* and Kohorn[5,6]. The endometrial cavity expands because of both retained blood and chorionic tissue. Excessive uterine size is usually associated with markedly elevated levels of human chorionic gonadotropin (hCG) from trophoblastic overgrowth.

8.1.3 THECA LUTEIN OVARIAN CYSTS

The reported frequency of theca lutein ovarian cysts varies depending upon whether the diagnosis is established by clinical or ultrasound examination. Montz *et al.* reported that theca lutein cysts were clinically palpable in 102 (26.4%) of 386 patients with molar pregnancy[7]. Kohorn also observed theca lutein cysts in 20% of patients with molar pregnancy[6]. However, Santos-Ramos *et al.*, using ultrasound observed theca lutein ovarian cysts >5 cm in diameter in 23 (46%) of 50 patients with molar pregnancy[8].

Theca lutein ovarian cysts are usually bilateral and multicystic, containing amber-colored or serosanguineous fluid. Though usually in the 6–12 cm range, they may reach substantial proportions of larger than 20 cm in size. While theca lutein cysts are generally noted at the time of presentation, they may enlarge substantially after uterine evacuation.

Theca lutein cysts result from hyperstimulation of the ovaries by high circulating blood levels of hCG and are detected almost exclusively in patients with very high serum hCG values.[9,10]. Infrequently these patients may develop other signs of ovarian hyperstimulation such as ascites or pleural effusions. When this occurs, fluid and electrolyte disturbances may require management.

Montz *et al.* reviewed the clinical records of 102 patients with molar pregnancy and theca lutein ovarian cysts to define their natural history[7]. The mean regression time for these cysts was eight weeks. Only two patients experienced an acute surgical complication involving ovarian torsion or rupture. Similarly, Kohorn reported that three (2.3%) of 127 patients with molar pregnancy developed torsion of ovarian theca lutein cysts[11]. If patients have severe symptoms of respiratory compromise, pelvic pressure or pain, theca lutein cysts may be decompressed by either ultrasound-directed percutaneous or laparoscopic aspiration. Laparoscopy may also be utilized to successfully manage cases of incomplete ovarian torsion or rupture[12].

8.1.4 TOXEMIA

Pre-eclampsia including hypertension, edema and/or proteinuria was observed in 27% of our patients with complete mole. Curry *et al.* reported pre-eclampsia in 12% of patients with molar disease in the Duke series[5]. Eclamptic convulsions occur rarely. In our experience toxemia was limited almost exclusively to patients with markedly elevated hCG values and excessive uterine enlargement. Curry *et al.* also noted that 81% of their patients with toxemia had excessive uterine size.

8.1.5 HYPEREMESIS GRAVIDARUM

Hyperemesis requiring antiemetic therapy developed in 26% and 20% of patients with molar pregnancy treated at our Center and at the Yale Center[11,13]. Five (2%) of our patients required hospitalization for correction of marked electrolyte disturbances. Hyperemesis also appears to be associated with high hCG levels and excessive uterine size. Depue *et al.* have proposed that hyperemesis results from elevated serum estrogen levels[14].

8.1.6 HYPERTHYROIDISM

Clinically evident hyperthyroidism was detected in 7% of our patients with complete mole. However, laboratory evidence for hyperthyroidism is more common. Galton *et al.* measured thyroid function tests in 11 patients with molar pregnancy before and after evacuation[15]. Pre-evacuation, all patients had elevated values for thyroidal ^{131}I uptake and serum free thyroxine; the thyroid function tests rapidly returned to normal after evacuation even before the hCG level became undetectable.

Hyperthyroidism occurs almost exclusively in patients with very high hCG levels. Some authors have suggested that hCG is the thyroid stimulator in patients with molar pregnancy[16]. Kenimer *et al;*. reported that highly purified hCG appeared to have intrinsic thyroid-stimulating activity[17]. Positive correlations have been reported in some studies between serum hCG levels and serum total thyroxine (T_4) or triiodothyronine (T_3) concentrations. However, Nagataki *et al.* found no correlation between serum hCG and free T_4 in 10 patients with molar pregnancy[18]. Similarly Amir *et al.* measured thyroid function tests in 47 patients with complete mole and observed no significant correlation between serum hCG levels and free T_4 or T_3 index values[19]. The identity of the thyrotropic factor in molar pregnancy is therefore still controversial.

Patients with untreated or poorly controlled hyperthyroidism may develop thyroid storm at the time of anesthesia induction and evacuation. Thyroid storm is characterized by hyperthermia, delirium, coma, atrial fibrillation and cardiovascular collapse. While blood samples should be drawn for laboratory confirmation, the diagnosis of thyroid storm must be made clinically so that treatment can be promptly instituted. The administration of β-adrenergic blocking agents prevents or rapidly reverses many of the cardiovascular and metabolic complications of thyroid storm. A pulmonary artery catheter may also be helpful to monitor cardiovascular status and guide fluid replacement.

8.1.7 RESPIRATORY INSUFFICIENCY

Two per cent of our patients with complete mole developed respiratory insufficiency. Pulmonary compromise is usually observed in patients with high hCG levels, excessive uterine size and very large theca lutein cysts. Twiggs *et al.* reported that 12 (27%) of 44 patients with a molar pregnancy of at least 16 weeks size developed pulmonary complications[20].

Patients may present with tachycardia, tachypnea and anxiety or confusion in the recovery room after molar evacuation. Arterial blood gases may show evidence of hypoxia and respiratory alkalosis. Auscultation of the chest usually reveals diffuse rales and chest roentgenogram may show bilateral pulmonary infiltrates. The signs and symptoms of respiratory distress usually resolve within 72 h with appropriate cardiovascular and respiratory support. However, it is important to recognize that some patients may require temporary mechanical ventilation to provide adequate oxygenation. While embolization of molar tissue to the pulmonary vasculature may contribute to respiratory distress, it may also result from the cardiovascular complications of toxemia, thyroid storm and massive fluid replacement.

In recent years, patients with complete mole are being more frequently managed at our Center before they develop the classic signs and symptoms. Recent changes in the clinical presentation of complete mole may be due to changing clinical practice such as the frequent use of hCG measurement and vaginal probe ultrasound in early pregnancy in women with vaginal staining and even in asymptomatic women.

Dr Valena Soto-Wright, a Fellow in Gynecologic Oncology at our Center, has reviewed the presentation of 74 patients with complete mole who underwent uterine evacuation at the NETDC between 1988 and 1993. Vaginal bleeding continued to be the most common presenting symptom, occurring in 62 (84%) patients. However, excessive uterine size (size > gestational age) , anemia (hemoglobin <10 g/dl) and toxemia were noted in only 21 (28%), four (5%) and one (1.3%) patient, respectively. Additionally, hyperemesis was observed in only six (8%) patients and no patient had clinical hyperthyroidism or respiratory insufficiency. Patients with complete mole in the recent series were diagnosed earlier in gestation. The mean gestation age at diagnosis in the earlier (1965–1975) and current series was 16.5 and 11.8 weeks, respectively. It is important to emphasize that the incidence of post-molar gestational trophoblastic tumor did not change in the recent series; 15 of 64 (23%) patients with complete mole, who did not receive chemoprophylaxis, developed post-molar persistent tumor. Among the entire group of 74 patients, 19 (25.7%) patients developed post-molar persistent tumor.

8.2 PRESENTATION OF PARTIAL MOLAR PREGNANCY

Patients with partial mole usually do not present with the classical features of complete mole. We reviewed the medical records of 81 consecutive patients with partial mole to delineate its clinical presentation and natural history[21]. Excessive uterine size was noted in only three (4%) patients and hyperemesis, hyperthyroidism, prominent theca lutein ovarian cysts and respiratory insufficiency were not encountered. Toxemia was observed in only one patient. The clinical diagnosis preoperatively was incomplete or missed abortion in 74 (91%) patients and molar pregnancy in only five (6%).

Other investigators have noted similar findings. Szulman and Surti and Czernobilsky *et al.* reported excessive uterine enlargement in nine (11%) of 81 patients and in two (8%) of 25 patients with partial mole[22,23]. Toxemia was reported in both studies in only 4% of patients. Other medical complications of complete mole such as hyperthyroidism and theca lutein cysts are uncommon with partial mole. Szulman and Surti also observed that the clinical diagnosis prior to evacuation was incomplete or missed abortion in 92% of their patients. Characteristically, the diagnosis of partial mole is made after histological review of curettage specimens from presumed incomplete or missed abortions.

8.3 DIAGNOSIS

8.3.1 ULTRASOUND

Ultrasonography has proved to be an accurate and sensitive technique for the diagnosis of complete mole. Complete mole produces a characteristic vesicular pattern due to generalized swelling of the chorionic villi (Figure 8.1) However, in the first trimester, ultrasound may be unable to identify small molar villi or distinguish an early mole from degenerating chorionic villi[24]. The specificity of the sonographic findings in complete molar pregnancy may be increased by correlation with the hCG level[25]. A complete mole may be better differentiated from a missed abortion by considering the hCG value at the time of the ultrasound.

Ultrasonography may also contribute to the detection of partial hydatidiform mole. Naumoff *et al.* reviewed the ultrasound findings in 19 patients with partial mole who underwent ultrasound examination prior to

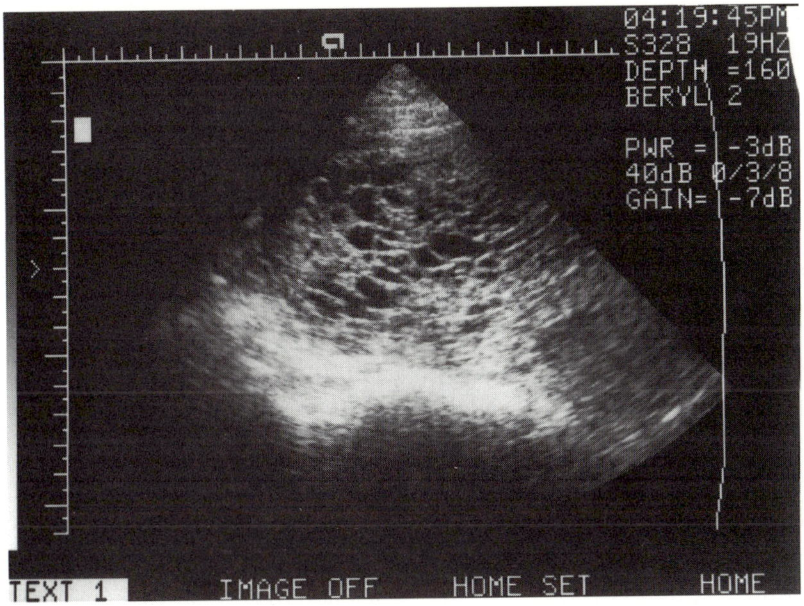

Figure 8.1 Ultrasound of a complete molar pregnany showing diffuse vesicular change in the chorionic tissue.

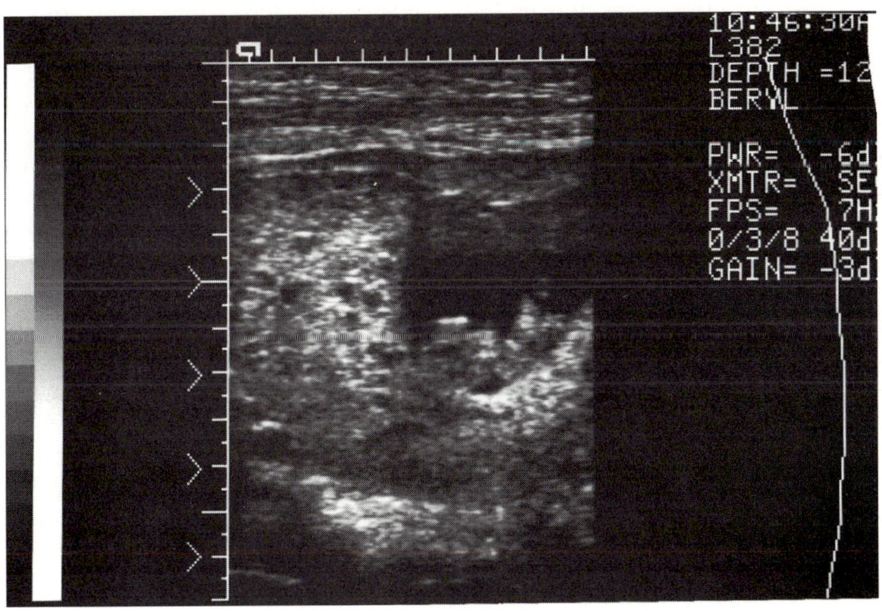

Figure 8.2 Ultrasound of a partial molar pregnancy showing a fetus and focal cystic spaces in the placenta.

curettage[26]. The following ultrasound findings were observed in these cases: excessively enlarged placenta, cystic spaces within the placenta, gestational sac which was either empty or contained amorphous echoes and growth-retarded fetus. Fine *et al.* studied ultrasound in patients with partial mole to determine if sonographic criteria could be established to detect partial mole before evacuation[27]. Ultrasound from 22 partial moles and 33 first-trimester missed abortions were reviewed independently by three radiologists who were unaware of the pathological diagnoses. Each radiologist evaluated the appearance of the placenta, the shape, dimensions and contents of the gestational sac and the presence or absence of ovarian cysts. Two sonographic findings were significantly associated with the diagnosis of partial hydatidiform mole: cystic spaces in the placenta and ratio of transverse to anteroposterior dimension of the gestational sac >1.5 (Figure 8.2). These changes in the shape of the gestational sac may be part of the embryopathy of triploidy. There was high inter-observer correlation for both criteria. When both criteria were present, the positive predictive value for partial mole was 87%. When both criteria were absent, the positive predictive value for missed abortion was 90%.

8.3.2 hCG MEASUREMENT

Markedly elevated hCG levels are commonly seen in patients with complete molar pregnancy. Genest *et al.* reviewed the clinical and pathological characteristics of 153 cases of complete mole managed at the NETDC between 1980 and 1990[28]. Pre-evacuation hCG levels were greater than 100 000 U/l in 46% of the patients. Similarly, Menczer *et al.* reported that 30 (41%) of 74 patients with molar pregnancy had pre-evacuation hCG values greater than 100 000 U/l[29]. The measurement of a high hCG level (>100 000 Ul) may therefore suggest the diagnosis of a complete molar pregnancy, particularly when associated with vaginal bleeding and uterine enlargement.

In contrast, partial hydatidiform mole is less commonly associated with markedly elevated hCG values. Only two (6%) of 30 patients with partial mole at our center had pre-evacuation hCG levels greater than 100 000 U/l[21]. Czernobilsky *et al.* also reported that only one (6%) of 17 patients with partial mole had a pre-evacuation urinary hCG level greater than 300 000 U/l[23].

Studies using monoclonal antibodies with high sensitivity and specificity for measuring hCG and its free subunits suggest that trophoblastic cells in complete and partial moles differ significantly in the manner in which they secrete the free subunits of hCG[30,31]. Complete moles have higher serum levels of percentage free βhCG than do partial moles (2.4 versus 1.0; $p<0.005$). In contrast, partial moles have higher serum levels of percentage free αhCG than do complete moles (0.85 versus 0.17: $p\leq0.005$). The mean ratios of percentage free βhCG to αhCG in complete and partial mole are 20.9 and 2.4, respectively ($p<0.005$).

8.4 TREATMENT

When a diagnosis of complete or partial molar pregnancy has been made, the patient should be evaluated for the presence of medical complications, including anemia, toxemia, hyperthyroidism and respiratory insufficiency. All patients should have baseline hCG and thyroid tests performed in addition to routine blood work and urinalysis. After the patient has been medically evaluated and stabilized, a decision must be made concerning the most appropriate method of evacuation.

If the patient no longer desires to preserve fertility, hysterectomy may be performed with the mole *in situ*. Prominent ovarian theca lutein cysts can be aspirated at the time of surgery and the ovaries conserved. It is important to inform the patient that while hysterectomy eliminates the complications of local invasion, it does not prevent metastatic disease and therefore gonadotropin follow-up is required.

In patients who wish to retain fertility, suction curettage is the preferred method of evacuation regardless of uterine size[32]. An oxytocin infusion should be started before anesthesia induction to increase myometrial tone and facilitate contraction and thus decrease blood loss. Concern has been expressed that oxytocin may promote metastasis of trophoblastic tissue. However, Flam *et al.* reported that uterine stimulation before evacuation did not increase the risk of persistent tumor[33]. The cervix should be carefully dilated to accommodate a cannula appropriate for the volume of trophoblastic tissue. A 12 mm cannula is generally satisfactory because it allows rapid evacuation and involution of the uterus. During dilatation, brisk bleeding may be encountered due to passage of copious amounts of blood retained in the endometrial cavity. However, it is best to proceed promptly to uterine evacuation. After the initiation of suction evacuation, the uterus generally shrinks rapidly and bleeding is well controlled. If the uterus is larger than 14 weeks size, one hand may be placed on top of the fundus to assess uterine size and to massage the uterus. When suction evacuation is thought to be complete sharp curettage should be performed to remove any residual chorionic tissue. Patients who are Rh negative should receive Rh immune globulin at the time of evacuation because the RhD factor is expressed on trophoblast.

8.4.1 CHEMOPROPHYLAXIS

The use of prophylactic chemotherapy at the time of molar evacuation remains controversial. However, several investigators have reported that chemoprophylaxis reduces the incidence of post-molar tumor. Goldstein reported that chemoprophylaxis reduced the risk of persistent tumor from 20% to 8% and eliminated metastases[34]. Similarly, Kashimura *et al.* noted that chemoprophylaxis in patients with complete mole reduced the frequency of post-mole tumor from 18% to 7%[35]. Fasoli *et al.* also observed that prophylactic chemotherapy reduced the risk for post-molar disease from 9% to 3%[36]. However, one of the main objections of exposing all patients with molar pregnancy to chemoprophylaxis is that only a small minority are at risk for persistence.

Kim *et al.* conducted a prospective, randomized trial of the use of prophylactic chemotherapy in patients with complete mole[37]. Seventy-one patients with complete mole were randomized to be treated with either molar evacuation alone or molar evacuation with prophylactic methotrexate and folinic acid. Patients were categorized as either high or low risk based upon prognostic factors for the development of persistent disease (a thorough discussion of these prognostic factors will be given later in this chapter). Among patients with high-risk complete mole, prophylactic chemotherapy reduced the incidence of post-molar tumor from 47% to 14%. Among patients with low-risk complete mole, prophylactic chemotherapy did not influence the incidence of persistent disease (7.7% versus 5.6%). However, patients who developed persistent tumor after prophylactic methotrexate subsequently required more courses of therapeutic methotrexate to attain remission.

At our Center, 93 patients with high-risk complete mole were treated with prophylactic actinomycin D and only 10 (11%) developed persistent disease[38]. All 10 patients had non-metastatic tumor. Six patients were treated with methotrexate for persistent tumor and five required only one course of methotrexate to attain remission. In order to avoid drug resistance, it may be important to use a different chemotherapeutic agent for therapy following failed chemoprophylaxis. The risk for chemoprophylaxis failure was increased in patients with particularly high pre-evacuation hCG levels.

Chemoprophylaxis may be particularly useful in patients with high-risk complete mole when hormonal follow-up is either unavailable or unreliable. Molar pregnancy is more prevalent in certain global regions such as Asia and Africa where medical follow-up may be less available[39].

8.4.2 FOLLOW-UP

Patients with both complete and partial molar pregnancy should be monitored with serial hCG values after evacuation to assure that they achieve complete sustained remission. Patients are followed with weekly hCG levels until non-detectable for three weeks and then monthly hCG levels until non-detectable for six months. Patients with partial mole are at a lower risk of developing post-molar tumor. Therefore, in patients with partial mole who rapidly attain non-detectable weekly hCG values (less than seven weeks post-evacuation), monthly hCG follow-up may be discontinued after three months.

Patients with molar pregnancy must be encouraged to use reliable contraception during the entire interval of hCG monitoring. An intrauterine device should be avoided before gonadotropin remission because of the risk of uterine perforation with invasive tumor. Therefore, patients are confronted with the choice of barrier methods or steroidal contraception when they desire to preserve fertility.

Stone and Bagshawe reported in 1979 that the use of oral contraceptives prior to gonadotropin remission increased the frequency of post-molar tumor two- to three-fold[40]. However, data from our center, the Gynecologic Oncology Group, and the University of Southern California all indicate that oral contraceptives do not increase the risk for post-molar persistent tumor[41–43]. Importantly, the Gynecologic Oncology Group study was a randomized prospective trial. Interestingly, Ho Yuen and Burch also reported that the use of oral contraceptives containing 50 μg or less of estrogen was not associated with an increased risk of post-molar persistent tumor[44]. However, they observed that oral contraceptives containing more than 50 μg of estrogen may be associated with an increased risk of post-molar disease. Ho Yuen and Burch speculated that the conflicting data concerning the use of oral contraceptives and the risk of developing post-molar tumor may be explained by differences in the dosage of estrogen. Deicas *et al.* reviewed the experience from the John I. Brewer Trophoblastic Disease Center and concluded that the use of oral contraceptives significantly reduced the incidence of post-molar tumor[45]. Additionally, the dose of estrogen used was not significantly associated with a risk of developing gestational trophoblastic tumor. Therefore, we believe that following molar evacuation patients may be safely prescribed oral contraceptives during the entire interval of hormonal follow-up. Current formulations of oral contraceptives generally contain 50 μg or less of estrogen in the form of ethinyl estradiol or mestranol.

8.5 PERSISTENT GESTATIONAL TROPHOBLASTIC TUMOR AFTER COMPLETE MOLAR PREGNANCY

Complete molar pregnancy is well recognized to have a risk of developing persistent gestational trophoblastic tumor. However, the incidence of persistent tumor after complete mole has been reported from 8% to 29%[1,5,13,46–48]. This marked variation in the reported incidence of post-molar tumor results from differences in diagnostic criteria.

On the basis of the follow-up of more than 7000 patients, Bagshawe reported that

Table 8.1 Postmolar gestational trophoblastic tumor (GTT) in the USA

Authors	*No. of patients*	*Non-metastatic GTT (%)*	*Metastatic GTT (%)*	*Total GTT (%)*
Goldstein and Berkowitz [1]	858	14.7	4.0	18.7
Lurain *et al.* [47]	738	16.3	3.0	19.3
Curry *et al.* [5]	347	16.6	3.5	20.1
Morrow *et al.* [48]	121	23.1	3.3	26.4
Kohorn [11]	127	26.0	3.1	29.1

only 7.9% of patients with molar pregnancy required chemotherapy at the Charing Cross Hospital[46]. The criteria for diagnosing post-molar tumor were as follows: hCG>20 000 U/l more than four weeks after evacuation, progressively rising hCG values with a minimum of three rising values over two to three weeks, metastasis to the brain, liver, kidney, gastrointestinal tract or lungs larger than 2 cm in diameter or three or more in number or persistent hCG level four to six months after evacuation. Using similar criteria, Fasoli *et al.* from Italy and Franke *et al.* from Holland reported that 9% and 10% of patients respectively developed post-molar tumor[36,49]. Importantly, the data from England, Italy and Holland represent the experience when patients with molar disease are followed with an organized and systematic regional or national registry and health care system.

In the USA the incidence of post-molar tumor is reported from 18% to 29% (Table 8.1). Most centers in the USA define persistent post-molar disease by the presence of a re-elevation or persistent plateau in hCG for at least three consecutive weeks. However, it is important to acknowledge that even amongst American centers there is some variation in the definition of persistence[50]. The criteria for diagnosing persistent tumor after mole in the USA are therefore considerably less stringent than the criteria followed in England or elsewhere in Europe. Clearly, some patients who receive chemotherapy for post-molar tumor in the USA would have achieved remission if gonadotropin follow-up continued in the absence of therapy. The use of less stringent diagnostic criteria for post-molar tumor in the USA is partly motivated by the concern that some patients may be lost to follow-up. Schlaerth *et al.* reported that 19 (19%) of 99 patients with molar pregnancy were lost to follow-up at the University of Southern California[51]. Similarly, Kim *et al.* noted that 36 (27%) of 133 patients with complete mole were lost to follow-up in Korea[37].

Several studies have shown that the risk for developing post-molar tumor is increased in patients with signs and symptoms of marked trophoblastic proliferation: excessive uterine enlargement, markedly elevated hCG values and prominent ovarian theca lutein cysts as well as associated medical factors such as toxemia, hyperthyroidism and respiratory insufficiency. Curry *et al.* reported that post-molar disease developed in 49% of patients with prominent theca lutein ovarian cysts and in 57% of patients with ovarian cysts and large-for-dates uteri[5]. These findings were confirmed and extended by other investigators. Morrow also observed the occurrence of post-molar tumor in 55% of patients with theca lutein ovarian cysts or uterine size greater than 20 weeks[52].

At the NETDC, we reviewed the outcome of 858 patients with complete mole to assess prognostic factors for persistent tumor. Signs of marked trophoblastic growth such as excessive uterine size, theca lutein cysts >6 cm in diameter and pre-evacuation hCG level >100 000 U/l were present in 352 (41%) patients. Non-metastatic and metastatic gestational trophoblastic tumor developed in 31% and 8.8% respectively of these patients. In contrast, 506 (59%) patients with complete mole did not present with signs and symptoms of marked trophoblastic proliferation. Non-metastatic and metastatic disease developed in only 3.4% and 0.6% respectively of these patients. Patients with complete mole who present with excessive uterine size, ovarian cysts and/or markedly elevated hCG values are therefore considered as high risk for developing post-molar tumor. Similarly, Kim *et al.* observed post-molar persistent disease in 47.4% of high-risk and only 7.7% of low-risk complete moles using the same clinical risk criteria[37].

The risk for post-molar tumor has also been observed to be increased in patients of older age. Tow[53] and Xia *et al.*[54] reported that 37% and 33% respectively of women over 40 with molar pregnancy developed persistent tumor. Tsukamoto *et al.* also observed that 56% of women over 50 developed post-molar tumor[55]. Complete moles in older women are more commonly aneuploid, and aneuploidy may be a risk factor for persistent tumor[56]. Martin *et al.* reported that 10 (77%) of 13 aneuploid complete moles developed persistent tumor[57].

Patients with repetitive molar pregnancy are also at increased risk of developing persistent tumor in their later episodes of molar pregnancy. Parazzini *et al.* reported a three-fold increased risk of post-molar tumor in patients with repetitive molar pregnancy[58]. Between June 1965 and July 1993, we treated 24 patients with repeat molar gestations at our Center[59]. Each patient had at least two documented molar pregnancies and each molar gestation was diagnosed as either partial or complete on the basis of established histopathological criteria. Persistent tumor developed following the first mole in two (13.3%) of 15 complete moles. However, post-molar tumor occurred following the second mole in seven (50%) of 14 complete moles.

Conflicting data exist concerning the potential prognostic significance of the histopathological features of complete molar pregnancy. While some authors have indicated that histological features significantly predict the risk of persistent tumor, other investigators have suggested that histological grading has no prognostic value[60–63]. Genest *et al.* reviewed the histopathological characteristics and clinical outcome of 153 complete moles who were managed at our Center between 1980 and 1990[28]. No patient received prophylactic chemotherapy and all histological material was reviewed independently by two pathologists. The histological grade of the complete mole did not correlate significantly with any index of clinical outcome evaluated.

Khazaeli *et al.* reported that a high free βhCG value was predictive of an increased risk of post-molar tumor but the study did not distinguish between complete and partial moles[64]. However, we observed that the measurement of free βhCG did not identify our patients with complete mole who were particularly at risk of developing persistent tumor[31]. The mean percentage free βhCG and βhCG level did not differ significantly between patients with complete mole who attained spontaneous remission and those who developed post-molar tumor.

Wake *et al.* noted that the risk of persistent tumor was increased in complete moles with a heterozygous genotype[65]. Post-molar disease was observed in heterozygous and homozygous complete moles in 50% and 4% of cases, respectively. However, other investigators have not confirmed that heterozygous complete moles are associated with an increased risk of persistent tumor[66, 67].

8.6 PERSISTENT GESTATIONAL TROPHOBLASTIC TUMOR AFTER PARTIAL MOLAR PREGNANCY

Between January 1979 and January 1989, 16 (6.6%) of 240 patients who were followed for partial mole at our Center developed persistent tumor[68]. Our experience with partial mole is consistent with other published data. Table 8.2 summarizes the data from eight studies: 40 (2.2%) of 1823 patients with partial mole developed persistent tumor[2,22,23,69–74].

All of our patients with persistent tumor following partial mole had non-metastatic disease. Similarly, in the collected series in Table 8.2, only five (13%) patients had metastases. While Goto *et al.* reported three patients with pulmonary metastases, all three patients had barely detectable metastases on computed tomography[74].

Our patients with partial mole who developed persistent disease did not have pathological or clinical features that distinguished them from other patients with partial mole[68]. Fifteen (94%) of the patients were thought to have a missed abortion prior to evacuation. Only one patient presented with the classic signs and symptoms of molar disease, including excessive uterine size, high hCG levels and ovarian theca lutein cysts.

Teng and Ballon reported three patients with diploid partial mole who developed persistent tumor and suggested that diploid partial moles may have a high risk for post-molar disease[75]. Lage *et al.* studied the DNA content of 14 partial moles that developed persistent tumor[73]. Eleven (85%) partial moles were triploid, two (15%) were diploid and one DNA histogram was uninterpretable. All patients with triploid partial moles achieved remission after one course of chemotherapy. The two with diploid partial moles required multiple courses of chemotherapy to achieve remission. While the DNA content of most partial moles with persistent tumor was triploid, diploid partial moles with persistent tumor may be less sensitive to single-agent chemotherapy.

8.7 MULTIPLE CONCEPTION WITH COMPLETE OR PARTIAL MOLAR PREGNANCY AND COEXISTING FETUSES

The estimated incidence of twin pregnancy consisting of a complete mole and a

Table 8.2 Persistent gestational trophoblastic tumor after partial hydatidiform mole

Series	*No. of patients*	*No. with post-molar tumor*	*No. with metastases*
Vassilakos *et al.* [2]	56	0	0
Czernobilsky *et al.* [23]	25	1	0
Szulman and Surti [22]	49	2	0
Wong *et al.* [69]	35	4	2
Ohama *et al.* [70]	56	0	0
Bolis *et al.* [71]	86	2	0
Bagshawe *et al.* [72]	857	4	0
Lage *et al.* [73]	310	17	0
Goto *et al.* [74]	349	10	3
Total	1823	40 (2.2%)	5 (0.3%)

coexisting fetus is one per 22 000–100 000 pregnancies[76]. We recently described our experience with eight cases of twin pregnancy with complete mole and a coexisting fetus and reviewed 14 additional published cases by other investigators[77]. Additionally, we described one case of a partial mole coexisting with a normal placenta and fetus. As compared with singleton complete moles, pregnancies consisting of complete moles and coexisting fetus are diagnosed later, have more markedly enlarged uteri and have higher pre-evacuation hCG values. Importantly, persistent tumor developed in 12 (55%) of 22 patients. There are limited data to guide antenatal management of multiple gestations consisting of complete mole and coexisting fetuses. Five (23%) fetuses survived and no fetal anomalies have been described. Prompt termination of pregnancy may be necessary if severe toxemia or other medical complications arise. The occurrence of multiple gestation containing a molar pregnancy may increase with greater use of ovulation induction.

8.8 PREGNANCIES AFTER MOLAR PREGNANCY

Since our Center was established in 1965, we have been committed to collecting data about later pregnancy experience. All patients and referring physicians are requested to keep us informed about subsequent pregnancies when they complete gonadotropin follow-up. Questionnaires are mailed to all of our patients every two to three years concerning later pregnancies and general health problems.

Our patients who were treated for complete mole had 1205 subsequent pregnancies between June 1965 and December 1992[59]. These later conceptions resulted in 826 (68.5%) term live births, seven (0.5%) stillbirths, 90 (7.5%) premature deliveries and 11 (0.9%) ectopic pregnancies. Spontaneous abortion occurred in 216 (17.9%) conceptions and major and minor congenital anomalies were detected in 38 (4.1%) infants. Primary Cesarean section was performed in 56 (17.6%) of 318 later term and premature deliveries between January 1979 and December 1992. Importantly, chemoprophylaxis had no adverse effect on later pregnancy experience. Similarly, Ho *et al.* and Kashimura *et al.* reported that patients receiving chemoprophylaxis have a normal later reproductive experience[35,78].

After partial mole, our patients had 149 later gestations between June 1965 and December 1992[59]. These subsequent pregnancies resulted in 109 (73.2%) term live births, one (0.7%) stillbirth, four (2.7%) premature deliveries and one (0.7%) ectopic pregnancy. Spontaneous abortion occurred in 23 (15.5%) pregnancies and major and minor congenital anomalies were diagnosed in only three (2.6%) infants. Primary Cesarean section was performed in 19 (16.8%) of 113 term or premature deliveries. Therefore, in general patients with both complete and partial mole can anticipate normal future reproductive outcomes.

However, patients with molar disease are at increased risk of developing molar pregnancy in subsequent conceptions[79]. After one molar pregnancy, the risk of having molar disease in a future conception is about 1%[80,81]. Between June 1965 and July 1993, we treated 24 patients with repeat molar pregnancy at our center[59]. We observed every possible combination of repeat complete and partial molar gestation. In five cases, the medical records clearly indicated that the patient had a different partner at the conception of different molar pregnancies.

Following two episodes of molar pregnancy, our 24 patients had 20 later conceptions resulting in 13 full-term deliveries, four complete moles, two spontaneous abortions and one ectopic pregnancy. Therefore, among our patients with two molar pregnancies, the risk of developing molar disease in a subsequent conception was 20%. Bagshawe *et al.* also reported that the risk of molar disease following two episodes of molar pregnancy was 15%[80]. However, patients with repeat mole can achieve normal full-term pregnancies. Similarly, Lurain *et al.* reported that five of eight patients with repetitive mole later achieved normal term gestation[82].

Because of the increased risk of later molar disease, we advise our patients with molar pregnancy to undergo ultrasound in the first trimester of subsequent pregnancies to confirm normal gestational development. A careful pathological review should also be performed on the placenta or products of conception from later pregnancies. Additionally, hCG should be measured six weeks after the completion of any future pregnancy to exclude choriocarcinoma.

REFERENCES

1. Goldstein D.P. and Berkowitz, R.S. (1982) The diagnosis and management of molar pregnancy, in *Gestational Trophoblastic Neoplasms: Clinical Principles of Diagnosis and Management*, Saunders, Philadelphia, Ch. 7, pp. 143–75.
2. Vassilakos, P., Riotton, G. and Kajii, T. (1977) Hydatidiform mole: two entities. *Am. J. Obstet. Gynecol.*, **127**, 167–70.
3. Szulman, A.E. and Surti, U. (1978) The syndromes of hydatidiform mole. I. Cytogenetic and morphologic correlations. *Am. J. Obstet. Gynecol.*, **131**, 665–71.
4. Szulman, A.E. and Surti, U. (1978) The syndromes of hydatidiform mole. II. Morphologic evolution of the complete and partial mole. *Am. J. Obstet. Gynecol.*, **132**, 20–7.
5. Curry, S.L., Hammond, C.B., Tyrey, L. *et al.* (1975) Hydatidiform mole: diagnosis, management, and long-term follow up of 347 patients. *Obstet. Gynecol.*, **45**, 1–8.
6. Kohorn, E.I. (1984) Molar pregnancy: presentation and diagnosis. *Clin. Obstet. Gynecol.*, **27**, 181–91
7. Montz, F.J., Schlaerth, J.B. and Morrow, C.P. (1988) The natural history of theca lutein cysts. *Obstet. Gynecol.*, **72**, 247–51.
8. Santos-Ramos, R., Forney, J.P. and Schwartz, B.E. (1980) Sonographic findings and clinical correlations in molar pregnancy. *Obstet. Gynecol.*, **56**, 186–92.
9. Osathanondh, R., Berkowitz, R., de Cholnoky, C. *et al.* (1986) Hormonal measurements in patients with theca lutein cysts and gestational trophoblastic disease. *J. Reprod. Med.*, **31**, 179–82.
10. Ho, P.C., Wong, L.C. and Ma, H.K. (1986) Plasma prolactin, progesterone, estradiol and human chorionic gonadotropin in complete and partial moles before and after evacuation. *Obstet. Gynecol.*, **67**, 99–106.
11. Kohorn, E.I. (1982) Hydatidiform mole and gestational trophoblastic disease in Southern Connecticut. *Obstet. Gynecol.*, **59**, 78–84.
12. Berkowitz, R.S., Goldstein D.P. and Bernstein, M.R. (1980) Laparoscopy in the management of gestational trophoblastic neoplasms. *J. Reprod. Med.*, **24**, 261–4.
13. Berkowitz, R.S. and Goldstein, D.P. (1993) The management of molar pregnancy and gestational trophoblastic tumors, in *Gynecologic Oncology*, 2nd edn (eds R.C. Knapp and R.S. Berkowitz), McGraw-Hill, New York, 1993, pp. 328–38.
14. Depue, R.H., Bernstein, L., Ross, R.K. *et al.* (1987) Hyperemesis gravidarum in relation to estradiol levels, pregnancy outcome and other maternal factors: a seroepidemiologic study. *Am. J. Obstet. Gynecol.*, **156**, 1137–41.
15. Galton, V.A., Ingbar, S.H., Jimenez-Fonseca, J. *et al.* (1971) Alterations in thyroid hormone economy in patients with hydatidiform mole. *J. Clin. Invest.*, **50**, 1345–54.
16. Nisula, B.C. and Taliadouros, G.S. (1980) Thyroid function in gestational trophoblastic neoplasia: evidence that the thyrotropic activity of chorionic gonadotropin mediates the thyrotoxicosis of choriocarcinoma. *Am. J. Obstet. Gynecol.*, **138**, 77–85.
17. Kenimer, J.G., Hershman, J.M. and Higgins, H.P. (1975) The thyrotropin in hydatidiform moles is human chorionic gonadotropin. *J. Clin. Endocrinol. Metab.*, **40**, 482–91.
18. Nagataki, S., Mizuno, M., Sakamoto, S. *et al.* (1977) Thyroid function in molar pregnancy. *J. Clin. Endocrinol. Metab.*, **44**, 254–63.
19. Amir, S.M., Osathanondh, R., Berkowitz, R.S. *et al.* (1984) Human chorionic gonadotropin and thyroid function in patients with hydatidiform mole. *Am. J. Obstet. Gynecol.*, **150**, 723–8.

20. Twiggs, L.B., Morrow, C.P. and Schlaerth, J.B. (1979) Acute pulmonary complications of molar pregnancy. *Am. J. Obstet. Gynecol.*, **135**, 189–94.
21. Berkowitz, R.S., Goldstein, D.P. and Bernstein, M.R. (1986) Natural history of partial molar pregnancy. *Obstet. Gynecol.*, **66**, 677–81.
22. Szulman, A.E. and Surti, U. (1982) The clinicopathologic profile of the partial hydatidiform mole. *Obstet. Gynecol.*, **59**, 597–602.
23. Czernobilsky, B., Barash, B. and Lancet, M. (1982) Partial moles: a clinicopathologic study of 25 cases. *Obstet. Gynecol.*, **59**, 75–7.
24. Munyer, T.P., Callen, P.W., Filly, R.A. *et al.* (1981) Further observations on the monographic spectrum of gestational trophoblastic diseases. *J. Clin. Ultrasound*, **9**, 349–58.
25. Romero, R., Horgan, J.G., Kohorn, E.I. *et al.* (1985) New criteria for the diagnosis of gestational trophoblastic disease. *Obstet. Gynecol.*, **66**, 553–8.
26. Naumoff, P., Szulman, A.E., Weinstein, B. *et al.* (1981) Ultrasonography of partial hydatidiform mole. *Radiology*, **140**, 467–70.
27. Fine, C., Bundy, A.L., Berkowitz, R.S. *et al.* (1989) Sonographic diagnosis of partial hydatidiform mole. *Obstet. Gynecol.*, **73**, 414–18.
28. Genest, D., Laborde, O., Berkowitz, R.S. *et al.* (1991) A clinicopathologic study of 153 cases of complete hydatidiform mole (1980–1990): histologic grade lacks prognostic significance. *Obstet. Gynecol.*, **78**, 402–9.
29. Menczer, J., Modan, M. and Serr, D.M. (1980) Prospective follow-up of patients with hydatidiform mole. *Obstet. Gynecol.*, **55**, 346–9.
30. Ozturk, M., Berkowitz, R., Goldstein, D. *et al.* (1988) Differential production of human chorionic gonadotropin and free subunits in gestational trophoblastic disease. *Am. J. Obstet. Gynecol.*, **158**, 193–8.
31. Berkowitz, R., Ozturk, M., Goldstein, D. *et al.* (1989) Human chorionic gonadotropin and free subunits' serum levels in patients with partial and complete hydatidiform moles. *Obstet. Gynecol.*, **74**, 212–16.
32. Goldstein, D.P. and Berkowitz, R.S. (1994) Current management of complete and partial molar pregnancy. *J. Reprod. Med.*, **39**, 139–46.
33. Flam, F., Lundstrom, V. and Pettersson, F. (1991) Medical induction prior to surgical evacuation of hydatidiform mole: is there a greater risk of persistent trophoblastic disease? *Eur. J. Obstet. Gynecol. Reprod. Biol.*, **42**, 57–60.
34. Goldstein, D.P. (1971) Prophylactic chemotherapy of patients with molar pregnancy. *Obstet. Gynecol.*, **38**, 817–22.
35. Kashimura, Y., Kashimura, M., Sugimori, H. *et al.* (1986) Prophylactic chemotherapy for hydatidiform mole: five to 15 years follow-up. *Cancer*, **58**, 624–9.
36. Fasoli, M., Ratti, E., Francheschi, S. *et al.* (1982) Management of gestational trophoblastic disease: results of a cooperative study. *Obstet. Gynecol.*, **60**, 205–9.
37. Kim, D.S., Moon, H., Kim, K.T. *et al.* (1986) Effects of prophylactic chemotherapy for persistent trophoblastic disease in patients with complete hydatidiform mole. *Obstet. Gynecol.*, **67**, 690–4.
38. Berkowitz, R.S., Goldstein, D.P., Dubeshter, B. and Bernstein, M.R. (1987) Management of complete molar pregnancy. *J. Reprod. Med.*, **32**, 634–9.
39. Palmer, J.R. (1994) Advances in the epidemiology of gestational trophoblastic disease. *J. Reprod. Med.*, **39**, 155–62.
40. Stone, M. and Bagshawe, K.D. (1979) An analysis of the influences of maternal age, gestational age, contraceptive method, and the mode of primary treatment of patients with hydatidiform moles on the incidence of subsequent chemotherapy. *Br. J. Obstet. Gynecol.*, **86**, 782–92.
41. Berkowitz, R.S., Goldstein, D.P., Marean, A. and Bernstein, M.R. (1981) Oral contraceptives and postmolar trophoblastic disease. *Obstet. Gynecol.*, **58**, 474–7.
42. Curry, S., Schlaerth, J., Kohorn, E. *et al.* (1989) Hormonal contraception and trophoblastic sequelae after hydatidiform mole (a Gynecologic Oncology Group study). *Am. J. Obstet. Gynecol.*, **160**, 805–11.
43. Morrow, C.P., Nakamura, R., Schlaerth, J. *et al.* (1985) The influence of oral contraceptive on the postmolar human chorionic

gonadotropin regression curve. *Am. J. Obstet. Gynecol.*, **151**, 906–14.
44. Ho Yuen, B. and Burch, P. (1983) Relationship of oral contraceptives and the intrauterine contraceptive devices to the regression of concentrations of the beta subunit of human chorionic gonadotropin and invasive complications after molar pregnancy. *Am. J. Obstet. Gynecol.*, **145**, 214–17.
45. Deicas, R.E., Miller, D.S., Rademaker, A.W. and Lurain, J.R. (1991) The role of contraception in the development of postmolar gestational trophoblastic tumor. *Obstet. Gynecol.*, **78**, 221–6.
46. Bagshawe, K.D. (1993) Trophoblastic neoplasia, in *Cancer Medicine*, 3rd edn (eds J.F. Holland, E. Frei III, R. Bast, Jr *et al.*), Williams & Wilkins, Baltimore, pp. 1691–968.
47. Lurain, J.R., Brewer, J.I., Torok, E.E. and Halpern, B. (1983) Natural history of hydatidiform mole after primary evacuation. *Am. J. Obstet. Gynecol.*, **145**, 591–5.
48. Morrow, C.P., Kletzky, O.A., DiSaia, P.J. *et al.* (1977) Clinical and laboratory correlates of molar pregnancy and trophoblastic disease. *Am. J. Obstet. Gynecol.*, **128**, 424–30.
49. Franke, H.R., Risse, E.K.J., Kenemans, P. *et al.* (1983) Epidemiologic features of hydatidiform mole in the Netherlands. *Obstet. Gynecol.*, **62**, 613–16.
50. Kohorn, E.I. (1993) Evaluation of the criteria used to make the diagnosis of non-metastatic gestational trophoblastic neoplasia. *Gynecol. Oncol.*, **48**, 139–47.
51. Schlaerth, J.B., Morrow, C.P., Kletzky, O.A. *et al.* (1981) Prognostic characteristics of serum human chorionic gonadotropin titer regression following molar pregnancy. *Obstet. Gynecol.*, **58**, 478–82.
52. Morrow, C.P. (1984) Postmolar trophoblastic disease: diagnosis, management and prognosis. *Clin. Obstet. Gynecol.*, **27**, 211–20.
53. Tow, W.S.H. (1966) The influence of primary treatment of hydatidiform mole on subsequent course. *J. Obstet. Gynaecol. Br. Commonw.*, **73**, 544–52.
54. Xia, Z., Song, H. and Tang, M. (1980) Risk of malignancy and prognosis using a provisional scoring system in hydatidiform mole. *Chin. Med. J.*, **93**, 605–12.
55. Tsukamoto, N., Iwasaka, T., Kashimura, Y. *et al.* (1985) Gestational trophoblastic disease in women aged 50 or more. *Gynecol. Oncol.*, **20**, 53–61.
56. Tsuji, K., Yagi, S. and Nakano, R.I. (1981) Increased risk of malignant transformation of hydatidiform moles in older gravidas: a cytogenetic study. *Obstet. Gynecol.*, **58**, 351–5.
57. Martin, D.A., Sutton, G.P., Ulbright, T.M. *et al.* (1989) DNA content as a prognostic index in gestational trophoblastic neoplasia. *Gynecol. Oncol.*, **34**, 383–8.
58. Parazzini, F., Mangili, G., Belloni, C. *et al.* (1988) The problem of identification of prognostic factors for persistent trophoblastic disease. *Gynecol. Oncol.*, **30**, 57–62.
59. Berkowitz, R.S., Bernstein, M.R., Laborde, O. and Goldstein, D.P. (1994) Subsequent pregnancy experience in patients with gestational trophoblastic disease: New England Trophoblastic Disease Center, 1965–1992. *J. Reprod. Med.*, **39**, 228–32.
60. Hertig, A.T. and Sheldon, W.H. (1947) Hydatidiform mole: a pathologico-clinical correlation of 200 cases. *Am. J. Obstet. Gynecol.*, **53**, 1–36.
61. Driscoll, S.G. (1977) Gestational trophoblastic neoplasms: morphologic considerations. *Hum. Pathol.*, **8**, 529–39.
62. Elston, C.W. and Bagshawe, K.D. (1972) The value of histological grading in the management of hydatidiform mole. *J. Obstet. Gynaecol. Br. Commonw.*, **79**, 717–24.
63. Tow, W.S. and Yung, R.H. (1967) The value of histologic grading in the prognostication of hydatidiform mole. *J. Obstet. Gynaecol. Br. Commonw.*, **74**, 292–3.
64. Khazaeli, M.B., Hedayat, M.M., Hatch, K.D. *et al.* (1986) Radioimmunoassay of free-beta subunit of human chorionic gonadotropin as a prognostic test for persistent trophoblastic disease in molar pregnancy. *Am. J. Obstet. Gynecol.*, **155**, 320–4.
65. Wake, N., Fujino, T., Hoshi, S. *et al.* (1987) The propensity to malignancy of dispermic heterozygous moles. *Placenta*, **8**, 319–26.
66. Lawler, S., Fisher, R. and Dent, J. (1991) A prospective genetic study of complete and partial hydatidiform moles. *Am. J. Obstet. Gynecol.*, **164**, 1270–7.
67. Mutter, G.L., Pomponio, R.J., Berkowitz, R.S.

and Genest, D.R. (1993) Sex chromosome composition of complete hydatidiform moles: Relationship to metastasis. *Am. J. Obstet. Gynecol.*, **168**, 1547–51.
68. Rice, L.W., Berkowitz, R.S., Lage, J.M. and Goldstein, D.P. (1990) Persistent gestational trophoblastic tumor after partial hydatidiform mole. *Gynecol. Oncol.*, **36**, 358–62.
69. Wong, L.C. and Ma, H.K. (1984) The syndrome of partial mole. *Arch. Gynecol.*, **234**, 161–6.
70. Ohama, K., Ueda, K., Okamoto, E. *et al.* (1986) Cytogenetic and clinicopathologic studies of partial moles. *Obstet. Gynecol.*, **68**, 259–62.
71. Bolis, G., Belloni, C., Bonazzi, C. *et al.* (1988) Analysis of 309 cases after hydatidiform mole: different follow-up program according to biologic behavior. *Tumori*, **74**, 93–6.
72. Bagshawe, K.D., Lawler, S.D., Paradinas, F.J. *et al.* (1990) Gestational trophoblastic tumours following initial diagnosis of partial hydatidiform mole. *Lancet*, **335**, 1074–6.
73. Lage, J.M., Berkowitz, R.S., Rice, L.W. *et al.* (1991) Flow cytometric analysis of DNA content in partial hydatidiform moles with persistent gestational trophoblastic tumor. *Obstet. Gynecol.*, **77** 111–15.
74. Goto, S., Yamada, A., Ishizuka, T. and Tomoda, Y. (1993) Development of postmolar trophoblastic disease after partial molar pregnancy. *Gynecol. Oncol.*, **48**, 165–70.
75. Teng, N. and Ballon, S.C. (1984) Partial hydatidiform mole with diploid karyotype: report of three cases. *Am. J. Obstet. Gynecol.*, **150**, 961–4.
76. Vejerslev, L.O. (1991) Clinical management and diagnostic possibilities in hydatidiform mole with coexistent fetus. *Obstet. Gynecol. Surv.*, **46**, 577–88.
77. Steller, M.A., Genest, D.R., Bernstein, M.R. *et al.* (1994) Clinical features of multiple conception with partial or complete molar pregnancy and coexisting fetuses. *J. Reprod. Med.*, **39**, 147–54.
78. Ho, P.C., Wong, L.C. and Ma, H.K. (1985) Return to ovulation after evacuation of hydatidiform mole. *Am. J. Obstet. Gynecol.*, **153**, 638–42.
79. Brandes, J.A. and Peretz, A. (1965) Recurrent hydatidiform mole. *Obstet. Gynecol.*, **25**, 398–400.
80. Bagshawe, K.D., Dent, J. and Webb, J. (1986) Hydatidiform mole in England and Wales 1973–1983. *Lancet*, **ii**, 673–7.
81. Rice, L.W., Lage, J.M., Berkowitz, R.S. *et al.* (1989) Repetitive complete and partial hydatidiform mole. *Obstet. Gynecol.*, **74**, 217–19.
82. Lurain, J.R., Sand, P.K., Carson, S.A. and Brewer, J.I. (1982) Pregnancy outcome subsequent to consecutive hydatidiform moles. *Am. J. Obstet Gynecol.*, **142**, 1060–1.

PRESENTATION AND MANAGEMENT OF PERSISTENT GESTATIONAL TROPHOBLASTIC DISEASE AND GESTATIONAL TROPHOBLASTIC TUMORS IN THE UK

9

Edward Newlands

9.1 INTRODUCTION

Gestational trophoblastic tumors (GTT) can occur after any type of antecedent pregnancy (Table 9.1). The most frequent antecedent pregnancy is that of a patient presenting with a hydatidiform mole. Depending on the selection criteria for treatment, approximately 8% of these patients will need chemotherapy because of persistent trophoblastic activity which is usually referred to as persistent trophoblastic disease (PTD). A small proportion of patients who have had a hydatidiform mole can develop choriocarcinoma, which probably happens with an incidence of approximately 3%. Accurate figures are not available since histological confirmation of the progression of hydatidiform mole to choriocarcinoma is only occasionally obtained as the disease is usually eliminated with chemotherapy without resorting to major surgery. Patients with hydatidiform mole form a reasonably homogeneous cohort of patients in terms of initial diagnosis, management, follow-up and treatment, and they will be considered as one group. The presentation and management of patients presenting after a non-molar pregnancy are much more diverse and will be considered separately.

9.2 PRESENTATION AND MANAGEMENT OF PATIENTS PRESENTING WITH A HYDATIDIFORM MOLE

As discussed in the chapters on genetics and pathology (Chapters 2 and 4), hydatidiform

Table 9.1 Gestational trophoblastic tumors

Antecedent pregnancy	*Outcome*
Hydatidiform mole	Spontaneous regression Persistent trophoblastic disease (also → Choriocarcinoma)
Normal pregnancy Ectopic pregnancy Stillbirth Spontaneous abortion	Choriocarcinoma Placental site trophoblastic tumor

Gestational Trophoblastic Disease.
Edited by B.W. Hancock, E.S. Newlands and R.S. Berkowitz.
ISBN 0 412 63100 8

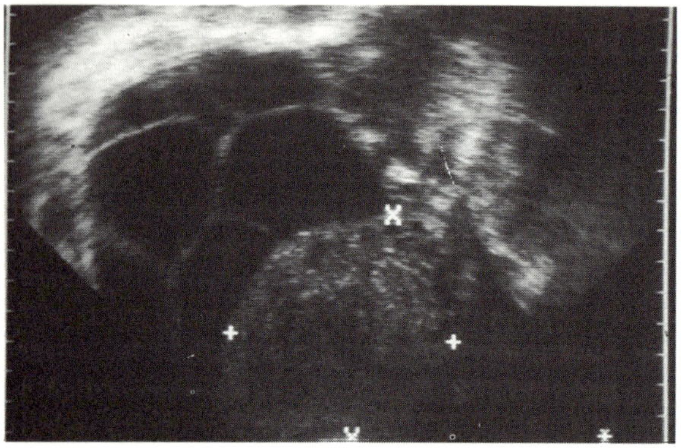

Figure 9.1 Approximately 30% of patients with PTD requiring chemotherapy have ovarian cysts on ultrasound at the time of starting chemotherapy. In this patient the ovarian cysts were unusually large: during chemotherapy the cysts torsioned and required surgical removal.

moles are either complete (diploid and androgenetic)[1,2] or partial (triploid conceptuses with two paternal and one maternal haplotypes)[3,4]. Although their genetic, pathological and biological behavior differs in a number of respects, overall the clinical management for both syndromes is essentially very similar since both can be followed by PTD or a GTT[5–9].

Patients with a complete mole usually present with varying amounts of vaginal bleeding which usually occurs between eight and 12 weeks into the pregnancy. With a complete molar pregnancy, patients may be large for dates and have more nausea and vomiting than in a normal pregnancy. The high concentration of hormones produced (including human chorionic gonadotropin (hCG)) quite commonly induces ovarian cysts (Figure 9.1). In some patients, where the hCG level is over $>10^6$ U/l, biochemical and clinical hyperthyroidism may develop[10,11]. The main differential diagnosis in these patients is between a threatened abortion and a hydatidiform mole. Partial moles tend to have considerably less trophoblastic proliferation, with much less uterine enlargement and with lower concentrations of hCG being produced. Again they usually present with varying degrees of vaginal bleeding and the main differential diagnosis is of threatened or incomplete abortion.

Provided ultrasound is available, a presumptive preoperative diagnosis can usually be made on the basis of characteristic sonographic appearances detecting the hydropic villi and the absence of a fetus (Figure 9.2)[12–14]. The initial management of the patient is evacuation of the uterine cavity by dilatation and curettage (D&C). The recommended method of evacuating the uterine cavity is by suction evacuation since this minimizes the chance of uterine perforation. Molar pregnancies are very vascular and commonly invade into the myometrium, making this susceptible to perforation with metal curettes. The initial D&C is clearly essential in all patients to confirm the diagnosis and to reduce the chance of further bleeding by evacuating the uterine cavity. We have analyzed our series by the numbers of D&Cs that have been performed (Table 9.2). The incidence of chemotherapy requirement in patients who had a single D&C is low. If molar tissue is detected in the uterine cavity after the initial evacuation, on ultrasound or

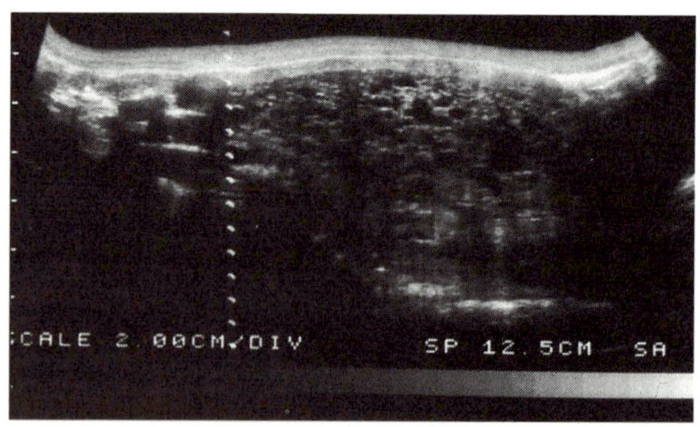

Figure 9.2 Ultrasound appearance of an unevacuated complete hydatidiform mole showing the characteristic echo pattern detecting the multiple hydropic villi of the mole and confirming the absence of a fetus.

Table 9.2 Hydatidiform moles and number of uterine evacuations, Charing Cross Hospital (1973–1986)

No. of evacuations	*Patients not treated*	*Patients treated*	*Patients treated (%)*
1	4481	109	2.4
2	1495	267	18
3	106	106	50
4	5	22	81
5	3	0	0

if there is vaginal bleeding, a second D&C may be indicated in selected patients. However, from the figures in Table 9.2 it is clear that further D&Cs are normally contraindicated, since a high proportion of these patients will need chemotherapy because the molar proliferation is deep in the myometrium or has invaded further into the pelvic tissues or even metastasized.

Once the diagnosis has been confirmed on histology that the patient has either a complete or a partial mole, she needs to be registered for follow-up to determine whether or not the molar tissue is going to die out spontaneously or persist as gestational trophoblastic disease (GTD)[6]. In the UK a nationwide service has been established since 1973 under the auspices of the Royal College of Obstetrics and Gynaecologists and the Department of Health. Patients are registered at three reference laboratories for serial hCG estimations, based at Dundee, Sheffield and the Charing Cross Hospital in London. The current number of registrations of these patients is shown in Table 9.3. The follow-up is now computerized and the frequency of samples for hCG measurements is shown in Table 9.4.

In a detailed analysis of the first decade of this registration scheme[6], it was clear that in patients whose hCG fell rapidly to normal by eight weeks following evacuation of the molar pregnancy it was extremely rare to have any further reactivation of the abnormal trophoblast. Therefore, in this group the follow-up was shortened to six months. Since molar tissue can die out over quite a prolonged period of time, in the UK we have been prepared to follow these patients up to six months provided their hCG is continuing to fall. We have been very conservative in treating only those patients whose disease is clearly active or is persisting beyond six months from the evacuation of the mole, since it is important that the minimum number of patients is exposed to cytotoxic chemotherapy. This approach results in between 7% and 8% of patients registered on the hydatidiform mole follow-up requiring chemotherapy. Since patients on this register include those with both complete and partial moles, and also some patients with uncertain or suspicious histology, this is clearly a composite figure. When analysed by histological criteria, approximately 15% of patients with complete moles and 0.5% of patients with partial moles required chemotherapy[15].

9.2.1 INDICATIONS FOR TREATMENT

The indications for treatment that have been used in the UK for a number of years are shown in Table 9.5. Since the concentration of hCG is a semi-quantitative estimate of the amount of abnormal trophoblast present in

Table 9.3 Hydatidiform mole registration centres: number of patients registered

Year	*London*	*Sheffield*	*Dundee*	*Total*
1981	548	289	59	896
1982	644	280	66	346
1983	679	327	76	1082
1984	566	374	83	1023
1985	625	358	98	1081
1986	676	356	90	1122
1987	663	390	78	1131
1988	634	413	82	1129
1989	582	358	75	1015
1990	684	377	89	1150
1991	690	404	77	1171
1992	693	383	97	1173
1993	758	384	93	1235
1994	781	365	102	1248

Table 9.4 Charing Cross Hospital: hydatidiform mole follow-up

Serum samples for hCG	2-weekly until normal;
Then urine samples for hCG	4-weekly until 1 year post evacuation;
Then urine samples for hCG	3-monthly until 2 years post evacuation.

1. hCG follow-up will range from 6 months to 2 years after evacuation of hydatidiform mole
2. If the patient's hCG values reach normal range within 8 weeks of evacuation, follow-up will be limited to 6 months
3. Patients who do not have normal hCG values within 8 weeks of evacuation should have 2-year follow-up
4. Further estimations of hCG 6 weeks and 10 weeks *after any future* pregnancies are requested because of a small increase in risk of choriocarcinoma developing in such patients

the patient, a high hCG more than four weeks after evacuation of the mole carries a risk of uterine perforation and major hemorrhage. Clinical experience has indicated that a serum hCG of >20 000 U/l is a satisfactory cut-off point for defining patients at greater risk of uterine perforation. Patients with histological evidence of choriocarcinoma already have a frank malignancy which will not regress spontaneously and will require

Table 9.5 Indications for chemotherapy

Indications
Serum hCG above 20 000 U/l more than 4 weeks after evacuation, because of the risk of uterine perforation
Histological evidence of choriocarcinoma
Evidence of metastases in brain, liver or gastrointestinal tract, or radiological opacities greater than 2 cm on chest X-ray
Long-lasting uterine hemorrhage
Rising hCG values
hCG in body fluids 4–6 months after evacuation

treatment. Those with clearly aggressive disease with widespread metastases clearly also need treatment. It should be noted, however, that not all small pulmonary metastases are associated with clinically progressive disease provided the hCG is falling (Figure 9.3). Patients with PTD in the uterus commonly have varying amounts of vaginal bleeding. If this is severe, a combination of bed rest and chemotherapy will usually control the bleeding within 72 h. However, a small proportion of patients will have significant arteriovenous malformations induced by their trophoblastic disease and occasionally these can present significant problems in controlling the hemorrhage (Table 9.6). If the hCG is clearly rising, confirming that the PTD is not dying out, the patient will need chemotherapy. The last indication for treatment is the time cut-off point following evacuation of the mole. We are prepared to wait up to six months following these patients with serial hCG estimations provided the hCG is falling. After six months, clinical experience has confirmed that PTD can become increasingly drug-resistant. Therefore, patients are treated at six months if the hCG is still raised. We analyzed the indications for treatment in 552 patients treated between 1982 and 1992 and, using the criteria in Table 9.5, on average patients had two of these indications for requiring treatment (Table 9.7). The commonest reason for

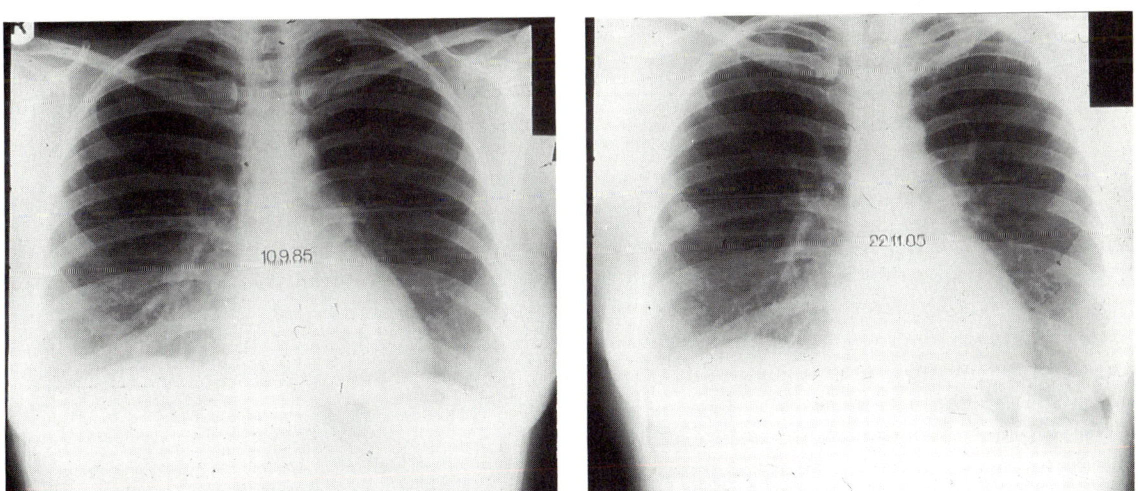

Figure 9.3 Chest X-ray of a patient on follow-up after a hydatidiform mole who developed a clear-cut pulmonary lesion, but as her hCG was falling satisfactorily she never received treatment and the chest X-ray cleared spontaneously. The lesion detected was presumed to be an embolus of dying molar tissue.

Table 9.6 Hemorrhagic complications in patients after treatment for PTD 1978–1992

Total number of patients treated	946	(%)
Hysterectomy for severe vaginal bleeding	5	(0.5)
Hysterectomy for intra-abdominal bleeding	3	(0.3)
Embolization of uterine arteries to control severe vaginal bleeding[a]	7	(0.7)

[a]These patients wanted to preserve their fertility.

Table 9.7 Indications for treatment for patients with post-molar trophoblastic disease at Charing Cross Hospital (1 January 1982 to 26 March 1992)

Total number of patients treated	552	(%)
1. High hCG >4/52 post evacuation/delivery	261	(47)
2. Heavy hemorrhage	66	(12)
3. Rising hCG	390	(71)
4. hCG raised >4/12 post evacuation not falling	125	(23)
5. hCG raised post 6 months	82	(15)
6. Pulmonary, vulval, vaginal metastases, hCG not falling	78	(14)
7. Metastases other than lung, vulval, vaginal	9	(2)
8. Histology; choriocarcinoma with raised hCG	25	(4)
9. Irregular or persistent bleeding	72	(13)
10. Other	25	(4)
Total number of indications	1133[a]	

[a]Some had more than one reason for starting treatment.

requiring chemotherapy was a rising hCG, followed by patients with a high hCG more than four weeks after delivery, and then patients whose hCG was not falling between four and six months after evacuation of the hydatidiform mole.

The effect of exogenous hormones (usually the oral contraceptive) on PTD is a controversial area[16,17]. In the Charing Cross series we think that there are two patient populations. In those patients whose hCG falls rapidly to normal within eight weeks of evacuation of the mole, once the hCG is normal there is no major effect that we can detect in patients receiving the oral contraceptive. However, in a subgroup of patients whose hCG is still raised more than eight weeks post evacuation of the mole, there is a population that appears to be at risk of stimulating their PTD if they are exposed to the oral contraceptive at this stage. A recent analysis of our data is shown in Table 9.8. Our interpretation of this data is that PTD that is persisting beyond eight weeks may have evolved biologically towards progressive trophoblastic disease. The ex-

Table 9.8 Effects of taking oral contraceptives within six months of evacuation of a hydatidiform mole: Charing Cross Hospital (1973–1989)

Total number of patients	8882	(%)
Total number of patients requiring chemotherapy	663	(7.5)
Numbers who received oral contraceptive	1384	(15.6)
A. Patients with normal hCG prior to oral contraceptive	1049	
Number requiring chemotherapy	5[a]	(0.0047)
B. Patients with raised hCG given oral contraceptives	335	
Number requiring chemotherapy	103	(30.7)
A versus B, $p < 0.001$		

[a]Three patients required chemotherapy after a subsequent pregnancy; one patient required chemotherapy after a subsequent hydatidiform mole: one patient required chemotherapy after 18 months post hydatidiform mole.

posure of this abnormal tissue to exogenous hormones (usually the contraceptive pill) stimulates its growth in a proportion of patients, increasing the number who need chemotherapy. On the basis of our data we continue to recommend that patients do not take the oral contraceptive until the hCG is clearly normal. This subgroup of patients would not be clinically apparent using criteria for treating all patients with PTD at eight weeks if the hCG is still raised. This may explain the different results reported from different centers[17– 21].

Patients who have had a previous molar pregnancy are more at risk of having a subsequent one and the incidence of a second molar pregnancy is approximately one in 70[6]. These patients are also more at risk of having a trophoblastic tumor after a subsequent normal pregnancy. It is therefore important to check that their hCG returns to normal six and 10 weeks after delivery of each subsequent pregnancy (Figure 9.4). We have recently been able to prove what has been suspected for some years, that a tumor following a subsequent term pregnancy is not necessarily related to that most recent pregnancy and may derive from a previous molar pregnancy[22]. This provides additional evidence that hormonal changes associated with a pregnancy can potentially stimulate the regrowth of a nest of dormant abnormal trophoblast.

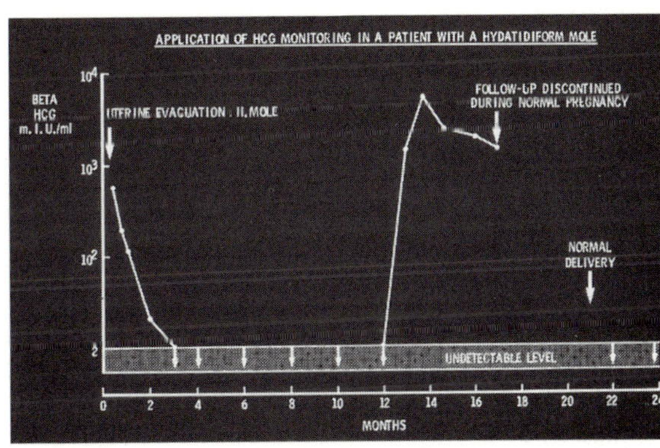

Figure 9.4 Patient on follow-up after a hydatidiform mole. The hCG fell to the normal range after evacuation of the mole. When the hCG remained normal for six months there was no contraindication to the patient becoming pregnant. Once the pregnancy was confirmed to be normal on ultrasound, hCG follow-up was discontinued until after delivery, and confirmation that the hCG was normal after the birth was done at six and 10 weeks.

9.3 PRESENTATION AND MANAGEMENT OF PERSISTENT GESTATIONAL TROPHOBLASTIC DISEASE AND TUMORS AFTER NON-MOLAR PREGNANCIES

GTT can occur after non-molar abortions, ectopic pregnancies and full term live births. Although rare from the point of view of the individual gynecologist, this mode of presentation accounts for just under 17% of patients treated at the Charing Cross Hospital. These patients present considerably more diagnostic difficulties than patients presenting with a hydatidiform mole. An awareness of a potential trophoblastic tumor is very important since most of these patients are curable with appropriate treatment.

We have analyzed 602 patients treated between 1985 and 1994 at the Charing Cross Hospital: there were 100 cases (16.6%) where the antecedent pregnancy was either a non-molar abortion or a live birth; there were 62 cases of choriocarcinoma occurring after a live birth; six patients who had had a prior molar pregnancy whose tumor developed after a subsequent live birth; and 32 patients developed choriocarcinoma after a non-molar abortion[23]. Approximately two-thirds of these patients presented with varying degrees of abnormal vaginal bleeding but in one-quarter of the patients the primary complaint was associated with symptoms from metastatic disease involving lung, brain or abdomen (Table 9.9). Histological evidence of choriocarcinoma was found in over 50% of patients. In the other patients, histological confirmation was not available but the presence of a high hCG level in the absence of a pregnancy together with metastatic disease was taken as a presumptive diagnosis of gestational choriocarcinoma in women of childbearing age.

In some cases the question of whether the tumor is gestational in origin can present a major management problem. Provided samples are available from the patient's tumor, and blood from the patient and her

Table 9.9 Symptoms and distribution of disease in 100 women presenting with choriocarcinoma after a non-molar pregnancy [23]

Symptoms	
Irregular vaginal bleeding	43%
Postpartum hemorrhage	11%
Dyspnoea	9%
Central nervous system symptoms	8%
Abdominal pain	7%
Sites of disease	
Uterus	56%
Vagina	11%
Abdomen	5%
Lung	40%
Brain	17%
Liver	7%
Other	13%

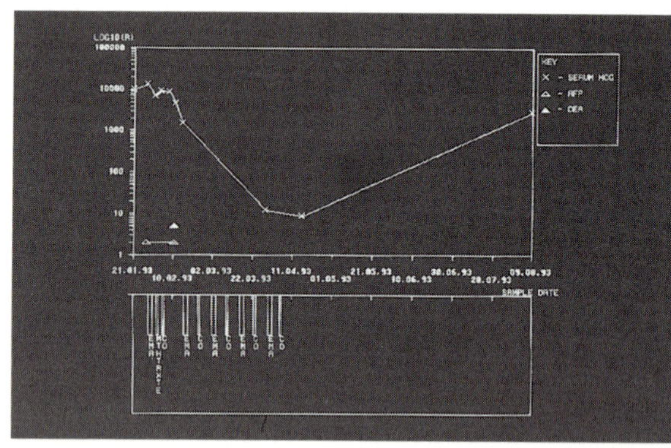

Figure 9.5 A 33-year-old female who smoked 20 cigarettes per day presenting with a breast mass during pregnancy with an initial diagnosis of an abscess. Computed tomography scan and histological review were compatible with a bronchial primary. On genetic analysis there was no evidence of paternal genes in the tumor. EMA/CO chemotherapy was administered on a palliative basis and she had a good partial response to this, lasting 10 months.

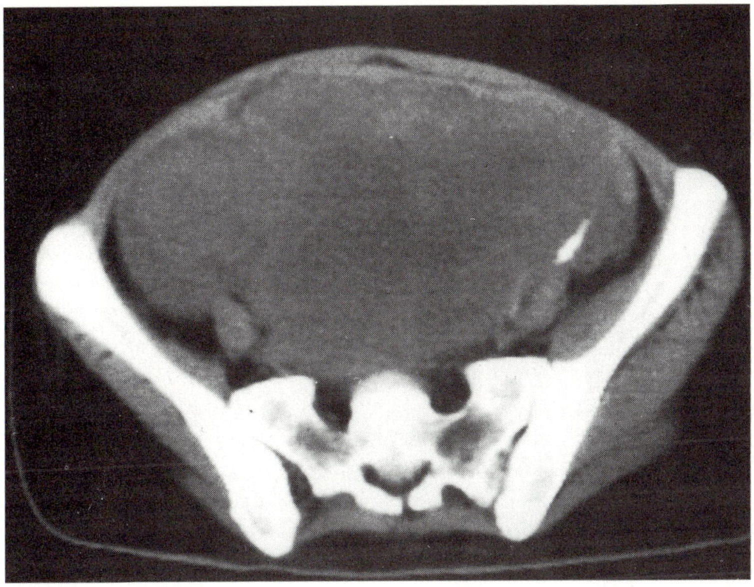

Figure 9.6 Massive uterine enlargement in a patient who had miscarried six months previously. Clinical presentation included investigation of severe abdominal pain and thyrotoxicosis. Her initial hCG level at the start of treatment was 1.6×10^6 U/l.

partner, modern molecular genetics can sometimes help resolve this dilemma[24]. The presence of paternal alleles in the tumor clearly defines the tumor as gestational and these patients should be treated appropriately and the majority can be cured. However, a range of other primary tumors can masquerade as choriocarcinoma with trophoblastic differentiation and hCG production. Examples include carcinomas of the bronchus, stomach, bladder, colon and occasionally other tumor types. Here the absence of paternal genes adds additional weight to an unusual clinical pattern of disease which is not typical of a GTT. Curiously, these non-gestational tumors with trophoblastic differentiation can be reasonably chemosensitive although not curable with current therapy[25]. Regressions lasting between six months and two years can sometimes be obtained. Treatment appropriate for a high-risk GTT can be clinically useful to the patient (Figure 9.5).

The outcome in patients who develop a GTT after a non-molar abortion is less satisfactory than for patients who have had a hydatidiform mole[23]. In the small group

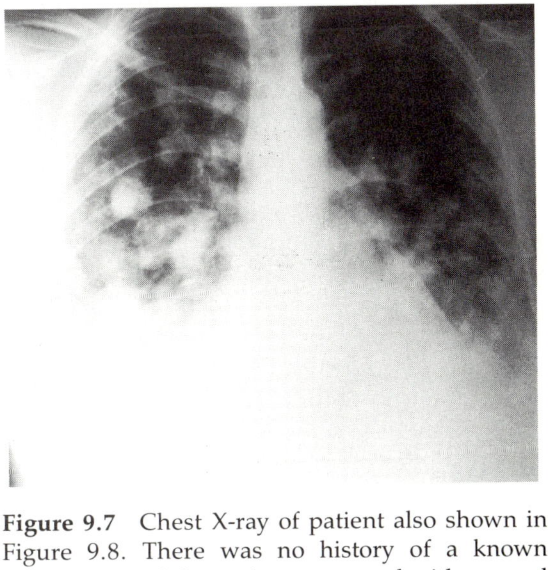

Figure 9.7 Chest X-ray of patient also shown in Figure 9.8. There was no history of a known pregnancy and the patient presented with a grand mal fit associated with an intracerebral hemorrhage and a cerebral metastasis (Figure 9.8). She was breathless at rest and was not considered fit for an anesthetic until chemotherapy had improved her pulmonary function. Interestingly, her pulmonary function did not deteriorate at the start of treatment[27], which may be associated with the high-dose dexamethasone she was on for the intracranial lesion.

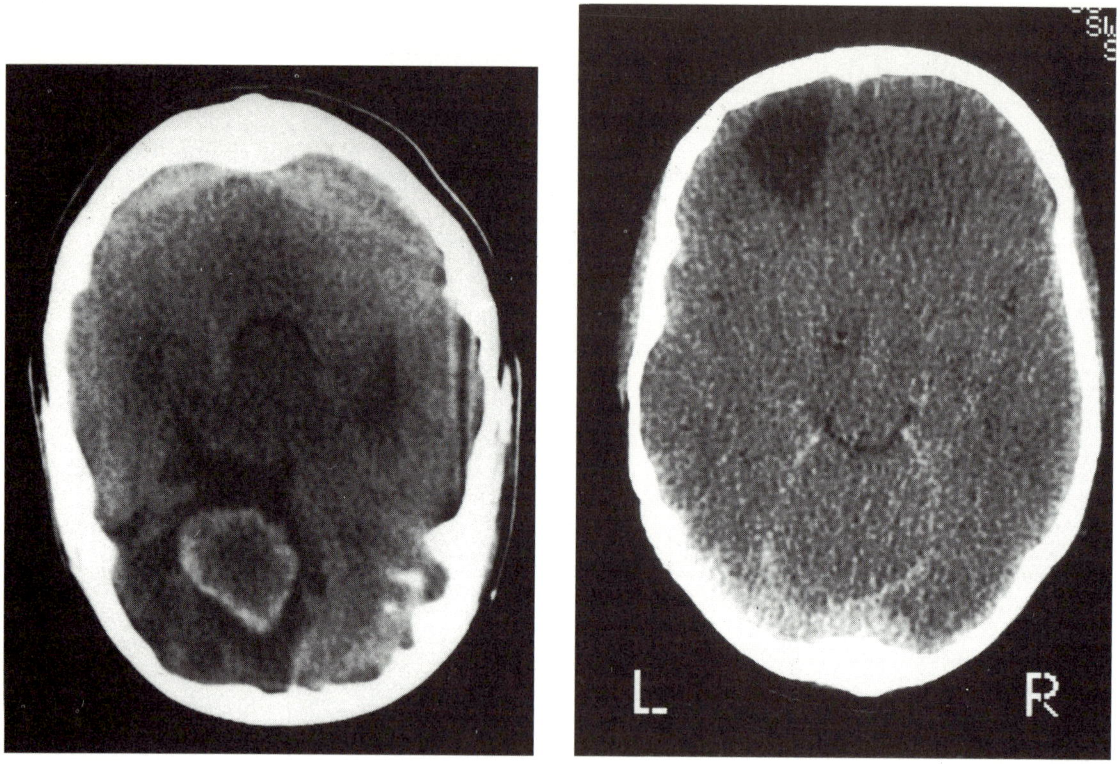

Figure 9.8 Computed tomography scans of the head of a patient also illustrated in Figure 9.7. (a) Scan at presentation showing a hemorrhagic deposit in the frontal lobe. Since this was a single deposit and there was a major risk of further hemorrhage, the metastasis was excised as soon as her pulmonary function improved sufficiently for her to have an anesthetic. (b) Postoperative scan.

of six patients who had a prior mole followed by a full term pregnancy, three of these were detected by hCG screening and all six of these patients were salvaged with appropriate treatment. In patients presenting with non-molar abortions, two (6.3%) died from their disease. The biggest problem was associated with the patients who developed choriocarcinoma following a live birth, 13 (21%) of the 62 patients dying from their disease[23]. It has long been recognized that patients presenting with choriocarcinoma after a live birth have an aggressive tumor. Clinically there are two patterns of presentation: those who present with varying amounts of vaginal hemorrhage in the first four months after delivery – in these patients the tumor is frequently highly aggressive and widely metastatic; the second pattern is of slower tumor growth and presentation at a later stage after delivery. In both these groups the problem at the time of diagnosis can be disease extent (Figures 9.6–9.8). There is still a mortality in patients presenting with respiratory failure from pulmonary metastases, pulmonary artery hypertension and embolism, multiple cerebral metastases and massive liver metastases (Table 9.10)[26–28].

One rare variant of trophoblastic tumor that presents specific diagnostic and management problems is the placental site

Table 9.10 Early deaths[26][a]

Patient	Antecedent pregnancy (AP)	Interval from AP (months)	Days from admission to death	Cause of death
1	Miscarriage	6	7	Respiratory failure
2	Miscarriage	6	14	Respiratory failure
3	Live birth	7	6	Respiratory failure
4	Live birth	180[b]	4	Respiratory failure
5	Miscarriage	48	15	Respiratory failure
6	Live birth	4	2	Cerebral metastases
7	Live birth	7	8	Cerebral metastases
8	Stillbirth	12	7	Cerebral infarct
9	Live birth	24	4	Hepatic failure
10	Live birth[c]	24	2	Pulmonary embolus

[a]Deaths occuring within 3 weeks of starting chemotherapy.
[b]Hysterectomy 15 years prior to admission.
[c]Hydatidiform mole 72 months prior to chemotherapy, then two normal pregnancies following the mole.

Table 9.11 Placental site trophoblastic tumors: Charing Cross Hospital 1975–1994

	Range	Mean
Interval from antecedent pregnancy	5–180 (months)	47.7
hCG concentration at diagnosis	15–20 710(U/l)	1849

trophoblastic tumor (PSTT)[29] and this will also be discussed in chapter 11. PSTT can present after both full term and molar pregnancies[30]. The interval from the antecedent pregnancy can be long and in our small series of 18 patients this varied between five and 180 months (mean 47.2) (Table 9.11). Pathologically these are predominantly cytotrophoblastic tumors which produce relatively small amounts of hCG and the older tumors can calcify (Figure 9.9). PSTT are more commonly limited to the uterus but can invade locally in the pelvis. Six of our 18 patients had pulmonary metastases (Table 9.12). The mode of diagnosis of PSTT is variable: an alert pathologist may make a diagnosis on either D&C or on a hysterectomy specimen (Table 9.13). However, some are only identified on review. An important but rare phenomenon in diagnosing a PSTT is unexpected resistance of PTD

Table 9.12 Placental site trophoblastic tumors: Charing Cross Hospital 1975–1994. Sites of disease at diagnosis in 18 patients

Site	No.	(%)
Uterus	18	(100)
Lungs	6	(33)
Pelvic nodes	2	(11)
Ovary	1	(6)
Multiple nodes	1	(6)

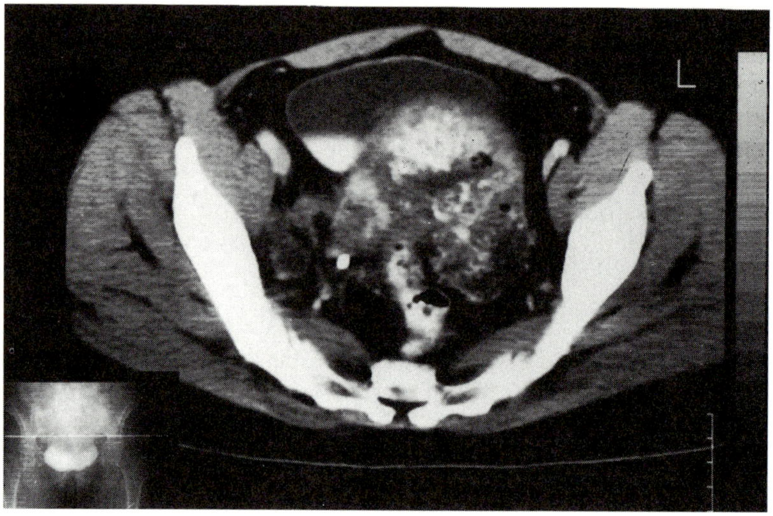

Figure 9.9 Patient presenting with irregular vaginal bleeding, pelvic and back pain. A large calcified lesion was removed at hysterectomy and histology confirmed PSTT. The last known pregnancy was 14 years previously. Genetic analysis confirmed that the tumor was derived from a biparental pregnancy[30]. She had metastases in the pelvis, para-aortic region, lungs and supraclavicular nodes. Despite treatment with EMA/CO (chapter 11), surgery and radiotherapy, her disease relapsed through treatment and she rapidly died from her disease.

to chemotherapy (Table 9.13 and Figure 9.10). PSTTs have quite variable chemosensitivity. Of the 17 patients who have completed treatment, only three (43%) out of seven with metastatic disease are alive. For those patients with disease limited to the pelvis, the combination of surgery and chemotherapy has resulted in nine (90%) out of 10 complete remissions. This gives an overall survival at present of 12 (71%) out of 17 patients. In addition one patient refused hysterectomy

Table 9.13 Placental site trophoblastic tumors: Charing Cross Hospital 1975–1994. Mode of initial diagnosis in 18 patients

Mode	*No.*	*(%)*
D&C	6	(33)
Hysterectomy	4	(22)
Unexpected drug resistance on treatment for PTD	4	(22)
Retrospective review of slides	4	(22)

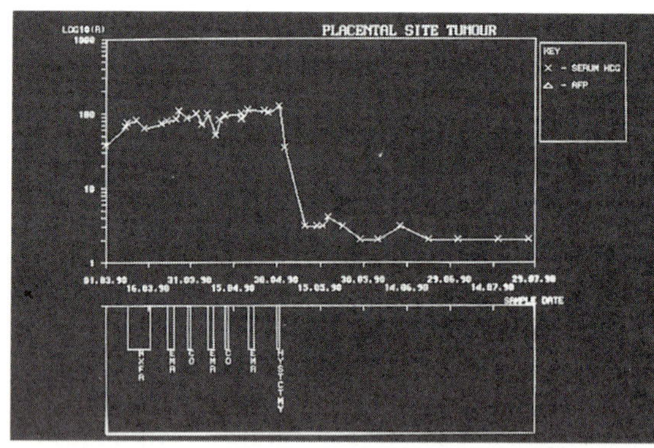

Figure 9.10 Patient on follow-up after a complete hydatidiform mole. She was treated because the hCG level was rising but was low risk on prognostic score (chapter 11). There was unexpected resistance to methotrexate, then EMA/CO chemotherapy. D&C confirmed placental site trophoblastic tumor and following a hysterectomy she has remained in remission. Genetic analysis of her tumor confirmed that it was androgenetic and therefore originated from her hydatidiform mole.

and the disease remitted spontaneously; this patient subsequently had an uneventful normal pregnancy. The rarity of this tumor, together with variable biological behavior and chemosensitivity, makes it difficult to identify the optimum management for this variant of trophoblastic tumor.

REFERENCES

1. Kajii, T. and Omaha, K. (1977) Androgenetic origin of hydatidiform mole. *Nature*, **268**, 633–4.
2. Wake, N, Takaqi, N. and Sasaki, M. (1978) Androgenesis as a cause of hydatidiform mole. *Nat. Cancer Inst.*, **60**, 51–7.
3. Szulman, A., and Surti, U. (1978) The syndrome of hydatidiform mole. I. Cytogenetic and morphologic correlations. *Am. J. Obstet. Gynecol.*, **131**, 665–71.
4. Szulman, A. and Surti, U. (1978) The syndrome of hydatidiform mole. II. Morphologic evidence of the complete and partial mole. *Am. Obstet. Gynecol.*, **132**, 20–7.
5. Berkowitz, R.S., Goldstein, D.P., Dubeshter, B. and Bernstein, M.R. (1987) Management of complete molar pregnancy. *J. Reprod. Med.*, **32**, 634–9.
6. Bagshawe, K.D., Dent, J. and Webb, J. (1986) Occasional survey: hydatidiform mole in England and Wales 1973–83. *Lancet*, **ii**, 673–7.
7. Bagshawe, K.D., Lawler, S.D., Paradinas, F.J. *et al.* (1990) Gestational trophoblasic tumours following initial diagnosis of partial hydatidiform mole. *Lancet*, **335**, 1074–6.
8. Lawler, S.D., Fisher, R.A. and Dent, J. (1991) A prospective study of hydatidiform mole. *Am. J. Obstet. Gynecol.*, **164**, 1270–7.
9. Goldstein, D.P. and Berkowitz, R.S. (1994) Current management of complete and partial molar pregnancy. *J. Reprod. Med.*, **39**, 139–46.
10. Nisula, B.C. and Taliadouros, G.S. (1980) Thyroid function in gestational trophoblastic neoplasia: evidence that the thyrotropic activity of chorionic gonadotrophin mediates the thyrotoxicosis of choriocarcinoma. *Am. J. Obstet. Gynecol.*, **138**, 77–85.
11. Amir, S.M., Osathanondh, R., Berkowitz, R.S. *et al.* (1984) Human chorionic gonadotrophin and thyroid function in patients with hydatidiform mole. *Am. J. Obstet. Gynecol.*, **150**, 723–8.
12. Fine, C., Bundy, A.L., Berkowitz, R.S. *et al.* (1989) Sonographic diagnosis of partial hydatidiform mole. *Obstet. Gynecol.*, **73**, 414–18.
13. Long, M.G., Boultbee, J.E. and Langley, R. (1992) Doppler assessment of uterine circulation and clinical behaviour of gestational trophoblastic tumours requiring chemotherapy. *Br. J. Cancer*, **66**, 883–7.
14. O'Reilly, S.M., Boultbee, J.M., Langley, R. *et al.* (1995) Pelvic ultrasound can help to predict the development of drug resistance in patients with low risk gestational trophoblastic disease. *Int. J. Gynaecol. Cancer*, in press.
15. Paradinas, F.J. (1994) The histological diagnosis of hydatidiform moles. *Curr. Diagn. Pathol.*, **1**, 24–31.
16. Stone, M., Dent, J., Kardana, A. *et al.* (1976) Relationship of oral contraception to development of trophoblastic tumour after evacuation of a hydatidiform mole. *Br. J. Obstet. Gynaecol.*, **83**, 913–16.
17. Deicas, R.E., Miller, D.S., Rademaker, A.W. and Lurain, J.R. (1981) The role of contraception in the development of postmolar gestational trophoblastic tumor. *Obstet. Gynecol.*, **78**, 221–6.
18. Berkowitz, R.S., Goldstein, D.P., Marean, A. and Bernstein, M.R. (1981) Oral contraceptives and post-molar trophoblastic disease. *Obstet. Gynecol.*, **58**, 474–7.
19. Ho Yuen, B. and Burch, P. (1983) Relationship of oral contraceptives and the intrauterine contraceptive devices to the regression of concentrations of the beta subunit of human chorionic gonadotrophin and invasive complications after molar pregnancy. *Am. J. Obstet. Gynecol.*, **145**, 214–17.
20. Curry, S., Schlaerth, J., Kohorn, E. *et al.* (1989) Hormonal contraception and trophoblastic sequelae after hydatidiform mole (a Gynecologic Oncology Study Group study). *Am. J. Obstet. Gynecol.*, **160**, 805–11.
21. Morrow, C.P., Nakamura, R., Schlaerth, J. *et al.* (1985) The influence of oral contraceptive on the postmolar human chorionic gonadotrophin regression curve. *Am. J. Obstet. Gynecol.*, **151**, 906–14.

22. Fisher, R.A., Soteriou, B., Meredith, L. *et al.*(1994) Previous hydatidiform mole identified as the causative pregnancy of choriocarcinoma following birth of normal twins. *Int. J. Gynaecol. Cancer*, **5**, 64–70.
23. Tidy, J.A., Rustin, G.J.S., Newlands, E.S. *et al.* (1995) The presentation and management of women with choriocarcinoma after nonmolar pregnancy. *Br. J. Obstet. Gynaecol.*, **102**, 715–19.
24. Fisher, R.A., Newlands, E.S., Jeffreys, A.J. *et al.* (1992) Gestational and non-gestational trophoblastic tumours distinguished by DNA analysis. *Cancer*, **69**, 839–45.
25. Crawford, S.M., Ledermann, J.A., Turkie, W. *et al.* (1986) Is ectopic production of human chorionic gonadotrophin (hCG) or alphafoetoprotein (AFP) by tumours a marker of chemosensitivity? *Eur. J. Clin. Oncol.*, **22**, 1483–7.
26. Newlands, E.S., Bagshawe, K.D., Begent, R.H.J. *et al.* (1991) Results with the EMA/CO (etoposide, methotrexate, actinomycin D, cyclophosphamide, vincristine) regimen in high risk gestational trophoblastic tumours, 1979 to 1989. *Br. J. Obstet. Gynaecol.*, **98**, 550–7.
27. Kelly, M.P., Rustin, G.J.S., Ivory, C. *et al.* (1990) Respiratory failure due to choriocarcinoma: a study of 103 dyspnoeic patients. *Gynaecol. Oncol.*, **38**, 149–54.
28. Sasaki S., Katayama, P.K., Roesler, M. *et al.* (1982) Cytogenetic analysis of choriocarcinoma cell lines. *Acta Obstet. Gynaecol. Jpn.*, **34**, 2253–6.
29. Cole, L.A., Kardana, A., Andradegordon, P. *et al.* (1991) The heterogeneity of human chorionic gonadotrophin (hCG). 3. The occurrence and biological and immunological activities of nicked hCG. *Endocrinology*, **129**, 1559–68.
30. Fisher, R.A., Paradinas, F.J., Newlands, E.S. and Boxer, G.M. (1992) Genetic evidence of placental site trophoblastic tumours originating from hydatidiform mole or a normal conceptus. *Br. J. Cancer*, **65**, 355–8.

PRESENTATION AND MANAGEMENT OF PERSISTENT GESTATIONAL TROPHOBLASTIC DISEASE AND GESTATIONAL TROPHOBLASTIC TUMORS IN THE USA

10

Ross S. Berkowitz and Donald P. Goldstein

Persistent gestational trophoblastic disease (GTD) and tumors (GTT) are one of the rare human malignancies that are highly curable even with widespread dissemination[1–3]. GTD encompasses a group of interrelated diseases including partial and complete molar pregnancy, placental site trophoblastic tumor (PSTT) and choriocarcinoma (CC) that have varying propensities for invasion and dissemination. While GTT most commonly occurs after molar gestation, it may develop after any type of pregnancy. The current chapter will review the presentation and management of GTT based primarily upon our experience at the New England Trophoblastic Disease Center (NETDC). Further detailed discussion of investigation and treatment will be provided in chapters by Dr Newlands and Drs Lurain and Homesley. Additionally, the role of surgery will be reviewed in depth by Dr Millar and the long-term effect of chemotherapy upon fertility and secondary cancers will be addressed by Dr Rustin.

10.1 PRESENTATION

Following molar pregnancy, GTT may have the histological pattern of either molar tissue or CC. However, after a non-molar antecedent pregnancy, GTT always has the histological features of CC. PSTT is an uncommon variant of CC which is composed almost entirely of mononuclear intermediate trophoblast.

10.1.1 PRESENTATION OF NON-METASTATIC GTT

Locally invasive GTT occurs in about 15% of patients after complete hydatidiform mole and infrequently after other gestations[4]. These patients may present with irregular vaginal bleeding, uterine subinvolution or asymmetric enlargement, theca lutein ovarian cysts and persistently elevated human chorionic gonadotropin (hCG) levels. Bulky necrotic tumors may be a focus for uterine infection and cause purulent discharge and pelvic pain. Trophoblastic tumor may perforate through the myometrium producing intra-abdominal bleeding or erode into uterine vessels causing vaginal hemorrhage.

10.1.2 PRESENTATION OF METASTATIC GTT

Metastases develop in about 4% of patients after complete mole and infrequently after other pregnancies[4]. Metastases are com-

Gestational Trophoblastic Disease.
Edited by B.W. Hancock, E.S. Newlands and R.S. Berkowitz.
ISBN 0 412 63100 8

monly CC which has a propensity for early vascular invasion and dissemination. Patients may present with signs and symptoms of bleeding from metastases such as hemoptysis or hepatic rupture.

The lungs are the most common site of metastasis. Eighty per cent of our patients with metastatic GTT have pulmonary involvement on chest radiographs[5]. Patients with pulmonary metastases may have cough, chest pain, hemoptysis, dyspnea or an asymptomatic lesion on chest radiograph. Pulmonary hypertension and right heart strain may develop due to pulmonary arterial occlusion by trophoblastic emboli[6]. Because respiratory symptoms may be dramatic and striking, the patient may be thought to have a primary pulmonary disease. Importantly, gynecological symptoms may be minimal or absent. Regrettably, the diagnosis of GTT may only be considered after the patient has undergone thoracotomy. It is important to emphasize that the diagnosis of GTT should be considered in any woman in the reproductive age group with unexplained pulmonary or systemic symptoms.

GTT may produce four principal pulmonary radiographic patterns: (1) discrete rounded densities; (2) an alveolar or 'snowstorm' pattern; (3) pleural effusion, or (4) embolic pattern caused by pulmonary arterial occlusion[7–10]. Importantly, patients may have pulmonary hypertension in the absence of substantial parenchymal disease. The extent of pulmonary involvement can vary greatly amongst centers due to differences in the frequency of early diagnosis. At our center, patients with pulmonary metastases rarely present with respiratory symptoms and have comparatively small pulmonary nodules on chest radiographs. In contrast, Bakri *et al*. described 75 patients from Saudi Arabia with pulmonary metastases and observed pleural effusion and greater than 50% opacification of the lungs in 48% and 33% of the patients respectively[11].

Patients with extensive pulmonary involvement may develop early respiratory failure requiring mechanical ventilation within one month of presentation. Risk factors for developing early respiratory failure include cyanosis, pulmonary hypertension, anemia, dyspnea and greater than 50% lung opacification[11,12]. Bakri *et al*. and Kelly *et al*. reported a 100% mortality in eight and 11 patients, respectively, with early respiratory failure. Importantly, Kelly *et al*. observed that reducing the initial dose of chemotherapy did not protect against the development of early respiratory failure, and therefore recommended the use of intensive chemotherapy at the outset.

Vaginal metastases occur in 30% of our patients with metastatic GTT. Vaginal lesions are most commonly located suburethrally or in the fornices and present with a purulent discharge or irregular bleeding. These lesions are highly vascular and may bleed vigorously if biopsied.

Cerebral and hepatic metastases occur in about 10% of our patients with metastatic GTT. Cerebral and hepatic involvement are most commonly seen in patients with a non-molar antecedent pregnancy with protracted delays in diagnosis and high hCG levels. Virtually all patients with cerebral and hepatic lesions have concurrent pulmonary and/or vaginal involvement.

Most patients with cerebral metastases are symptomatic and present with headache, hemiparesis, vomiting, seizures, visual disturbance or slurred speech[13,14]. Neurological symptoms were present in all 34 patients reported by Liu *et al*. and in 66 of 69 patients (96%) and in 20 of 23 patients (87%) described by Athanassiou *et al*. and Bakri *et al*., respectively[15–17].

Patients with hepatic metastases less frequently present with symptoms that are attributable to hepatic involvement. Bakri *et al*. reported that only five (26%) of 19 patients with liver involvement presented with epigastric pain, jaundice and/or intraperitoneal bleeding. Most of these patients presented with symptoms related to other sites of involvement[18].

10.2 DIAGNOSIS

After a molar gestation, the diagnosis of GTT is usually made by a persistent plateau or re-elevation in the hCG level. As discussed in Chapter 8 the criteria for diagnosing post-molar GTT varies amongst centers. At the NETDC, we consider a persistent plateau in hCG as the presence of hCG levels within the range of inter-assay variation over a period of at least three weeks. A persistently elevated hCG measurement without evidence of either an intrauterine or ectopic pregnancy is also strongly suggestive of GTT in any woman in the reproductive age group. Patients may present with gynecological and/or systemic symptoms. Biopsy of metastases should be avoided because it may induce exsanguinating hemorrhage. Patients with otherwise unexplained elevated hCG values should also be considered to potentially have a germ cell tumor of the ovary or other site or a non-trophoblastic gonadotropin-producing tumor.

10.3 DIAGNOSTIC EVALUATION

The optimal management of GTT requires a thorough assessment of the extent of disease prior to the initiation of treatment. All patients should undergo a careful pretreatment evaluation including a complete history and physical examination, measurement of hCG, hepatic, renal and thyroid function tests, and determination of the complete blood count. The metastatic work-up should include a chest radiograph, ultrasound or computed tomography (CT) scan of the abdomen and pelvis, and CT or magnetic resonance imaging (MRI) scan of the head.

If the chest radiograph and pelvic examination are negative, it is uncommon to have metastases to other sites. MRI or CT scans of the liver will document most metastases in patients with abnormal liver function tests. Head CT scan has successfully facilitated the early diagnosis of asymptomatic cerebral lesions[16]. Chest CT scans may demonstrate micrometastases in the presence of a normal chest radiograph. Mutch *et al.* reported that 16 (41%) of 39 patients with presumed non-metastatic GTT had pulmonary micrometastases on chest CT scan[19].

Patients with metastatic GTT may have hCG levels measured in the cerebrospinal fluid (CSF) to exclude cerebral involvement if the head CT is normal. The plasma/CSF hCG ratio tends to be <60 in the presence of cerebral metastases[20]. However, rapid changes in plasma hCG levels may not be promptly reflected in the CSF such that a single plasma/CSF hCG ratio may be misleading[21]. Bakri *et al.* reported that the serum/CSF hCG ratio was >60 in five of nine patients with cerebral metastases[17].

Pelvic ultrasonography may be useful in detecting extensive uterine involvement and in identifying sites of resistant uterine tumor[22]. The sensitivity of ultrasonography in detecting uterine tumor may be further enhanced by the use of a vaginal probe as well as color flow Doppler[23–26]. Ultrasonography may help to select patients who may benefit from hysterectomy because it can accurately and non-invasively detect extensive uterine tumor.

10.4 STAGING

The International Federation of Gynecology and Obstetrics (FIGO) has adopted an anatomical staging system for GTT (Table 10.1). Stage I includes all patients with tumor confined to the uterine corpus and persistently elevated hCG values. Stage II comprises all patients with tumor outside of the uterus but localized to the pelvis and/or vagina. Stage III disease includes all patients with pulmonary metastases with or without uterine, pelvic or vaginal involvement. Stage

Table 10.1 Staging of GTT

Stage	*Description*
I	Disease confined to uterus
IA	Disease confined to uterus with no risk factors
IB	Disease confined to uterus with one risk factor
IC	Disease confined to uterus with two risk factors
II	GTT extending outside uterus but limited to genital structures (adnexa, vagina, broad ligament)
IIA	GTT involving genital structures without risk factors
IIB	GTT extending outside uterus but limited to genital structures with one risk factor
IIC	GTT extending outside uterus but limited to genital structures with two risk factors
III	GTT extending to lungs with or without known genital tract involvement
IIIA	GTT extending to lungs with or without genital tract involvement and with no risk factors
IIIB	GTT extending to lungs with or without genital tract involvement and with one risk factor
IIIC	GTT extending to lungs with or without genital tract involvement and with two risk factors
IV	All other metastatic sites
IVA	All other metastatic sites without risk factors
IVB	All other metastatic sites with one risk factor
IVC	All other metastatic sites with two risk factors

Risk factors affecting staging include the following: (1) hCG >100 000 U/l and (2) duration of disease >6 months from termination of antecedent pregnancy.

The following factors should be considered and noted in reporting: (1) prior chemotherapy has been given for known GTT; (2) placental site tumors should be reported separately; (3) histological verification of disease is not required.

IV patients have extensive tumor burdens with involvement of the brain, liver, kidneys or gastrointestinal tract. Stage IV tumors commonly follow a non-molar antecedent pregnancy and generally have the histological pattern of CC. Patients with stage IV disease are at highest risk of being resistant to chemotherapy and succumbing to their disease.

It is also helpful to use prognostic variables to predict the likelihood of drug resistance and to assist selecting appropriate chemotherapy[27]. The World Health Organization (WHO) has published a prognostic scoring system which reliably predicts the potential for chemotherapy resistance (Table 10.2)[28]. Most of the prognostic factors relate to sites of metastases, tumor burden (hCG level, number and size of metastases), duration of disease, and the degree of prior chemotherapy exposure and resistance. When the prognostic score is 8 or greater, the patient is considered high-risk and requires intensive combination chemotherapy to attain remission. Patients with stage I GTT generally have a low-risk score and patients with stage IV GTT have a high-risk score. The distinction between low- and high-risk therefore primarily applies to stages II and III disease.

Table 10.2 Scoring system based on prognostic factors

	Score[b]			
Prognostic factors	*0*	*1*	2	4
Age (years)	≤39	>39		
Antecedent pregnancy	hydatidiform mole	Abortion	Term	
Interval[a]	4	4–6	7–12	12
hCG (U/l)	10^3	10^3–10^4	10^4–10^5	10^5
ABO groups (female × male)		O × A A × O	B AB	
Largest tumor, including uterine tumor		3–5 cm	5 cm	
Site of metastases		Spleen Kidney	Gastrointes-tinal tract Liver	Brain
No. of metastases identified		1–4	4–8	8
Prior chemotherapy			Single drug	2 or more drugs

[a]Interval time (months) between end of antecedent pregnancy and start of chemotherapy.
[b]The total score for a patient is obtained by adding the individual scores for each prognostic factor. Total score ≤4, low risk; 5–7, middle risk; ≥8, high risk.

The use of a prognostic scoring system is more predictive of clinical outcome than the use of individual high-risk factors. For example, DuBeshter *et al*. reported complete remission in all 21 patients with traditional high-risk factors whose WHO prognostic score was 7 or less; interestingly, 14 (67%) of these patients attained complete remission with single-agent chemotherapy[29]. Similarly, other investigators have reported that the WHO prognostic scoring system which integrates several prognostic variables is more predictive of patient outcome than reliance upon individual high-risk factors[30–33].

10.5 MANAGEMENT OF STAGE I GTT

The NETDC protocol for the management of stage I GTT and the results of treatment are reviewed in Tables 10.3 and 10.4. The selection of therapy is based primarily upon the patient's desire to retain fertility.

If the patient no longer wishes to preserve fertility, hysterectomy with adjuvant single-agent chemotherapy may be performed as primary treatment. Adjuvant chemotherapy is administered for three reasons: (1) to

Table 10.3 Treatment protocol for stage I GTT (New England Trophoblastic Disease Center)

Initial
Single-agent chemotherapy or
Hysterectomy with adjunctive chemotherapy

Resistant
Combination chemotherapy
Hysterectomy with adjunctive chemotherapy
Local resection
Pelvic infusion

Follow-up
hCG: Weekly until normal × 3
Monthly until normal × 12

Contraception
12 consecutive months of normal hCG levels

Table 10.4 New England Trophoblastic Disease Center, July 1965 to December 1993. Stage I: confined to uterine corpus

Remission therapy	*No. of patients*	*No. of remissions (%)*
Initial	422 (93.6%)	
Sequential MTX/ACTD		385 (91.2)
Hysterectomy		29 (6.9)
MAC		3 (0.7)
EMA		5 (1.2)
Resistant	29 (6.4%)	
MAC		10 (34.5)
EMA		14 (48.3)
Hysterectomy		2 (6.9)
Local uterine resection		2 (6.9)
Pelvic infusion		1 (3.4)
Total	451	451 (100)

MXT, methotrexate; ACTD, actinomycin D; MAC, methotrexate, actinomycin D, cyclophosphamide; EMA, etoposide, methotrexate, actinomycin D.

reduce the likelihood of disseminating viable tumor cells at surgery; (2) to maintain a cytotoxic level of chemotherapy in tissues and the bloodstream in case viable tumor cells are disseminated at surgery; and (3) to treat any occult metastases that may already be present. Chemotherapy may be safely administered at the time of hysterectomy without increasing operative morbidity. Primary hysterectomy and adjuvant chemotherapy was performed on 29 of our patients and all attained complete remission with no further therapy. None of our patients experienced any postoperative bleeding, infection or wound complications.

When patients are diagnosed as having PSTT, they should undergo a prompt and thorough metastatic evaluation. If the patient is found to have non-metastatic disease, hysterectomy should be performed, since PSTT is generally resistant to chemotherapy[34]. There are few long-term survivors with metastatic PSTT despite intensive multimodal therapy[35]. Because PSTT contains little syncytiotrophoblast, hCG levels tend to be low even in the presence of large tumor burdens. Measurement of hCG values is therefore not as sensitive as an indicator of disease status as in other trophoblastic tumors.

Single-agent chemotherapy is the preferred treatment in patients with stage I GTT who desire to preserve fertility. Primary single-agent chemotherapy induced complete remission in 385 (93%) of 414 patients with stage I disease. The remaining 29 resistant patients later achieved remission with either combination chemotherapy or surgical intervention. Local uterine resection may be considered if a patient is resistant to chemotherapy and wants to retain fertility. When local resection is considered, ultrasound, MRI scan and/or arteriography may identify the site of resistant tumor.

Table 10.5 Treatment protocol for stages II and III GTT (New England Trophoblastic Disease Center)

Low-risk[a]	
Initial:	Single-agent chemotherapy
Resistant:	Combination chemotherapy
High risk[a]	
Initial:	Combination chemotherapy
Resistant:	Second-line combination chemotherapy
Follow-up	
hCG:	Weekly until normal × 3 Monthly until normal × 12
Contraception:	
12 consecutive months of normal hCG levels	

[a]Local resection optional.

Eight of our patients with stage I disease were treated with primary combination chemotherapy because of a high prognostic score.

10.6 MANAGEMENT OF STAGE II AND III GTT

Tables 10.5–10.7 review the NETDC protocol for the management of stage II and III disease and the results of therapy. In general, low-risk patients are treated with primary single-agent chemotherapy and high-risk patients are managed with primary combination chemotherapy.

Twenty-seven patients with stage II GTT were treated at the NETDC and all attained remission. Single-agent chemotherapy induced complete remission in 16 (84.2%) of 19 low-risk patients but in only two (50%) of four high risk patients.

Several investigators have demonstrated that single-agent chemotherapy can induce a high remission rate in patients with low-risk metastatic GTT. Table 10.8 outlines the experience from four centers and collectively single-agent chemotherapy induced complete remission in 128 (87.1%) of 147 patients with low-risk metastatic GTT. All patients who were resistant to single-agent chemotherapy later attained remission with combination chemotherapy, except two patients reported by Ayhan *et al.*[29,32,36,37].

Vaginal metastases may bleed profusely because they are highly friable and vascular. Bleeding may be controlled by packing the vagina or performing wide local excision. Infrequently, angiographic embolization of the hypogastric arteries may be required to control hemorrhage from vaginal metastases.

Between July 1965 and December 1993, 130 patients with stage III GTT were managed at the NETDC and 129 (99.2%) achieved complete remission. Single-agent chemotherapy induced complete remission in 71 (83.5%) of 85 low-risk patients and in 13 (65%) of 20 high-risk patients. All patients, who

Table 10.6 New England Trophoblastic Disease Center, July 1965 to December 1993. Stage II: Metastases to pelvis and vagina

Remission therapy		*No. of patients*	*No. of remissions (%)*
Low risk		19 (70.4%)	
Initial:	Sequential MTX/ACTD		16 (84.2)
Resistant:	MAC		2 (10.5)
	EMA-CO		1 (5.3)
High risk		8 (29.6%)	
Initial:	Sequential MTX/ACTD		2 (25.0)
	MAC		4 (50.0)
Resistant:	MAC		1 (12.5)
	CHAMOCA		1 (12.5)
Total		27	27 (100)

MTX, methotrexate; ACTD, actinomycin D; MAC, methotrexate, actinomycin D, cyclophosphamide; CHAMOCA, Bagshawe multi-agent regimen; EMA-CO, etoposide, methotrexate, actinomycin D, cyclophosphamide, oncovin.

Table 10.7 New England Trophoblastic Disease Center, July 1965 to December 1993. Stage III: Metastases to lung

Remission therapy		*No. of patients*	*No. of remissions (%)*
Low risk		85 (65.4%)	
Initial:	Sequential MTX/ACTD		71 (83.5)
Resistant:	MAC		12 (14.1)
	EMA		2 (2.4)
High risk		45 (34.6%)	
Initial:	Sequential MTX/ACTD		13 (28.9)
	MAC		12 (26.6)
	EMA		12 (26.6)
Resistant:	MAC		2 (4.4)
	CHAMOCA		1 (2.2)
	5-FU–Adria		1 (2.2)
	VPB		2 (4.4)
	EMA		1 (2.2)
Total		130	129 (99.2)

MTX, methotrexate; ACTD, actinomycin D; MAC, methotrexate, actinomycin D, cyclophosphamide; EMA, etoposide, methotrexate, actinomycin D; CHAMOCA, Bagshawe multi-agent regimen; 5-FU–Adria, 5-fluorouracil, adriamycin; VPB, vinblastine, cisplatin, bleomycin.

were resistant to single-agent treatment subsequently attained remission with combination chemotherapy.

Thoracotomy has a limited role in the treatment of stage III disease. Thoracotomy should be performed if the diagnosis is seriously in doubt. Furthermore, pulmonary resection may be performed if a patient has

Table 10.8 Results of single-agent chemotherapy in low-risk metastatic GTT (WHO prognostic score ≤7)

Author	*Remission with single-agent chemotherapy*	*Eventual remission rate (%)*
DuBeshter *et al.*[29]	48/55 (87.3%)	55/55 (100)
Dubuc-Lissoir *et al.*[32]	21/25 (84%)	25/25 (100)
Ayhan *et al.*[36]	9/15 (60%)	13/15 (87)
Soper *et al.*[37]	50/52 (96.1%)	52/52 (100)
Total	128/147 (87.1%)	145/145 (98.6)

a persistent viable pulmonary nodule despite intensive chemotherapy[38–40]. Occult sites of resistant viable tumor may be identified by imaging with radioisotope-labeled antibody to hCG[41]. If surgery is considered to excise foci of resistant tumor, a thorough metastatic evaluation must be undertaken to exclude other sites of persistent disease. It is important to emphasize that fibrotic nodules may persist indefinitely on chest radiographs after complete gonadotropin remission is achieved.

Hysterectomy may be required in patients with metastatic disease to control uterine infection or hemorrhage[42]. Additionally, hysterectomy may substantially reduce the tumor burden in patients with bulky uterine tumor and thereby limit the need for chemotherapy.

10.7 MANAGEMENT OF STAGE IV GTT

The NETDC protocol for the management of stage IV disease and the results of therapy are reviewed in Tables 10.9 and 10.10. These patients are at the highest risk for developing rapidly progressive tumor despite intensive therapy. All patients with stage IV GTT should be treated with primary intensive combination chemotherapy and the selective use of radiation therapy and surgery[43]. Before 1975, only six (30%) of 20 patients with stage IV tumor achieved complete remission. However, after 1975, 14 (77.8%) of 18 patients with stage IV GTT attained remission. This dramatic improvement in survival results from the introduction of intensive multimodal therapy early in the course of treatment.

The management of liver metastases is particularly challenging. If a patient is resistant to systemic chemotherapy, hepatic arterial infusion of chemotherapy may induce complete remission in selected cases. Hepatic resection may occasionally be necessary to control bleeding or to excise resistant foci.

Whole brain irradiation is promptly instituted at our center if cerebral metastases are detected. Brace initially reported that brain irradiation may contribute to the eradication of trophoblastic cerebral involvement[44]. The risk of spontaneous intracranial hemorrhage may be reduced by the concurrent use of chemotherapy and brain irradiation[45]. Brain irradiation may be both hemostatic and tumoricidal. Yordan Jr *et al.* reported that deaths due to cerebral involvement occurred in 11 (44%) of 25 patients treated with chemotherapy alone but in none of 18 patients treated with brain irradiation and chemotherapy[46].

However, Rustin *et al.* have documented excellent remission rates in patients with brain involvement who were treated with

Table 10.9 Treatment protocol for stage IV GTT (New England Trophoblastic Disease Center)

Initial	
Combination chemotherapy	
Brain:	Whole head irradiation (3000 rad)
	Craniotomy to manage complications
Liver:	Resection to manage complications
Resistant[a]	
Second-line combination chemotherapy	
Follow-up	
hCG:	Weekly until normal × 3
	Monthly until normal × 24
Contraception	
24 consecutive months of normal hCG levels	

[a]Local resection optional.

Table 10.10 New England Trophoblastic Disease Center, July 1965 to December 1993. Stage IV: distant metastases

Remission therapy[a]		*No. of remissions (%)*	
<1975			
Initial:	Sequential MTX/ACTD	5	
Resistant	MAC	1	6/20 (30%)
>1975			
Initial:	Sequential MTX/ACTD	2	
	MAC	2	
Resistant:	HD MTX/ACTD	4	14/18 (77.8%)
	MAC	1	
	CHAMOCA	1	
	VPB	1	
	EMA	3	

[a]Radiotherapy and surgery utilized when indicated.
HD, high dose; MTX, methotrexate; ACTD, actinomycin D; MAC, methotrexate, actinomycin D, cyclophosphamide; CHAMOCA, Bagshawe multi-agent regimen; VPB, vinblastine, cisplatin, bleomycin; EMA, etoposide, methotrexate, actinomycin D.

chemotherapy alone[47]. Intensive combination chemotherapy including high-dose intravenous and intrathecal methotrexate (MTX) induced sustained remission in 13 (86%) of 15 patients with cerebral lesions. Excellent cure rates can therefore be achieved in patients with cerebral metastases with intensive chemotherapy alone.

Craniotomy may be necessary to provide acute decompression or to control bleeding. Craniotomy should be performed to manage life-threatening complications and thereby provide the opportunity for chemotherapy to induce complete remission. Infrequently, cerebral metastases may be resectable when they are resistant to chemotherapy. Fortunately, most patients with cerebral metastases who achieve remission generally have no residual neurological deficits.

10.8 CHEMOTHERAPY

10.8.1 SINGLE-AGENT CHEMOTHERAPY

Single-agent chemotherapy with either MTX or actinomycin-D (ACTD) has achieved excellent and comparable remission rates in both non-metastatic and low-risk metastatic GTT[48]. Several regimens using MTX and ACTD have been effectively used in the treatment of GTT but no study has compared all of these protocols. An optimal regimen would maximize response rate while minimizing morbidity and cost. Single-agent chemotherapy is administered either at a fixed time interval or on the basis of the hCG regression curve. At our center, after the first course of single-agent chemotherapy, further treatment is withheld as long as the hCG level is falling progressively. A second course of chemotherapy is administered under the following conditions: the hCG level plateaus for more than three consecutive weeks or re-elevates or the hCG level does not decline by 1 log within 18 days after completing the first treatment[49].

MTX with folinic acid (MTX–FA) has been the preferred single-agent regimen at our center[50]. MTX–FA induced complete remission in 147 (90.2%) of 163 patients with stage I GTT and in 15 (68.2%) of 22 patients with low-risk stage II and III GTT. One course of MTX–FA induced remission in 132 (81.5%) of these patients. After three consecutive weeks of non-detectable hCG values were attained, only two (1.1%) patients with non-metastatic disease developed tumor recurrence. Similarly, Hammond *et al.* reported that when single-agent chemotherapy was administered at a fixed time interval and induced remission in patients with non-metastatic GTT, relapse occurred in 2% of patients[51]. Resistance to MTX–FA was more common in patients with CC, metastases and pretreatment hCG levels >50 000 U/l. Following MTX–FA, granulocytopenia (white blood count <1500/mm^3), thrombocytopenia (platelets <100 000/mm^3) and hepatotoxicity (serum glutamic oxaloacetic transaminase (SGOT) >50 U/l) developed in three (1.6%), 11 (5.9%) and 26 (14.1%) patients, respectively. No patient developed sepsis or required platelet transfusion due to myelosuppression. MTX not only induced an excellent remission rate with minimal toxicity but also effectively limited chemotherapy exposure.

10.8.2 COMBINATION CHEMOTHERAPY

Triple therapy (MTX, ACTD and cyclophosphamide or chlorambucil) used to be the preferred combination drug regimen at our center[52]. However, triple therapy induces remission in only about half of patients with metastatic GTT and a high-risk WHO score. Table 10.11 reviews the response rate to primary triple therapy in patients with metastatic GTT and a high risk score from six centers[29,32–33,36,53]. Collectively, triple therapy induced a complete response in only 47 (51%) of 92 patients.

Etoposide (VP16) was first reported in 1977 to have antitumor activity in patients with GTT who were resistant to other chemotherapy[54]. When etoposide was administered as primary therapy, it induced complete remission in 56 (93%) of 60 patients with non-metastatic or low-risk metastatic GTT[55]. In 1984, Bagshawe described a new combination regimen that included etoposide, MTX, ACTD, cyclophosphamide

Table 10.11 Results of primary triple therapy in metastatic GTT with a high-risk WHO score (>7)

Author	*Complete response with triple therapy*	
DuBeshter *et al.*[29]	5/11	(45%)
Gordon *et al.*[31]	11/24	(46%)
Dubuc-Lissoir *et al.*[32]	11/22	(50%)
Mortakis and Braga[33]	12/20	(60%)
Ayhan *et al.*[36]	3/7	(43%)
Curry *et al.*[53]	5/8	(63%)
Total	47/92	(51%)

Table 10.12 Results of primary EMA-CO in metastatic GTT with a high-risk WHO score (>7)

Author	*Complete response with EMA-CO*	
Bolis *et al.*[57]	16/17	(94%)
Newlands *et al.*[58]	53/76	(70%)
Schink *et al.*[59]	3/5	(60%}
Soper *et al.*[60]	4/6	(67%)
Total	76/104	(73%)

and vincristine (EMA-CO) and reported 83% remission in patients with metastases and a high-risk score[56]. EMA-CO is currently the preferred primary treatment in patients with high-risk metastatic GTT. Table 10.12 reviews the results of primary EMA-CO therapy in high-risk metastatic GTT from four centers[57–60]. Collectively, primary EMA-CO induced complete remission in 76 (73%) of 104 patients with high-risk metastatic GTT. Similarly, Quinn *et al.* observed that primary EMA-CO induced complete sustained remission in 61 (94%) of 65 patients with a WHO score ≥5[61]. The EMA-CO regimen is generally well tolerated and treatment seldom has to be suspended because of toxicity.

If patients are resistant to EMA-CO, they are then treated with modification of this regimen by substituting cisplatin (75 mg/m^2) and etoposide (150 mg/m^2) on day 8 (EMA-CE). Newlands *et al.* reported that EMA-CE alone or in conjunction with surgery induced remission in nine (82%) of 11 patients and 14 (70%) of 20 patients, respectively, who were resistant to EMA-CO[58]. If patients are resistant to EMA-CO, surgical intervention may be necessary to remove sites of resistant disease.

Second-line therapy with cisplatin, vinblastine and bleomycin (PVB) may also be effective in patients with GTT. Gordon *et al.* reported that PVB induced complete sustained remission in two of 11 patients with prior resistance to triple therapy[62]. Additionally, DuBeshter *et al.* and Azab *et al.* reported complete remission with PVB in four of seven and five of eight patients, respectively, with drug-resistant GTT[63,64].

Patients who require combination chemotherapy must be treated intensively to achieve remission. We administer combination chemotherapy as frequently as toxicity permits until the patient attains three consecutive non-detectable hCG values. After the patient achieves non-detectable hCG levels, three additional courses of chemotherapy are administered to reduce the risk of relapse.

10.9 FOLLOW-UP

All patients with stages I, II and III GTT are followed with weekly hCG levels until undetectable for three weeks and then monthly hCG values until undetectable for 12 months. Patients with stage IV disease are monitored with monthly hCG levels until undetectable for 24 months because they have an increased risk for late relapse. After 12 or 24 months of follow-up, patients should be followed every six months for five years and then annually for life.

Mutch *et al.* reported recurrences after initial remission in 2% of patients with non-metastatic GTT, 4% of patients with good-prognosis metastatic GTT and 13% of patients with poor-prognosis disease[65]. Recurrences occurred within three and 18 months in 50% and 85% of patients, respectively.

Patients are encouraged to use reliable contraception during gonadotropin follow-up. Oral contraceptives may be of particular benefit for patients who receive intensive or prolonged chemotherapy. Intensive chemotherapy may induce ovarian dysfunction and thereby cause elevated serum levels of luteinizing hormone which may interfere with measurement of low levels of hCG.

REFERENCES

1. Goldstein, D.P. and Berkowitz, R.S. (1982) *Gestational Trophoblastic Neoplasms: Clinical Principles of Diagnosis and Management*, Saunders, Philadelphia.
2. Bagshawe, K.D. and Begent, R.H.J. (1981) Trophoblastic tumours: clinical features and management, in *Gynaecological Oncology* (ed. M. Coppleston), Chapman & Hall, London, pp. 757–72.
3. Xia, Z. and Wang, Y. (1983) 5-Fluorouracil in malignant trophoblastic tumors: report of 350 cases. *Chin. Med. J.*, **96**, 121–30.
4. Berkowitz, R.S. and Goldstein, D.P. (1993) Management of molar pregnancy and gestational trophoblastic tumors, in *Gynecologic Oncology*, (eds R. Knapp and R. Berkowitz), McGraw-Hill, New York, pp. 328–38.
5. Berkowitz, R.S. and Goldstein, D.P. (1981) Pathogenesis of gestational trophoblastic neoplasms. *Pathobiol. Ann.*, **11**, 391–411.
6. Bagshawe, K.D. and Noble, M.I.M. (1966) Cardio-respiratory aspects of trophoblastic tumours. *Q. J. Med.*, **137**, 39–54.
7. Sung, H.-C., Wu, P.-C., Hu, M-H. and Su, H.-T. (1982) Roentgenologic manifestations of pulmonary metastases in choriocarcinoma and invasive mole. *Am. J. Obstet. Gynecol.*, **142**, 89–97.
8. Bagshawe, K.D. and Garnett, E.S. (1963) Radiological changes in the lungs of patients with trophoblastic tumours. *Br. J. Radiol.*, **36**, 673–9.
9. Evans, K.T., Cockshott, W.P. and Hendrickse, P. (1965) Pulmonary changes in malignant trophoblastic disease. *Br. J. Radiol.*, **38**, 161–71.
10. Libshitz, H.I., Baber, C.E. and Hammond, C.B. (1977) The pulmonary metastases of choriocarcinoma. *Obstet. Gynecol.*, **49**, 412–16.
11. Bakri, Y.N., Berkowitz, R.S., Khan, J. *et al.* (1994) Pulmonary metastases of gestational trophoblastic tumor: risk factors for early respiratory failure. *J. Reprod. Med.*, **39**, 175–8.
12. Kelly, M.P., Rustin, G.J.S., Ivory, C. and Bagshawe, K.D. (1990) Respiratory failure due to choriocarcinoma: a study of 103 dyspneic patients. *Gynecol. Oncol.*, **38**, 149–54.

13. Jones, W.B., Wagner-Reiss, K.M. and Lewis, J.L., Jr (1990) Intracerebral choriocarcinoma. *Gynecol. Oncol.*, **38**, 234–43.
14. Song, H. and Wu, B. (1979) Brain metastasis in choriocarcinoma and malignant mole. *Chin. Med. J.*, **92**, 164–74.
15. Liu, T.-L., Deppe, G., Chang, Q.-T. and Tan, T.-T. (1983) Cerebral metastatic choriocarcinoma in the People's Republic of China. *Gynecol. Oncol.*, **15**, 166–70.
16. Athanassiou, A., Begent, R.H.J., Newlands, E.S. *et al.* (1983) Central nervous system metastases of choriocarcinoma: 23 years' experience at Charing Cross Hospital. *Cancer*, **52**, 1728–35.
17. Bakri, Y.N., Berkowitz, R.S., Goldstein, D.P. *et al.* (1994) Brain metastases of gestational trophoblastic tumor. *J. Reprod. Med.*, **39**, 179–84.
18. Bakri, Y.N., Subhi, J., Amer, M. *et al.* (1993) Liver metastases of gestational trophoblastic tumor. *Gynecol. Oncol.*, **48**, 110–13.
19. Mutch, D.G., Soper, J.T., Baker, M.E. *et al.* (1986) Role of computed axial tomography of the chest in staging patients with nonmetastatic gestational trophoblastic disease. *Obstet. Gynecol.*, **68**, 348–52.
20. Bagshawe, K.D. and Harland, S. (1976) Immunodiagnosis and monitoring of gonadotropin-producing metastases in the central nervous system. *Cancer*, **38**, 112–18.
21. Berkowitz, R.S., Osathanondh, R., Goldstein, D.P. *et al.* (1981) Cerebrospinal fluid human chorionic gonadotropin levels in normal pregnancy and choriocarcinoma. *Surg. Gynecol. Obstet.*, **153**, 687–9.
22. Berkowitz, R.S., Birnholz, J., Goldstein, D.P. and Bernstein, M.R. (1983) Pelvic ultrasonography and the management of gestational trophoblastic disease. *Gynecol. Oncol.*, **15**, 403–12.
23. Mangili, G., Spagnolo, D., Valsecchi, L. and Maggi, R. (1993) Transvaginal ultrasound in persistent trophoblastic tumor. *Am. J. Obstet. Gynecol.*, **169**, 1218–23.
24. Dobkin, G.R., Berkowitz, R.S., Goldstein, D.P. *et al.* (1991) Duplex ultrasonography for persistent gestational trophoblastic tumor. *J. Reprod. Med.*, **36**, 14–16.
25. Long, M.G., Boultbee, J.E., Begent, R.H.J. *et al.* (1990) Preliminary Doppler studies on the uterine artery and myometrium in trophoblastic tumors requiring chemotherapy. *Br. J. Obstet. Gynaecol.*, **97**, 686–9.
26. Hsieh, F.-J., Wu, C.-C., Chen, C.-A. *et al.* (1994) Correlation of uterine hemodynamics with chemotherapy response in gestational trophoblastic tumors. *Obstet Gynecol.*, **83**, 1021–5.
27. Bagshawe, K.D. (1976) Risk and prognostic factors in trophoblastic neoplasia. *Cancer*, **38**, 1373–85.
28. World Health Organization (1983) Trophoblastic diseases. *WHO Tech. Rep. Ser. 692*.
29. DuBeshter, B., Berkowitz, R.S., Goldstein, D.P. *et al.* (1987) Metastatic gestational trophoblastic disease: experience at the New England Trophoblastic Disease Center, 1965–1985. *Obstet. Gynecol.*, **69**, 390–5.
30. Lurain J.R., Casanova, L.A., Miller, D.S. and Rademaker, A.W. (1991) Prognostic factors in gestational trophoblastic tumors: a proposed new scoring system based on multivariate analysis. *Am. J. Obstet. Gynecol.*, **164**, 611–16.
31. Gordon, A.N., Gershenson, D.M., Copeland, L.J. *et al.* (1989) High-risk metastatic gestational trophoblastic disease: further stratification into two clinical entities. *Gynecol. Oncol.*, **34**, 54–6.
32. Dubuc-Lissoir, J., Sweizig S., Schlaerth, J.B. and Morrow, C.P. (1992) Metastatic gestational trophoblastic disease: a comparison of prognostic classification systems. *Gynecol. Oncol.*, **45**, 40–5.
33. Mortakis, A. and Braga, C.A. (1990) 'Poor prognosis' metastatic gestational trophoblastic disease: the prognostic significance of the scoring system in predicting chemotherapy failures. *Obstet. Gynecol.*, **76**, 272–7.
34. Finkler, N.J., Berkowitz, R.S., Driscoll, S.D. *et al.* (1988) Clinical experience with placental site trophoblastic tumors at the New England Trophoblastic Disease Center. *Obstet. Gynecol.*, **71**, 854–7.
35. Dessau, R., Rustin, G.J.S., Dent, J. *et al.* (1990) Surgery and chemotherapy in the management of placental site tumor. *Gynecol. Oncol.*, **39**, 56–9.
36. Ayhan, A., Yapar, E.G., Deren, O. and Kisnisci, H. (1992) Remission rates and significance of prognostic factors in gestational

trophoblastic tumors. *J. Reprod. Med.*, **37**, 461–5.

37. Soper, J.T., Clarke-Pearson, D.L., Berchuck, A. *et al.* (1994) 5-Day methotrexate for women with metastatic gestational trophoblastic disease. *Gynecol. Oncol.*, **54**, 76–9.
38. Shirley, R.L., Goldstein, D.P. and Collins, J.J., Jr (1972) The role of thoracotomy in management of patients with chest metastases from gestational trophoblastic disease. *J. Thorac. Cardiovasc. Surg.*, **63**, 545–50.
39. Edwards, J.L., Makey, A.R. and Bagshawe, K.D. (1975) The role of thoracotomy in the management of pulmonary metastases of gestational choriocarcinoma. *Clin. Oncol.*, **1**, 329–39.
40. Tomoda, Y., Arii, Y., Kaseki, S. *et al.* (1980) Surgical indications for resection in pulmonary metastases of choriocarcinoma. *Cancer*, **46**, 2723–30.
41. Begent, R.H., Bagshawe, K.D. and Green, A.J. (1987) The clinical value of imaging with antibody to human chorionic gonadotropin in the detection of residual choriocarcinoma. *Br. J. Cancer*, **55**, 657–60.
42. Soper, J.T. (1994) Surgical therapy for gestational trophoblastic disease. *J. Reprod. Med.*, **39**, 168–74.
43. Lurain, J.R. (1994) High-risk metastatic gestational trophoblastic tumors: current management. *J. Reprod. Med.*, **39**, 217–22.
44. Brace, K.C. (1968) The role of irradiation in the treatment of metastatic trophoblastic disease. *Radiology*, **91**, 540–4.
45. Weed, J.C. and Hammond, C.B. (1980) Cerebral metastatic choriocarcinoma: intensive therapy and prognosis. *Obstet. Gynecol.*, **55**, 89–94
46. Yordan, E.L., Jr, Schlaerth, J., Gaddis, O. and Morrow, C.P. (1987) Radiation therapy in the management of gestational choriocarcinoma metastatic to the central nervous system. *Obstet. Gynecol.*, **69**, 627–30.
47. Rustin, G.J.S, Newlands, E.S., Begent, R.H.J. *et al.* (1989) Weekly alternating etoposide, methotrexate, actinomycin-D/vincristine and cyclophosphamide chemotherapy for treatment of CNS metastases of choriocarcinoma. *J. Clin. Oncol.*, **7**, 900–3.
48. Homesley, H.D. (1994) Development of single-agent chemotherapy regimens for gestational trophoblastic disease. *J. Reprod. Med.*, **39**, 185–92.
49. Berkowitz, R.S. and Goldstein, D.P. (1979) Methotrexate with citrovorum factor rescue for nonmetastatic gestational trophoblastic disease. *Obstet. Gynecol.*, **54**, 725–8.
50. Berkowitz, R.S., Goldstein, D.P. and Bernstein, M.R. (1986) Ten years experience with methotrexate and folinic acid as primary therapy for gestational trophoblastic disease. *Gynecol. Oncol.*, **23**, 111–18.
51. Hammond, C.B., Weed, J.C., Jr and Currie, J.L. (1980) The role of operation in the current therapy of gestational trophoblastic disease. *Am. J. Obstet. Gynecol.*, **136**, 844–56.
52. Berkowitz, R.S., Goldstein, D.P. and Bernstein, M.R. (1984) Modified triple chemotherapy in the management of high-risk metastatic gestational trophoblastic tumors. *Gynecol. Oncol.*, **19**, 173–81.
53. Curry, S.L., Blessing, J.A., DiSaia, P.J. *et al.* (1989) A prospective randomized comparison of methotrexate, dactinomycin and chlorambucil versus methotrexate, dactinomycin, cyclophosphamide, doxorubicin, melphalan, hydroxyurea, and vincristine in 'poor prognosis' metastatic gestational trophoblastic disease: a Gynecologic Oncology Group Study. *Obstet. Gynecol.*, **73**, 357–62.
54. Newlands, E.S. and Bagshawe, K.D. (1977) Epipodophyllin derivative (VP16-213) in malignant teratomas and choriocarcinomas. *Lancet*, **ii**, 87.
55. Wong, L.C., Choo, Y.C. and Ma, H.K. (1986) Primary oral etoposide therapy in gestational trophoblastic disease, an update. *Cancer*, **58**, 14–17.
56. Bagshawe, K.D. (1984) Treatment of high-risk choriocarcinoma. *J. Reprod. Med.*, **29**, 813–20.
57. Bolis, G., Bonazzi, C., Landoni, F. *et al.* (1988) EMA/CO regimen in high-risk gestational trophoblastic tumor (GTT). *Gynecol. Oncol.*, **31**, 439–44.
58. Newlands, E.S., Bagshawe, K.D., Begent, R.H.J. *et al.* (1991) Results with the EMA/CO (etoposide, methotrexate, actinomycin D, cyclophosphamide, vincristine) regimen in high risk gestational trophoblastic tumours, 1979–1989. *Br. J. Obstet. Gynaecol.*, **98**, 550–7.

59. Schink, J.C., Singh, D.K., Rademaker, A.W. *et al.* (1992) Etoposide, methotrexate, actinomycin D, cyclophosphamide and vincristine for the treatment of metastatic, high-risk gestational trophoblastic disease. *Obstet. Gynecol.*, **80**, 817–20.
60. Soper, J.T., Evans, A.C., Clarke-Pearson, D.L. *et al.* (1994) Alternating weekly chemotherapy with etoposide methotrexate dactinomycin/ cyclophosphamide vincristine for high-risk gestational trophoblastic disease. *Obstet. Gynecol.*, **83**, 113–17.
61. Quinn, M., Murray, J., Friedlander, S. *et al.* (1994) EMACO in high risk gestational trophoblastic disease: the Australian experience. *Aust. N.Z. J. Obstet. Gynecol.*, **34**, 90–2.
62. Gordon, A.N., Kavanaugh, J.J., Gershenson, D.M. *et al.* (1986) Cisplatin, vinblastine and bleomycin combination therapy in resistant gestational trophoblastic disease. *Cancer*, **58**, 1407–10.
63. DuBeshter, B., Berkowitz, R.S., Goldstein, D.P. and Bernstein, M.R. (1989) Vinblastine, cisplatin and bleomycin as salvage therapy for refractory high-risk metastatic gestational trophoblastic disease. *J. Reprod. Med.*, **34**, 189–92.
64. Azab, M., Droz, J., Theodore C. *et al.* (1989) Cisplatin, vinblastine, and bleomycin combination in the treatment of resistant high-risk gestational trophoblastic tumors. *Cancer*, **64**, 1829–32.
65. Mutch, D.G., Soper, J.T., Babcock, C.J. *et al.* (1990) Recurrent gestational trophoblastic disease: experience of the Southeastern Regional Trophoblastic Disease Center. *Cancer*, **66**, 978–82.

INVESTIGATION AND TREATMENT OF PATIENTS WITH PERSISTENT GESTATIONAL TROPHOBLASTIC DISEASE AND GESTATIONAL TROPHOBLASTIC TUMORS IN THE UK

11

Edward S Newlands

11.1 INTRODUCTION

Since the treatment of patients with gestational trophoblastic disease (GTD) and gestational trophoblastic tumors (GTT) depends on a range of prognostic variables, the clinical history and examination are important. The majority of patients treated at a trophoblastic disease center will be patients who have been registered for follow-up after evacuation of a hydatidiform mole. Since these patients will have been monitored with serial human chorionic gonadotropin (hCG) estimations, they will normally have disease limited to the pelvis or early metastatic disease in the lungs. The main symptoms these patients have are varying amounts of vaginal bleeding and pelvic discomfort and the effects of hCG and the other hormones produced by the persistent trophoblastic disease (PTD). Patients presenting with GTD/GTT after term delivery or non-molar abortions have a much more diverse history (Chapter 9). They may have varying amounts of vaginal bleeding and some patients will have symptoms from metastatic disease. The interval from the prior pregnancy can also be difficult to determine and it can be many months.

Clinical examination of these patients will quite commonly detect uterine enlargement, sometimes with parametrial involvement and vaginal metastases (Figure 11.1). GTD and GTT rarely metastasize to lymph nodes. The exceptions to this general rule are the placental site trophoblastic tumors (PSTT) (Chapter

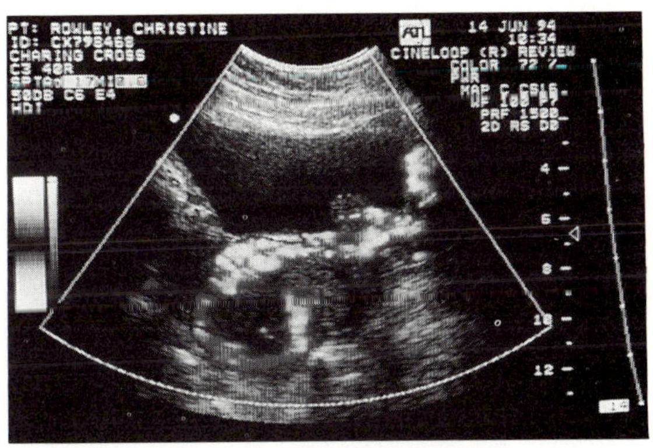

Figure 11.1 Ultrasound with Doppler of a patient with PTD post-hydatidiform mole with extension of the disease into the parametrial tissues and extending down between the bladder and vagina. Colour Doppler emphasizes the highly vascular nature of both PTD and GTD.

Gestational Trophoblastic Disease.
Edited by B.W. Hancock, E.S. Newlands and R.S. Berkowitz.
ISBN 0 412 63100 8

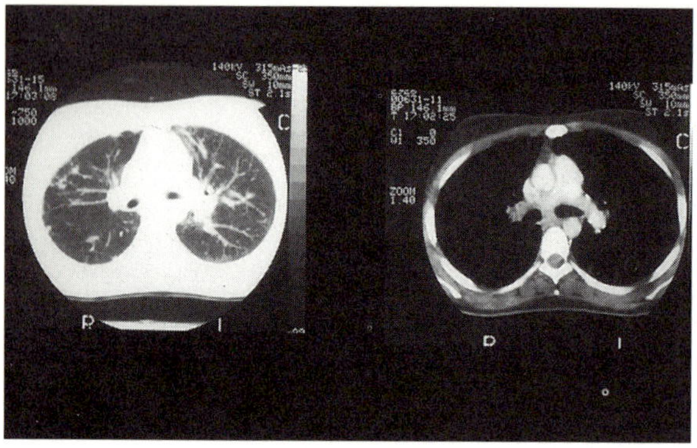

Figure 11.2 Patient presenting with symptoms compatible with multiple pulmonary emboli with progressive shortness of breath and recurrent episodes of pleuritic chest pain. The pulmonary arteriogram illustrates the extensive vascular occlusion from tumor growing in the pulmonary artery. Following successful treatment of her GTT, there was considerable revascularization of the pulmonary arteries and she had an uneventful subsequent pregnancy.

9). Clinical examination is unlikely to detect anything but gross pulmonary disease although it may pick up evidence of other metastatic sites such as brain and liver. One particular variant of GTT that can be detected clinically is when the tumor is growing in the pulmonary artery and there is evidence of pulmonary hypertension (Figure 11.2). This rare variant of the disease can mimic multiple pulmonary emboli[1]. Clinical evidence of hyperthyroidism is uncommon unless the hCG is >10^6 U/l and rarely needs treatment since this responds rapidly to the appropriate treatment of the tumor.

The principal investigations for these patients are listed below.

11.1.1 HISTOPATHOLOGY

This will normally be available for patients who have had a molar pregnancy and in most cases with non-molar pregnancies.

11.1.2 hCG ESTIMATIONS

This provides the key to monitoring the activity of the disease and its response to treatment.

11.1.3 ULTRASOUND

Ultrasound with Doppler assessment is now routine in managing these patients. In the pelvis the uterine size can be measured, providing an additional potential prognostic variable[2]. Doppler ultrasound can assess the vascularity of the disease (Figure 11.3).

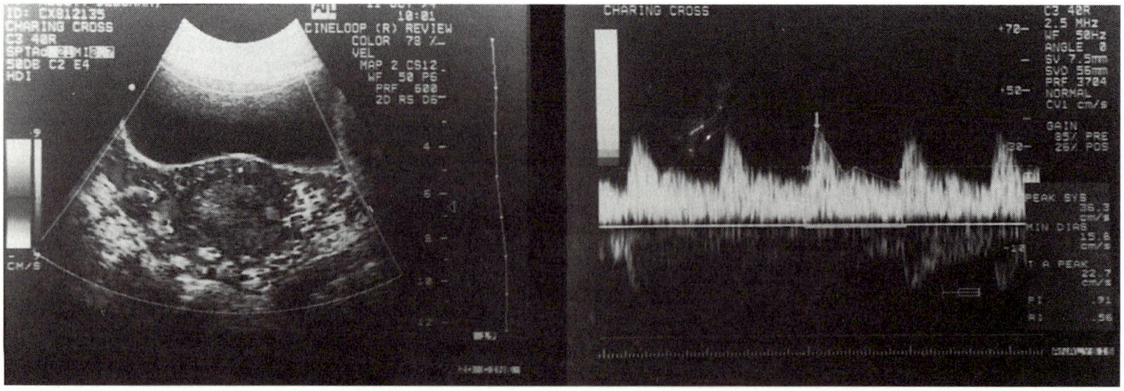

Figure 11.3 Ultrasound of patient with high-risk GTT with disease in the uterus with extensive abnormal vascularity around the tumor. On the right of the figure, Doppler shows the considerably increased blood flow in the uterine artery.

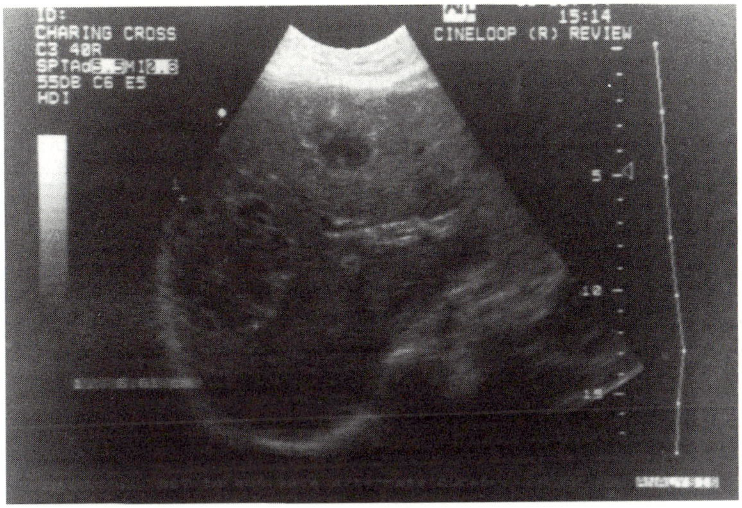

Figure 11.4 Ultrasound of the liver in a patient with high-risk GTT. The patient had an unusual distribution of disease involving liver, small bowel and uterus.

In addition we routinely ultrasound the liver for hepatic metastases (Figure 11.4).

We have analyzed the ultrasound results in several groups of patients with GTD and GTT. Uterine volume measured on ultrasound is clearly much more accurate than clinical examination. In an earlier analysis[2] we reported that a low pulsatility index in the uterine arteries (as measured by Doppler ultrasound) correlated with the development of drug resistance in the tumor. However, we repeated this analysis on a larger cohort and in this group of patients the closest correlation with treatment outcome was in patients with an hCG of $>10^4$ U/l and a uterine volume of >120 ml[3]. In patients with low-risk disease (Table 11.1) this combination of hCG and uterine volume predicted a 50% chance of developing drug resistance to methotrexate. Potentially this prognostic variable could be added to Table 11.1. However, given the long-term safety record of methotrexate (Chapter 16), we have continued treating these patients as low risk[4].

11.1.4 COMPUTED TOMOGRAPHIC SCANNING

Although computed tomography (CT) scanning of the chest is more sensitive than chest X-ray, we do not routinely CT scan the whole body unless there are clinical indications. Low-risk patients are usually managed on the basis of chest X-ray; however, in high-risk patients delineation of disease sites is important in determining overall management. All patients with high-risk disease and pulmonary metastases should also have a CT or magnetic resonance imaging (MRI) brain scan.

11.1.5 LUMBAR PUNCTURES

Patients with pulmonary disease are at risk of developing brain metastases and our experience is that cerebrospinal fluid (CSF) hCG estimations are useful in detecting tumor involvement of the neuraxis which can lead to the secretion of hCG into the CSF, reducing the serum CSF : hCG ratio to less than 65 : 1[5]. Despite advances in CT and MRI scanning, occasionally sites of metastatic disease can be detected by this simple technique when the scans are normal.

11.2 NURSING/COUNSELING

An important aspect of the management of these patients who are admitted to a trophoblastic disease unit is that they are treated by staff who have experience of this disease. They need to establish close rapport with the nursing and medical staff. There are a number of reasons why these patients have additional stresses in addition to the diagnosis of a disease that needs chemotherapy and which is either frankly malignant or evolving towards malignancy. The majority of these patients have young children and many have the additional distress of a recent pregnancy which has resulted in their disease rather than a child. These patients need counseling and considerable support from the staff. In addition it is important for patients to establish contact with other women with similar problems so that they do not feel isolated.

On admission, patients are naturally both anxious and depressed. Those who have had a recent pregnancy which has resulted in both a 'miscarriage' and their disease express feelings of loss and bereavement. The diagnosis of a disease which is either potentially malignant or frankly malignant causes anxiety. Fears about the side effects of chemotherapy are common, particularly alopecia and nausea and vomiting. There are commonly feelings of both anger and guilt between the patient and her partner. The majority of patients have very practical worries about how their families can cope during their treatment.

During treatment patients need continuing emotional support from the staff. While the side effects of methotrexate and folinic acid are frequently mild, more intensive chemotherapy will result in varying degrees of alopecia and other side effects. The stress of continuing on chemotherapy, particularly for the high-risk group, gets worse the longer the duration of treatment. Counseling and support from nursing and medical staff are important to persuade the patient that, despite the problems of the current treatment, the long-term outlook for most patients is excellent.

At the end of their treatment, patients can again feel anxious and depressed: anxious that on stopping chemotherapy their disease may relapse, and depressed because the support from the staff will be less. They need encouragement to re-establish their normal lifestyle and relationships with their families.

11.3 PROGNOSTIC FACTORS

A range of prognostic factors has been established which allow the adjustment of the intensity of treatment that an individual patient needs to eliminate her disease[4]. GTD and GTT form a spectrum of disease ranging from those whose disease can be eliminated with minimally toxic chemotherapy to highly aggressive tumors where intensive chemotherapy, sometimes with salvage surgery, is required.

Several staging classification systems have been devised (Chapter 6). At the Charing Cross Hospital we have continued to use a minor modification of the prognostic variables that were originally reported by Bagshawe in 1976[4] (Table 11.1). The major adverse prognostic variables are given a higher numerical score. Going through the variables in Table 11.1: age is a minor prognostic variable; the antecedent pregnancy is important since patients who have had a term pregnancy immediately prior to their GTT will have histological choriocarcinoma and an aggressive tumor to treat. The interval from the antecedent pregnancy to starting chemotherapy is a particularly important variable. Patients whose disease has been present

Table 11.1 Charing Cross Hospital scoring system for gestational trophoblastic disease

	Charing Cross scoring system			
Variable	*0*	*1*	*2*	*6*
Age (years)	<39	>39		
Antecedent pregnancy (AP)	Mole	Abortion or unknown	Term	
Interval (end of AP to chemotherapy at Charing Cross Hospital (months)	<4	4–7	7–12	>12
hCG (U/l)	10^3–10^4	<10^3	10^4–10^5	>10^4
ABO (female × male)		A × O O × A O or A × unknown	B × A or O AB × A or O	
Number of metastases	Nil	1–4	4–8	>8
Site of metastases	Not detected, lungs, vagina	Spleen, kidney	Gastrointestinal tract, liver	Brain
Largest tumor mass	<3 cm	3–5 cm	>5 cm	
Previous chemotherapy	Nil	Nil	Single drug	2 or more drugs

Low-risk = 0–5; medium risk = 6–9; high risk >9.
Modified 1983 from Bagshawe [4].

for more than 12 months from the antecedent pregnancy are more likely to develop drug-resistant disease. The concentrations of hCG reflect the quantity of viable tumor and it is widely accepted that a serum hCG of >10^5 U/l is an adverse prognostic variable. In the original analysis of Bagshawe[4], blood groups were a minor prognostic variable. The number, site and size of metastases, as might be expected, reflect the overall quantity of disease. The last prognostic variable is failure of prior chemotherapy. Drug resistance can be induced in GTD and GTT by failure to eliminate the disease promptly. Drug resistance remains one of the two significant causes of mortality in this patient population.

From the history, examination and investigations outlined above, patients can be allocated to one of the three risk groups: low, medium and high. The proportion of patients falling into each of these groups is shown in Table 11.2. We have analyzed patients both by the International Federation

Table 11.2 Risk factors in patients treated for gestational trophoblastic tumors. Charing Cross Hospital (1958–1994)

Risk group	*No. (%)*
Low	984 (62)
Medium	350 (22)
High	262 (16)
Total	1596

Table 11.3 Charing Cross Hospital treatment schedules for GTD

Low-risk: methotrexate/folinic acid	
Day 1	Methotrexate 50 mg i.m. at 1200 h
Day 2	Folinic acid 6 mg i.m. or p.o. at 1800 h
Day 3	Methotrexate 50 mg i.m. at 1200 h
Day 4	Folinic acid 6 mg i.m. or p.o. at 1800 h
Day 5	Methotrexate 50 mg i.m. at 1200 h
Day 6	Folinic acid 6 mg i.m. or p.o. at 1800 h
Day 7	Methotrexate 50 mg i.m. at 1200 h
Day 8	Folinic acid 6 mg i.m. or p.o. at 1800 h
Cycles are repeated after a 6-day drug-free interval	
Medium-risk	
1. Treatment a: etoposide	
Day 1	Etoposide 250 mg/m^2 i.v. in 500 ml N saline over 1 h
Day 2	No treatment
Day 3	Etoposide 250 mg/m^2 i.v. in 500 ml N saline over 1 h
2. Treatment b: HuMMP	
Day 1	Hydroxyurea 500 mg oral 12-hourly × 2 doses
Day 2	Methotrexate 50 mg i.m. at 1200 h
Day 3	6 Mercaptopurine 75 mg oral at 1200 h Folinic acid 6 mg i.m. or p.o. at 1800 h
Day 4	Methotrexate 50 mg i.m. at 1200 h
Day 5	6 Mercaptopurine 75 mg oral at 1200 h Folinic acid 6 mg i.m. or p.o. at 1800 h
Day 6	Methotrexate 50 mg i.m. at 1200 h
Day 7	6 Mercaptopurine 75 mg oral at 1200 h Folinic acid 6 mg i.m. or p.o. at 1800 h
Day 8	Methotrexate 50 mg i.m. at 1200 h
Day 9	6 Mercaptopurine 75 mg oral at 1200 h Folinic acid 6 mg i.m. or p.o. at 1800 h
3. Treatment c: Actinomycin D	
Actinomycin D 0.5 mg i.v. days 1–5 inclusive	
Sequence: a, b, c, b, a, b, c, b, with 6-day intervals between courses	
High-risk	
EMA-CO	
Week 1	
Day 1	Actinomycin D 0.5 mg i.v. bolus Etoposide 100 mg/m^2 i.v. in 500 ml N saline over 30 min Methotrexate 300 mg/m^2 i.v. in 1 litre N saline over 12 h
Day 2	Actinomycin D 0.5 mg i.v. bolus Etoposide 100 mg/m^2 i.v. in 500 ml N saline over 30 min Folinic acid 15 mg oral/i.m. 12-hourly × 4 doses starting 24 h after commencing methotrexate
Week 2	Vincristine 1.4 mg/m^2 i.v. bolus (max. 2 mg) Cyclophosphamide 600 mg/m^2 i.v. in 500 ml N saline over 30 min

of Gynecology and Obstetrics (FIGO) staging and prognostic scoring system and have confirmed that by using the FIGO staging alone there is a risk of both under- and overtreatment in some patients[6]. The treatment schedules used at the Charing Cross Hospital are shown in Table 11.3.

11.4 TREATMENT

The introduction of methotrexate in the management of GTT was a major landmark in the development of cancer chemotherapy. Hertz and Tullner[7,8] recognized that antifolates had antiproliferative effects. Li *et al.*[9] discovered the activity of methotrexate in patients with GTT. Initially methotrexate was administered by schedules which were quite toxic but with the introduction of folinic acid, which bypasses the metabolic block induced by methotrexate, this problem has been minimized. Actinomycin D was also introduced early in the management of GTT[10]. However, with the stratification of patients into prognostic groups[4] the majority of low-risk patients can be cured with methotrexate and folinic acid[11–13].

11.5 PROPHYLACTIC CHEMOTHERAPY

The role of prophylactic chemotherapy in patients at risk of PTD following a hydatidiform mole has been proposed as a method of eliminating PTD in patients who cannot be readily followed up with serial hCG estimations[14]. Follow-up of a large trial of 293 patients given prophylactic methotrexate therapy and 127 patients as controls has been reported[15]. The conclusion was that this approach did not eliminate the subsequent development of GTT. Provided that patients can be followed adequately with serial hCG estimations, there is no clinical justification for exposing women unnecessarily to cytotoxic chemotherapy. If follow-up is not possible, it is probably safer to treat the patient as having established GTD (see section 11.5.1). Incomplete chemotherapy carries the risk of inducing drug resistance.

11.5.1 LOW-RISK PATIENTS

The majority of low-risk patients have post-molar GTD limited to the pelvis. These patients are treated with methotrexate and folinic acid as shown in Table 11.3 and Figure 11.5. In general, this schedule is well tolerated provided the patient has normal renal function and high fluid intake, since methotrexate is excreted in the urine. Some patients will need an increase in the dose of folinic acid to either 9 or 12 mg if their mucosa is particularly sensitive to methotrexate. Occasionally patients develop methotrexate-induced hepatic damage with progressively rising transaminases, requiring a change of treatment. Some patients develop varying amounts of pleuritic chest pain and occasionally peritonism from a methotrexate-induced serositis. This unusual side effect rarely occurs with methotrexate except when it is used in this schedule. Methotrexate has two major advantages over other cytotoxic agents in that it does not induce alopecia and its long-term safety profile is excellent (Chapter 16).

In 1989[11] we reported the results using the methotrexate and folinic acid schedule shown in Table 11.3. Prior to 1974, when the prognostic variables (Table 11.1) were routinely introduced into the management of patients, we had treated 126 patients with an overall survival of 87%. When these patients were retrospectively stratified by the prognostic variables shown in Table 11.1, the survival fell from 96% in the low risk patients to 91% in the medium-risk patients and to only 31% in patients in the high-risk group. Although this was a retrospective analysis, it clearly showed that methotrexate as a single agent is inappropriate treatment for patients with high-risk disease. When the prognostic variables were used to stratify patients' treatment from

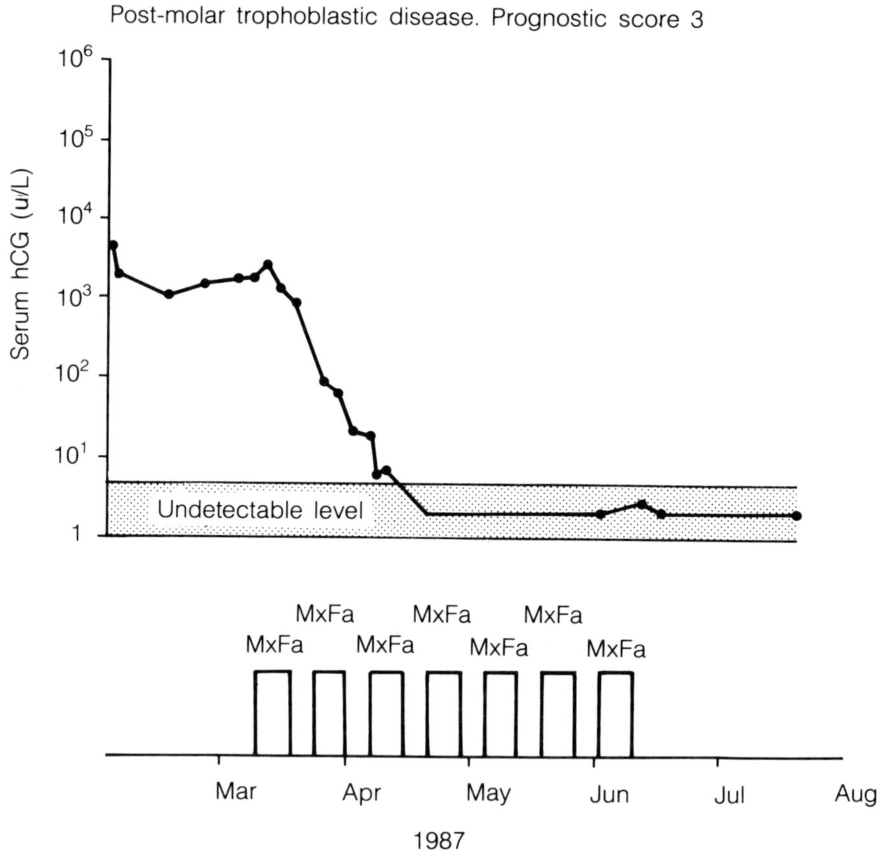

Figure 11.5 Patient with low-risk PTD treated successfully with methotrexate and folinic acid (see Table 11.3).

the start, the survival was 347 out of 348 (99.7%) (Table 11.4). The sole death in this group was due to a patient's concurrent non-Hodgkin's lymphoma (not therapy induced). Given its efficacy and safety profile, methotrexate/folinic acid remains the treatment of choice for patients in the low-risk category of GTD and GTT.

However, the same report also confirmed that 20% of patients would need to change from methotrexate and folinic acid because of the development of drug resistance and a further 5% because of intolerance to methotrexate. The cause of drug resistance to methotrexate does not appear to relate to different pharmacological profiles of methotrexate between patients and may reflect different genetic changes in the tumor cells[16]. The main causes of methotrexate toxicity requiring a change of treatment are drug-induced hepatitis and intractable pleuritic chest pain. Therefore, 25% of this patient population will need more intensive chemotherapy to eliminate their disease.

11.6 CENTRAL NERVOUS SYSTEM PROPHYLAXIS

In patients with pulmonary metastases we recommend central nervous system (CNS) prophylaxis using intrathecal methotrexate (12.5 mg total dose), given with the first three

Table 11.4 Survival of all patients treated with methotrexate and folinic acid

	Prognostic score				
	Low risk (0–5)	*Medium risk (6–9)*	*High risk (>9)*	*Total*	*Grand total (all patients)*
No. of patients before 1974 (survival %)	85/88 (96)	20/22 (91)	5/16 (31)	110/126 (87)	469/487 (96)
No. of patients 1974–1986 (survival %)	347/348 (99·7)	12/13 (92)	–	359/361 (99)	

courses of chemotherapy. CSF hCG concentrations should be measured each time. These patients are at risk of developing CNS metastases, and low-dose methotrexate has minimal penetration into the CNS.

11.7 RESPONSE TO THERAPY

Response to chemotherapy in GTD and GTT is monitored by serial hCG estimations. Since GTD and GTT never switch off hCG production, this can be used with a reliability not possible with tumor markers in other diseases. Serial hCG estimations show successful treatment outcome (Figure 11.5) and the identification of drug resistance and the need to change chemotherapy (Figure 11.6). However, it is not possible to use the initial rate of decay or half-life of hCG to predict for future drug resistance, as has been proposed by some groups[17,18]. When we analyzed 340 low-risk patients with GTD, the initial half-life of hCG in response to treatment would have resulted in 33.9% false positives (patients needing more intensive therapy) and 31.7% false negatives (patients not needing to change their treatment from methotrexate)[19]. This analysis confirmed that continuous reassessment of the rate of hCG fall using regression analysis gave the most reliable results (Figure 11.7). Using this approach, it is possible to calibrate the rate of response to treatment in the individual patient against a large cohort of previously treated patients, which can potentially refine clinical decision-making[19].

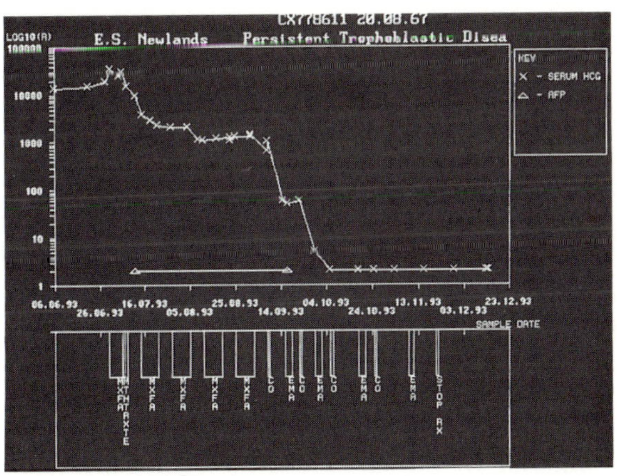

Figure 11.6 Patient with low-risk PTD treated initially with methotrexate and folinic acid but the hCG concentrations reached a plateau, confirming the presence of resistant disease. Prompt complete response obtained by changing the treatment to EMA-CO chemotherapy.

11.7.1 MEDIUM-RISK PATIENTS

Patients in the medium-risk category as shown in Table 11.1 have in the past been treated with the cycling regimen of chemotherapy shown in Table 11.3. This

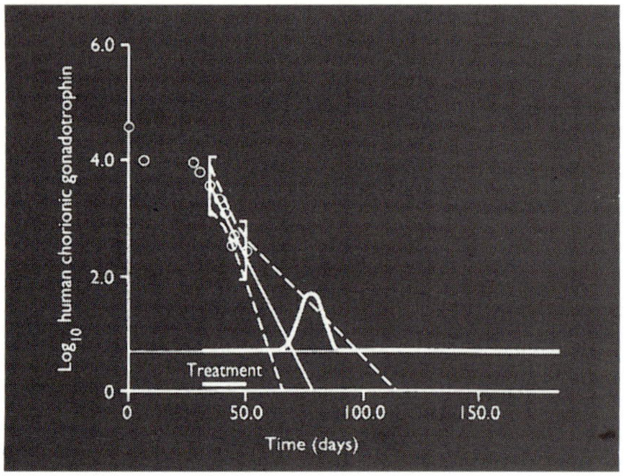

Figure 11.7 hCG regression analysis. The last six hCG concentrations are projected downwards and, as illustrated, the hCG is predicted to reach baseline before the mode of previous successfully treated patients (the hump on the baseline)[19]. Reproduced by kind permission of the *British Medical Journal*.

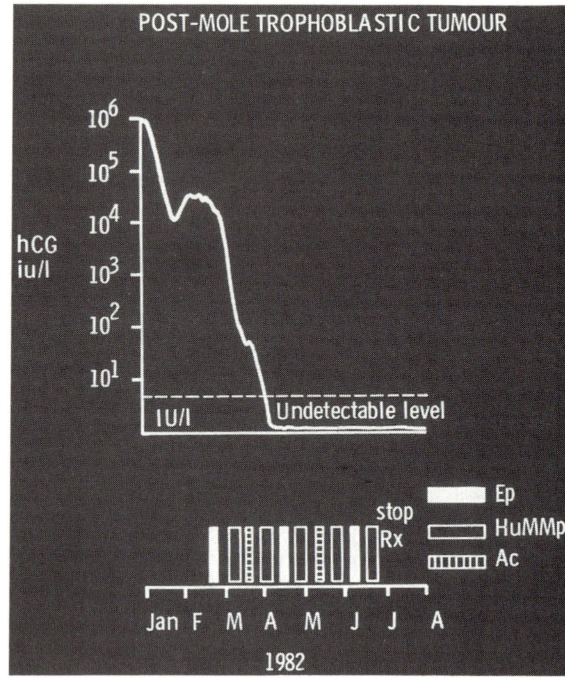

Figure 11.8 Patient treated with the cycling regimen (Table 11.3) for patients with medium-risk disease. This allows the assessment of response to etoposide as the initial treatment in a patient with a category of disease which now has 100% survival. In recent years these patients have been treated with the EMA-CO schedule which achieves remission more rapidly and with only one night's admission (for EMA) per two weeks.

schedule has the advantage of allowing assessment of a new promising cytotoxic agent such as etoposide as the initial treatment in a patient population who already have an excellent long-term survival (Figure 11.8)[20–22]. This approach of introducing a new agent early in the treatment of patients is important in clinical drug development since we need to develop newer, better and less toxic agents than the ones currently in the clinic[22–24]. If new agents are tested only in patients whose disease has become drug resistant, useful new drugs will be missed. We originally identified that etoposide is a highly active agent in this disease[25] and that it does not impair subsequent fertility[26], but it does carry a small risk of inducing acute myeloid leukaemia[27] (Chapter 16). We reported the results in patients treated with this medium-risk schedule in 1986[21]. The group of 76 patients treated between 1979 and 1983 are all alive and in remission. Several relapsed but have remained in complete remission after further, more intensive, treatment.

The principal problem with the schedules shown in Table 11.3 for the medium-risk group of patients is the number of days the patient needs to be in hospital or at the trophoblastic disease center. As experience of the EMA-CO schedule for high-risk patients has matured, we have increasingly switched patients in our medium-risk category, and those low-risk patients who become resistant to methotrexate, to the EMA-CO schedule (Figure 11.6). This results in patients receiving more intensive treatment over a shorter period of time than they would on the medium-risk schedule shown in Table 11.3.

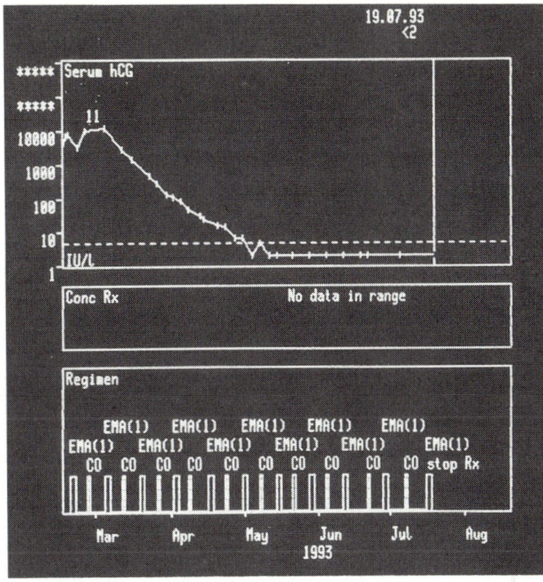

Figure 11.9 Patient with high-risk GTT also treated with the EMA-CO schedule. In most patients where the initial hCG is $<10^5$ U/l the fall in hCG is fairly linear, making clinical interpretation relatively easy.

11.7.2 HIGH-RISK PATIENTS

Clearly the most difficult therapeutic challenge in GTT is high-risk disease. A number of approaches to this problem have been made. Bagshawe developed a multidrug regimen, CHAMOCA, which produced a 76% survival[28]. However, cumulative myelosuppression was a problem with this schedule and in a randomized study against MAC (methotrexate, actinomycin D and chlorambucil) chemotherapy, the results using CHAMOCA were poor[29]. Wong *et al.*[30] reported better results with a modification of this chemotherapy (CHAMOMA) and obtained a survival of 41 (82%) of 50 patients. Cisplatin was identified as an active agent in GTT[31] and it has been used in combination with vincristine and bleomycin with somewhat disappointing results[32,33]. Better results were reported using etoposide/cisplatin combinations[34], producing sustained remissions in 19 (86%) of 22 patients.

Patients in the high-risk category need intensive chemotherapy. GTT appears to be more susceptible to chemotherapy which is administered frequently rather than the standard three- or four-week schedules that have been used in other diseases. This concept stimulated the development of the weekly EMA-CO schedule (Table 11.3). It allows relatively high dose intensity per week and, since the introduction of hemopoietic growth factors such as filgrastim, it is uncommon for patients to delay their chemotherapy because of neutropenia (Figures 11.9 and 11.10).

We reported our results using the EMA-CO schedule from 1979 to 1989[35] and in general these are reasonably good, giving an overall survival of 85% in 148 patients. There were two categories of treatment failure: in the 76 patients who had received no prior chemotherapy the principal cause of death (10 (71%) out of 14) was due to initial extent of disease in lung (five), brain (three), liver (one) and one case of pulmonary embolus. These patients died rapidly before adequate treatment could be given (Table 9.10). The antecedent pregnancies in this group of 10 patients were: live births six, miscarriage three, stillbirth one.

Respiratory failure presents a particular problem in these patients. They have stiff non-compliant lungs containing multiple metastases. The initiation of chemotherapy induces rapid tumor cell lysis and further inflammation in the lungs, reducing respiratory exchange still further. None of our patients who has been put on mechanical ventilation has survived. The pressures required to maintain respiratory exchange disrupts the residual functioning lung and the patients die of respiratory failure on the ventilator. We reported 103 cases presenting with dyspnea between 1960 and 1988 and there was a mortality of 11% overall[36,37]. It may be possible to reduce the inflammation induced by the initiation of chemotherapy by

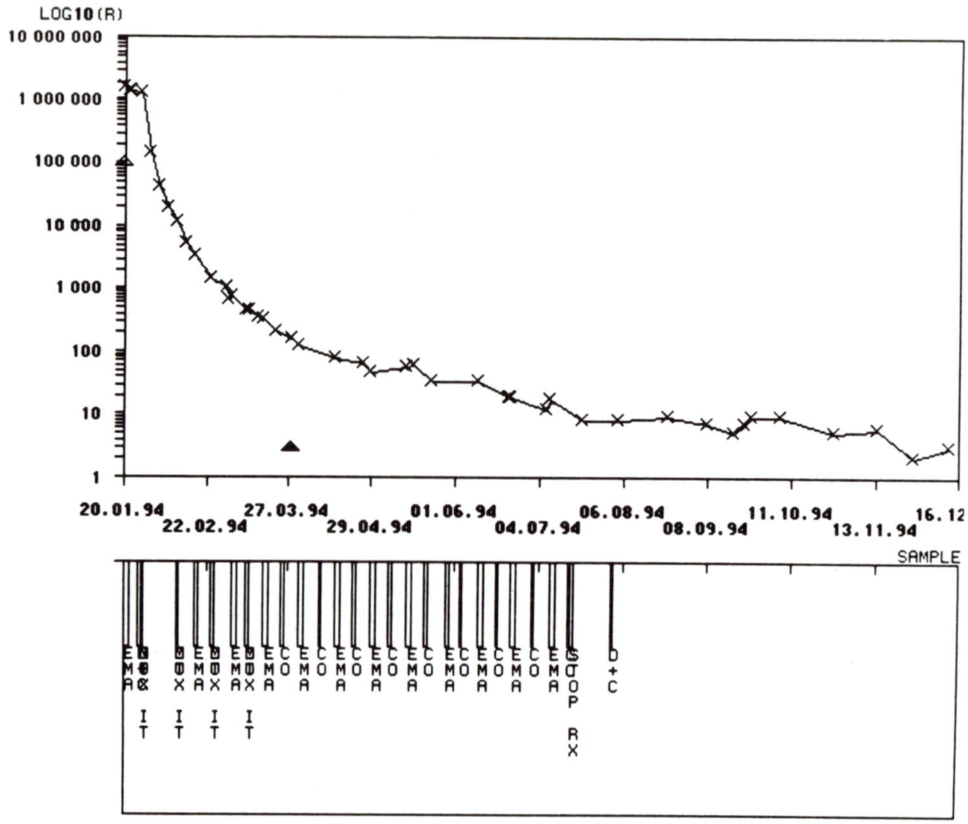

Figure 11.10 Patient with high-risk GTT also treated with the EMO-CO schedule. She had an enormous uterine mass (Figure 9.6) as the dominant site of disease and an initial hCG of $>10^6$ U/l. The hCG decay curve is clearly biphasic, making interpretation of the time to remission very difficult. This is a not uncommon problem in patients with large tumor masses and it is likely that hCG can leach out of dead tumor masses for some time. In this patient chemotherapy was stopped while the hCG was still above the normal range. D&C showed no tumor and she remains in remission. Continuing intensive chemotherapy >6 months increases the risk of inducing myeloid leukemia (Chapter 16).

high-dose dexamethasone (4 mg four times daily), which was successful in a recent case (Figure 9.8). An alternative approach for the future is the use of extracorporeal membrane oxygenation (ECMO) to support the patient through the initial few days until respiratory function recovers.

There were also 72 patients who had received prior chemotherapy, and were on regular hCG follow-up, in the report of EMA-CO chemotherapy[35]. They consisted of either our own treatment failures or patients referred from other centers, and here the survival was 89%. The principal cause of death was drug resistance. The apparent paradox of a better survival in this group is due to the early detection of reactivation of the disease by the rising hCG concentrations. Therefore the volume of disease at the start of further treatment was usually relatively small.

Salvage therapy is important in patients whose disease has progressed after their primary treatment for high-risk GTT. The main chemotherapeutic agent with established activity against this disease which is not included in the EMA-CO schedule is cisplatin[31]. We have usually used this in combination with etoposide (EP schedule: etoposide 150 mg/m^2; cisplatin 75 mg/m^2) given at weekly intervals alternating with the EMA schedule. This chemotherapy needs extremely careful monitoring of renal function since cisplatin is nephrotoxic and methotrexate is excreted in the urine. In our report of 1991[35], nine out of 11 (82%) patients achieved complete remission with the addition of cisplatin in this combination.

Salvage surgery is also important in these patients although the outcome is rather different from what one might anticipate from a tumor whose primary is normally in the uterus. When we retrospectively analyzed the success of surgery, only two (15%) out of 13 patients benefited from hysterectomy, in contrast to six (43%) out of 14 who benefited from thoracotomy and five (71%) out of seven patients who had a craniotomy. The surgical removal of the main active focus of disease with a limited amount of additional chemotherapy gives a surprisingly good outcome, with 14/20 (70%) complete remissions in this small subgroup of patients[35]. An important aspect of salvage surgery is identifying the main site of active disease. CT scans of brain, thorax and abdomen, together with ultrasound (with Doppler) of liver and pelvis, are the principal investigations. MRI of the brain and lumbar puncture for CSF hCG concentration may also be indicated. In patients with multiple residual radiological abnormalities, radioimmunolocalization with ^{131}I-labeled anti-hCG antibody can identify the active site in some patients[38].

The management of placental site trophoblastic tumors (PSTT) has also been discussed in Chapter 9. Here surgery plays an important role in the primary treatment of these patients either prior to chemotherapy if the disease is limited to the uterus or, following chemotherapy, if there is pelvic infiltration, making the initial hysterectomy difficult. The main chemotherapy we have used to treat patients with PSTT has been EMA-CO and, if drug resistance develops, the EP-EMA schedule[39]. The outcome in patients with disease limited to the pelvis has been quite good with either hysterectomy alone or chemotherapy followed by hysterectomy (nine out of 10 in complete remission). The outcome in patients with metastatic disease is poor: three (43%) out of seven patients remain alive.

11.8 ANTIEMETICS

The nausea and vomiting associated with intensive chemotherapy used to be one of the worst side effects for the patient. The introduction of the 5-HT$_3$ antagonists (ondansetron, granisetron, tropisetron) has made a major impact on this problem. These agents will usually control the nausea and vomiting induced by mildly and moderately emetic chemotherapy (e.g. the CO schedule in EMA-CO) on their own. However, more emetic schedules such as EMA or cisplatin frequently need the combination of a 5-HT$_3$ antagonist and dexamethasone[40]. This combination roughly doubles the proportion of patients who have their vomiting controlled. This combination was originally devised in 1988 to manage the uncontrollable nausea and vomiting experienced by a patient in her second relapse for high-risk GTT. Even her anticipatory vomiting resolved over several weeks with this combination. However, it is important to note that high-dose dexamethasone should not be used weekly since it increases the problems of Cushingoid appearance, adrenal suppression and the risk of *Pneumocystis carinii* pneumonia.

11.9 RADIOTHERAPY

The role of radiotherapy is uncertain in patients with drug-resistant GTT. Responses may be seen in individual lesions but the clinical problem is nearly always one of widely metastatic disease once drug resistance has developed. While the role of external beam radiotherapy in GTT remains unproven, there is a potential role for stereotactic radiotherapy in the occasional case where there is a single site of relapse. We have used this technique successfully in a patient who had a recurrence deep in the brain in the optic radiation. The combination of a single dose of stereotactically delivered radiotherapy followed by EMA-CO chemotherapy given with the modifications described below has achieved a sustained complete remission (section 11.11).

11.10 NEW DRUGS AND HIGH-DOSE CHEMOTHERAPY

At present there is a range of potentially new chemotherapeutic agents that need to be assessed in this patient population. These include the taxanes, taxol and taxotere; the camptothecans, topotecan and irinatecan; the new generation of antimetabolites (2-chlorodeoxyadenosine, tomudex); and temozolomide. The role of high-dose chemotherapy with autologous bone marrow or peripheral stem cell support so far has not been established in patients with drug-resistant disease. In the small number of patients treated with this approach, although responses have been seen these have not been durable. However, it may be appropriate to consider this approach in patients with ultra high-risk disease in remission at the end of their initial chemotherapy rather than reserve the high-dose chemotherapy for when drug resistance has been induced.

11.11 TREATMENT OF CENTRAL NERVOUS SYSTEM DISEASE

Patients with established CNS involvement at the start of treatment need special management. If there is an isolated brain metastasis that is superficial, our preference is for an initial craniotomy to remove the site of potential cerebral hemorrhage as early as possible in the patient's treatment (Figure 9.8). We have modified EMA-CO chemotherapy to increase the dose of methotrexate to 1 g/m^2 given as a 24 h infusion, followed by folinic acid 30 mg eight-hourly for 72 h, starting 32 h after the beginning of the methotrexate infusion. When methotrexate is given in this dose, normal baseline renal function needs to be confirmed by ethylenediaminetetraacetic acid (EDTA) clearance and monitored carefully so that the folinic acid dosage is adjusted appropriately. The high-dose methotrexate increases the penetration of the drug into the CNS from the systemic circulation. The other modification to the EMA-CO schedule in these patients is giving 12.5 mg (total dose) intrathecal methotrexate with the CO part of the schedule and this is continued until both serum and CSF hCG concentrations are normal. The initial CT scan and the hCG response in a patient is shown in Figures 11.11 and 11.12. We have reported our results in patients with CNS involvement and, in the most recent review, of 23 consecutive patients the survival was 65% [41,42].

11.12 REASONS FOR CURRENT SUCCESS AND CAUSES OF TREATMENT FAILURE

The main reasons for the successful outcome in patients with GTD and GTT are:

1. registration and follow-up of patients at risk;
2. GTD and GTT always produce hCG, allowing screening, monitoring treatment and follow-up;
3. inherent chemosensitivity of GTD and GTT;
4. centralization of expertise so that treatment can be optimized and further advances can be made.

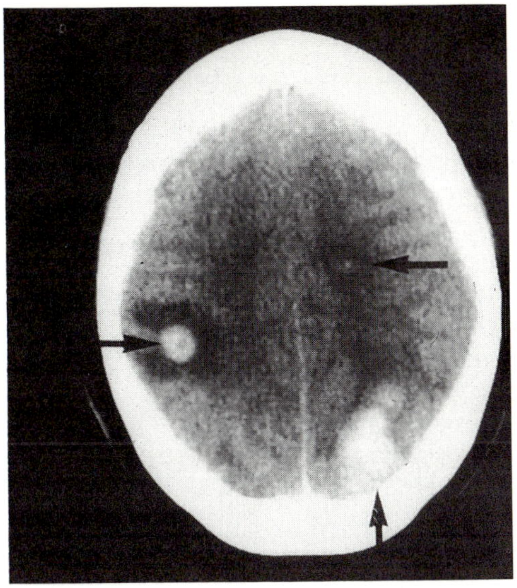

Figure 11.11 CT scan of a patient presenting with symptoms of subarachnoid hemorrhage (occipital lobe) and three CNS metastases. She had widespread disease including a pancreatic mass causing obstructive jaundice. The bile duct was stented and EMA-CO (modified for CNS disease) was given successfully.

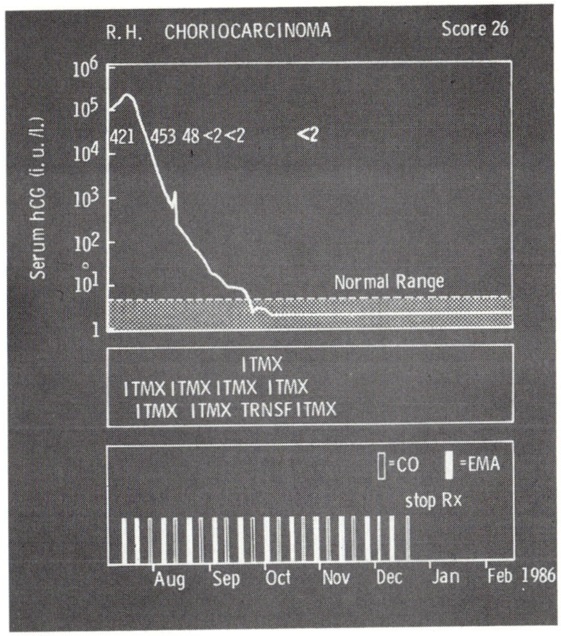

Figure 11.12 hCG response and treatment for patient shown in Figure 11.11

The main causes of treatment failure are:

1. early deaths from initial disease extent at the time of presentation;
2. development of drug resistance;
3. PSTTs behave unpredictably and are not very chemosensitive.

11.13 FOLLOW-UP

After completion of chemotherapy, patients are monitored by serial hCG estimations (Table 11.5). Since neither GTD nor GTT grow clinically without producing hCG, this is the key to the follow-up of these patients. We do not normally see them again clinically after a single outpatient appointment to check that all is well. Our recommendation following chemotherapy is that they do not become pregnant for 12 months, (1) to be reasonably certain that their disease has been eliminated and (2) to minimize the potential teratogenetic effects of the chemotherapy on the fetus (Chapter 16). The long-term results at the Charing Cross Hospital have confirmed the advantage of centralized management of a rare tumor in a limited number of centers with the appropriate expertise. In Figure 11.13 we have summarized our results from 1958. In the original cohort of 350 patients treated between 1958 and 1973 the survival was already close to 80%. The impact of the systematic application of prognostic factors in determining the patient treatment category is shown in the second group of patients treated between 1974 and 1978. In the late 1970s we introduced both etoposide and cisplatin into the chemotherapy for these patients. In addition CT and MRI scanning has allowed better localization of sites of resistant disease. The combination of these additional advances is the main explanation for the further improvement in survival in the last cohort of 944 patients treated between 1979 and 1992 who have an overall survival

Table 11.5 Follow-up for GTT patients who have received chemotherapy

Year 1:	Weekly serum and urine for 6 weeks serum and urine every 2 weeks until 6 months post treatment urine only every 2 weeks until 1 year post treatment
Year 2	urine sample every 4 weeks
Year 3:	urine sample every 8 weeks
Year 4:	urine sample every 12 weeks
Year 5:	urine sample every 16 weeks
Subsequently:	Every 6 months indefinitely

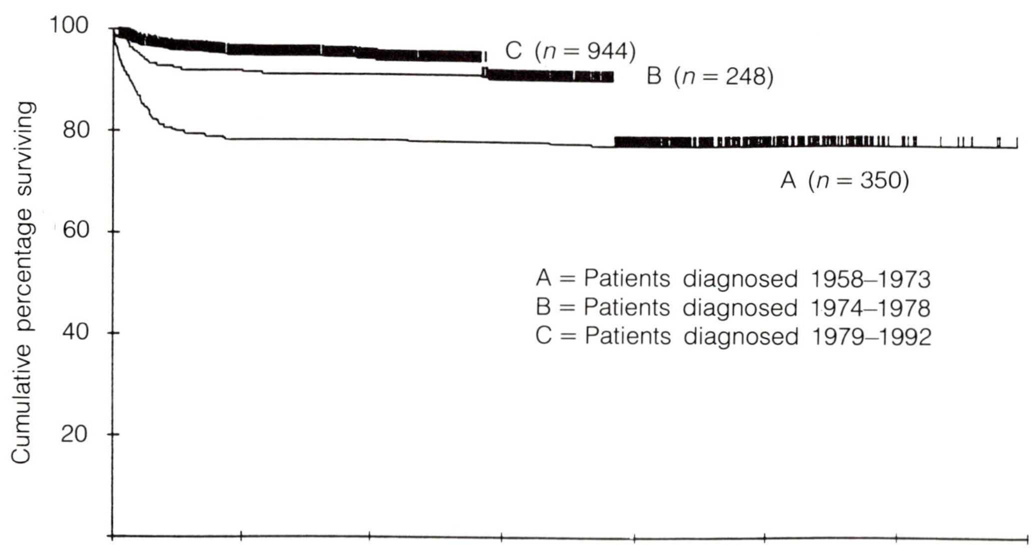

Figure 11.13 Patients with GTD treated at Charing Cross Hospital 1958–1992 (for details see text).

of 94% with a maximum follow-up at that analysis of 15 years.

REFERENCES

1. Seckl, M.J., Rustin, G.J.S., Newlands, E.S. *et al.* (1991) Pulmonary embolism, pulmonary hypertension and choriocarcinoma. *Lancet*, **338**, 1313–15.
2. Long, M.G., Boultbee, J.E., Langley, R. *et al.* (1992) Doppler assessment of the uterine circulation and its relationship to the clinical behaviour of gestational trophoblastic tumours requiring chemotherapy. *Br. J. Can-*

cer, **66**, 883–7.
3. O'Reilly, S.M., Boultbee, J.E., Gregory, W.M. *et al.* (1995) Pelvic ultrasound can help to predict the development of drug resistance in patients with low risk gestational trophoblastic disease. *Int. J. Gynaecol. Cancer*, in press.
4. Bagshawe, K.D. (1976) Risk and prognostic factors in trophoblastic neoplasia. *Cancer*, **38**, 1373–85.
5. Bagshawe, K.D. and Harland, S. (1976) Immunodiagnosis and monitoring of gonadotrophin producing metastases in the central nervous system. *Cancer*, **38**, 112–18.
6. Smith, D.B., Holden, L., Newlands, E.S. *et al.* (1993) Correlation between clinical staging (FIGO) and prognostic groups in gestational trophoblastic disease. *Br. J. Obstet. Gynaecol.*, **100**, 157–60.
7. Hertz, R. and Tullner, W.W. (1949) Inhibition of estrogen-induced growth in the genital tract of the female chick by a purine antagonist: reversal by adenine. *Science*, **109**, 539.
8. Hertz, R. and Tullner, W.W. (1950) Interference with hormonal effects by antivitamins and competition between structurally similar steroid hormones. *Ann. N.Y. Acad. Sci.*, **52**, 1260–73.
9. Li, M.C., Hertz, R. and Spencer, D.B. (1956) Effect of methotrexate therapy upon choriocarcinoma and chorioadenoma. *Proc. Soc. Exp. Biol. Med.*, **43**, 361–9.
10. Ross, G.T., Goldstein, D.P., Hertz, R. *et al.* (1965) Sequential use of methotrexate and actinomycin D in the treatment of metastatic choriocarcinoma and related trophoblastic diseases in women. *Am. J. Oncol.*, **93**, 223–9.
11. Bagshawe, K.D., Dent, J., Newlands, E.S. *et al.* (1989) The role of low-dose methotrexate and folinic acid in gestational trophoblastic tumours (GTT). *Br. J. Obstet. Gynaecol.*, **96**, 795–802.
12. Berkowitz, R.S., Goldstein, D.P. and Bernstein, M.R. (1986) Ten years experience with methotrexate and folinic acid as primary therapy for gestational trophoblastic disease. *Gynecol. Oncol.*, **23**, 111–18.
13. Soper, J.T., Clarke-Pearson, D.L., Berchuck, A. *et al.* (1994) 5-day methothrexate for women with metastatic gestational trophoblastic disease. *Gynecol. Oncol.*, **54**, 76–9.
14. Goldstein, D.P. (1971) Five years experience with the prevention of trophoblastic tumors by the prophylactic use of chemotherapy in patients with molar pregnancy. *Clin. Obstet. Gynecol.*, **13**, 945–61.
15. Kashimura, Y., Masamichi, K., Sugimori, H. *et al.* (1986) Prophylactic chemotherapy for hydatidiform mole. *Cancer*, **58**, 624–9.
16. Hilgers, R.D., Newlands, E.S., Hoffman, R. *et al.* (1991) Correlation of plasma methotrexate concentration with human chorionic gonadotrophin (hCG) and therapeutic response to low dose methotrexate–citrovorum factor in low-risk gestational trophoblastic tumors. *Gynecol. Oncol.*, **41**, 117–22.
17. Lange, H., Vogelzang, N., Goldman, A. *et al.* (1982) Marker half-life analysis as a prognostic tool in testicular cancer. *J. Urol.*, **128**, 708–11.
18. Picozzi, V., Hannigan, J., Freina, F. *et al.* (1984) Prognostic significance of a decline in serum human chorionic gonadotrophin levels after initial chemotherapy for advanced germ-cell carcinoma. *Ann. Intern. Med.*, **100**, 183–6.
19. Leaning, M.S., Gallivan, S., Newlands, E.S. *et al.* (1992) A computer system for assisting with clinical interpretation of tumour marker data. *BMJ*, **305**, 804–7.
20. Newlands, E.S. (1985) VP16 in combinations for first line treatment of malignant germ cell tumours and gestational choriocarcinoma. *Semin. Oncol.*, **12**, (Suppl. 2), 37–41.
21. Newlands, E.S., Bagshawe, K.D., Begent, R.H.J. *et al.* (1986) Developments in chemotherapy for medium and high risk patients with gestational trophoblastic tumours, 1979–84. *Br. J. Obstet. Gynaecol.*, **93**, 63–9.
22. Hitchins, R.N., Holden, L., Newlands, E.S. *et al.* (1988) Single agent etoposide in gestational trophoblastic tumours: experience at Charing Cross Hospital 1978–1987. *Eur. J. Cancer Clin. Oncol.*, **24**, 1041–6.
23. O'Reilly, S.M., Rustin, G.J.S., Smith, D.B. *et al.* (1992) Single agent activity of carboplatin in patients with previously untreated non-seminomatous germ cell tumours. *Ann. Oncol.*, **3**, 163–4.
24. Motzer, R.J., Bajorin, D.F., Schwartz, L.H. *et al.* (1994) Phase II trial of paclitaxel shows antitumor activity in patients with previously

treated germ cell tumors. *J. Clin. Oncol.*, **12**, 2277–83.

25. Newlands, E.S. and Bagshawe, K.D. (1980) Antitumour activity of the epipodophyllin derivative VP 16–213 (Etoposide: NRC-141540) in gestational choriocarcinoma. *Eur. J. Cancer*, **16**, 401.
26. Newlands, I.F., Rustin, G.J.S., Newlands, E.S. *et al.* (1986) Fertility in patients with gestational trophoblastic tumours treated with etoposide. *Eur. J. Clin. Oncol.*, **22**, 1479–82.
27. Newlands, E.S., Rustin, G.J.S., Lutz, J.-M. *et al.* (1995) Chemotherapy for gestational trophoblastic tumours (GTT) may increase the incidence of second tumours and may cause a premature menopause. *ASCO Abstract*, 744.
28. Bagshawe, K.D. and Begent, R.H.J. (1981) Trophoblastic tumours: clinical features and management, in *Gynaecological Oncology*, (ed. M. Coppleston), Churchill Livingstone, London, pp. 757–72.
29. Curry, S.L., Blessing, J.A., DiSaia, P.J. *et al.* (1989) A prospective randomized comparison of methotrexate, dactinomycin and chlorambucil versus methotrexate, dactinomycin, cyclophosphamide, doxorubicin, melphalan, hydroxyurea and vincristine in 'poor prognosis' metastatic gestational trophoblastic disease: a gynecologic oncology group study. *Obstet. Gynecol.*, **73**, 357–62.
30. Wong, L.C., Choo, Y.C. and Ma, H.K. (1986) Modified Bagshawe's regimen in high-risk gestational trophoblastic disease. *Gynecol. Oncol.*, **23**, 87–93.
31. Newlands, E.S. and Bagshawe, K.D. (1979) Activity of cis-platinum (NCI 119875) in drug-resistant gestational choriocarcinoma: a report of 17 cases. *Br. J. Cancer*, **40**, 943.
32. DuBeshter, B., Berkowitz, R.S., Goldstein, D.P. *et al.* (1989) Vinblastine, cisplatin and bleomycin as salvage therapy for refractory high-risk metastatic gestational trophoblastic disease. *J. Reprod. Med. Obstet. Gynecol.*, **34**, 189–92.
33. Azab, M., Droz, J.-P., Theodore, C. *et al.* (1989) Cisplatin, vinblastine and bleomycin combination in the treatment of resistant high-risk gestational trophoblastic tumors. *Cancer*, **64**, 1829–32.
34. Theodore, C., Azab, M., Droz, J.P. *et al.* (1989) Treatment of high-risk gestational trophoblastic disease with chemotherapy combinations containing cisplatin and etoposide. *Cancer*, **64**, 1824–8.
35. Newlands, E.S., Bagshawe, K.D., Begent, R.H.J. *et al.* (1991) Results with the EMA/CO (etopside, methotrexate, actinomycin D, cyclophosphamide, vincristine) regimen in high risk gestational trophoblastic tumours, 1979 to 1989. *Br. J. Obstet. Gynaecol.*, **98**, 550–7.
36. Kelly, M.P., Rustin, G.J.S., Ivory, C. *et al.* (1990) Respiratory failure due to choriocarcinoma: a study of 103 dyspneic patients. *Gynecol. Oncol.*, **38**, 149–54.
37. Bakri, Y.N., Berkowitz, R.S., Khan, J. *et al.* (1994) Pulmonary metastases of gestational trophoblastic tumour: risk factors for early respiratory failure. *J. Reprod. Med.*, **39**, 175–8.
38. Begent, R.H.J., Bagshawe, K.D., Green, A.J. *et al.* (1987) The clinical value of imaging with antibody to human chorionic gonadotrophin in the detection of residual choriocarcinoma. *Br. J. Cancer*, **55**, 657–60.
39. Dessau, R., Rustin, G.J.S., Dent, J. *et al.* (1990) Surgery and chemotherapy in the management of placental site tumor. *Gynecol. Oncol.*, **39**, 56–9.
40. Smith, D.B., Newlands, E.S., Rustin, G.J.S. *et al.* (1991) Comparison of ondansetron and ondansetron plus dexamethasone as antiemetic prophylaxis during cisplatin-containing chemotherapy. *Lancet*, **338**, 487–90.
41. Athanassiou, A., Begent, R.H.J., Newlands, E.S. *et al.* (1983) Central nervous system metastases of choriocarcinoma: 23 years experience at Charing Cross Hospital. *Cancer*, **52**, 1728–35.
42. Rustin, G.J.S., Newlands, E.S., Begent, R.H.J. *et al.* (1989) Weekly alternating etoposide, methotrexate and actinomycin/vincristine and cyclophosphamide chemotherapy for the treatment of CNS metastases of choriocarcinoma. *J. Clin. Oncol.*, **7**, 900–3.

TREATMENT OF NON-METASTATIC GESTATIONAL TROPHOBLASTIC DISEASE

12

Howard D. Homesley

12.1 INTRODUCTION

Despite the possible poor outcome of malignant gestational trophoblastic disease (GTD), most women can be successfully diagnosed and treated with preservation of normal reproductive potential. It is critical to manage hydatidiform mole properly to minimize acute complications, identify malignant sequelae and initiate therapy promptly. However, it is necessary to individualize therapy for women with malignant GTD based upon risk factor characterization, with patients at lower risk receiving less toxic therapy and aggressive multi-agent therapy reserved for patients with high-risk disease.

Even though GTD embraces varied neoplasms of the placenta, hydatidiform mole ordinarily can be managed by molar evacuation and expectant surveillance of quantitative serum human chorionic gonadotropin (hCG) levels. Approximately 80% of complete moles and more than 90–95% of partial moles go into complete remission without chemotherapy[1].

Malignant GTD can occur after any type of pregnancy. The prognosis is determined by several clinical risk factors including anatomical site of disease, duration of disease, hCG level and type of antecedent pregnancy. Patients with non-metastatic and low-risk metastatic (metastasis to lungs and/or vagina) GTD have an excellent outcome when treated with single-agent chemotherapy[2]. Non-metastatic GTD (NMGTD) is most amenable to single-agent therapy where patients have an antecedent molar pregnancy with a plateau, and elevation or a persistent hCG elevation after molar evacuation. For over 30 years, single-agent methotrexate (MTX) (20–25 mg intramuscularly every day for five days about every two weeks) has been associated with high cure rates for NMGTD[2]. MTX with citrovorum factor (CVF) rescue has a similar high remission rate with decreased toxicity[3–7].

12.2 GYNECOLOGIC ONCOLOGY GROUP

The Gynecologic Oncology Group (GOG) conducted clinical studies in patients with NMGTD with the intent to discover more convenient, less expensive and hopefully equally efficacious single-agent regimens[8–11].

12.2.1 DEFINITION OF NON-METASTATIC GESTATIONAL TROPHOBLASTIC DISEASE

The GOG criteria for inclusion of patients in the NMGTD trials are listed in Table 12.1.

Gestational Trophoblastic Disease.
Edited by B.W. Hancock, E.S. Newlands and R.S. Berkowitz.
ISBN 0 412 63100 8

Table 12.1 GOG definition for NMGTD

Factor	*Finding*
hCG level	No limit
Serial hCG levels	3
Percentage elevation	10%
Duration of elevation	3 weeks
Confirmation of elevation required	Yes – repeat once
Persistent elevation above normal	16 weeks

Table 12.2 GOG criteria for progression

Criterion	*Finding*
Metastasis	Yes
Decrease in hCG level	<10% over 2 weeks
One log hCG level decrease	Required over 6 weeks

Pelvic ultrasound to exclude intrauterine pregnancy was recommended for all patients treated more than two weeks after passage of a molar pregnancy. Computed tomography (CT) of the brain and liver was not mandatory in patients who strictly met the definition of non-metastatic, post-molar GTD without previous chemotherapy. In the USA patients seldom undergo pretreatment uterine curettage. Nearly all patients were placed on oral contraceptives after molar evacuation.

12.2.2 TREATMENT FAILURE

In a clinical trial, the definition of progression or failure has to be inflexible for there to be standardized assessment of response to chemotherapy (Table 12.2). Individualized therapy where one has the discretion to follow hCG levels that regress in a desultory manner over a prolonged interval is not practical. Thus, in the GOG collaborative trial, treatment flexibility was not possible and may have resulted in technically higher failure rates than where patients may be followed for longer periods of observation, especially at near-normal hCG levels.

12.2.3 PROGNOSTIC FACTORS

Identification of various prognostic factors at the start of chemotherapy allows patients with GTT to be categorized into low- and high-risk groups so that they can be given the minimal treatment necessary to achieve the highest efficacy.

Persistent GTD patients had twice as high (85.9 versus 48.3 U/ml) CA-125 levels prior to suction of molar evacuation[12]. These CA-125 level measurements may help predict which molar patients will develop persistent disease. Likewise higher progesterone at molar evacuation and continued levels higher than 5 ng/ml predict persistent mole[13].

The 1991 International Federation of

Table 12.3 FIGO staging for trophoblastic tumor

Stage I	Disease confined to uterus
Stage II	Metastasis limited to adnexa, vagina or vulva
Stage III	Metastasis to lungs
Stage IV	All other metastatic sites

Each stage is subcategorized into A, B and C
A: No risk factors
B: One risk factor
C: Two risk factors

Risk factors:
1. hCG with >100 000 U/l
2. Duration of disease greater than 6 months from termination of antecedent pregnancy

Society of Gynecologic Oncologists Staging Handbook [41].

Gynecology and Obstetrics (FIGO) staging for trophoblastic disease tumor combined anatomical and risk factor considerations in staging the non-metastatic patients (Table 12.3). The NMGTD patients would be those in stage IA or IB if the risk factor present was only a serum hCG >100 000 U/l. Yet, stages I, II and III less than 6 months from the antecedent pregnancy would all be considered low-risk disease patients.

It is noteworthy that for the GOG clinical trials there was no restriction for entry by hCG level. Analysis of hCG level in many studies reveals this to be a significant prognostic factor. The pretreatment hCG level in the GOG studies was found subsequently not to be prognostically significant and the hCG level was not found to relate to response[14]. The hCG regression curve serves as a reliable guide for the administration of chemotherapy, but also can be a means to identify patients who are going to develop a persistent mole[15].

A consecutive series of 454 women treated between 1968 and 1992 were analyzed by multivariant analysis and indicated pretherapy hCG levels were not significantly associated with survival[16]. Prior therapy, type of antecedent pregnancy, number of metastatic sites and duration of disease were identified as independent prognostic factors.

In comparing the available GTD staging and classification systems, all are able to identify low- and high-risk subsets of patients with similar efficiency[17]. The addition of FIGO substages enhances discrimination between prognostic groups in stage III. Others prefer a non-anatomical scoring system that predicts drug resistance and offers more specific therapy[18].

It is unclear whether or not chemoprophylaxis reduces the incidence of persistent trophoblastic disease in patients at high risk[19]. Following chemoprophylaxis to prevent persistent molar disease, more courses (2.5 versuss 1.4) of chemotherapy were required until remission was complete in the group who received prophylactic therapy compared to the untreated group.

The GOG has completed a prospective randomized study using traditional criteria for patients at high risk of developing persistent molar disease. The study is undergoing analysis but it is clear that there may be only a few factors that might predict high risk for persistent molar disease. It is still unclear as to whether patients can be identified to be at high risk and, if so, whether or not prophylactic chemotherapy is efficacious.

Although partial and complete hydatidiform moles are distinct clinicopathological entities that can be distinguished histologically, it does not appear that clinical management of partial mole should be any different from complete mole[20].

12.3 SONOGRAPHY

A number of investigators have assessed the reliability of transvaginal ultrasonography in the detection of uterine involvement in patients with GTT to determine the role of this procedure in management[21–27]. Uterine localization of disease can be detected appearing as hypoechoic areas and myometrial nodules. Favorable response to chemotherapy can be imaged by regressions of nodules noted by transvaginal ultrasonography. The transvaginal color flow Doppler sonography has also been noted to correlate with prognosis and hCG levels[23,25,26]. Color flow Doppler can be a non-invasive, reproducible, useful and highly reliable diagnostic approach for the diagnosis and management of patients suffering from uterine GTD.

12.4 METHOTREXATE WITH FOLINIC ACID RESCUE

In the NMGTD patient, MTX with folinic acid rescue is often preferred[28]. There is a high complete remission rate (90.2%) and often (81.5%) this can be obtained following only one course of chemotherapy. Between 1964 and 1986, 487 patients with gestational trophoblastic tumor were treated with MTX and folinic acid[29]. From 1974, all patients were stratified into prognostic groups on admission. Of the true low-risk patients, 347 of 348 (99.7%) survived. Of 13 patients underscored and treated as low risk when they should have been treated as medium risk, 12 (92%) were alive, but nine (69%) needed to change treatment because of drug resistance. Although the survival in these patients was excellent, 69 of 348 (20%) low-risk patients had to change treatment because of the development of drug resistance, and a further 23 (6%) needed to change treatment because of drug-induced toxicity. The 20% first-line failure rate is similar to that found with weekly intramuscular MTX, which has negligible toxicity. Others have concluded that high-dose MTX does not appear to offer any clinical advantage over conventional-dose MTX in low-risk patients[30].

12.5 GOG NMGTD CLINICAL TRIALS

In the two GOG intramuscular MTX trials, 125 patients were evaluable for response[8, 9]. There was no correlation noted between response and age, performance status or initial hCG values. With the weekly MTX, the time to response was a median of seven weeks with a range of 3–19 weeks – no different from the non-responders. In the initial study, using lower MTX levels, there was an 81% complete response rate in 53 patients. In the second study, with rapid escalation to 50 mg/m^2, the complete response rate was 74%. In both studies there were no delays in therapy related to myelotoxicity. No patients required hysterectomy during treatment.

In the single-dose actinomycin D (ACTD) GOG study of NMGTD, the same criteria for entry were used except no patient had an hCG titer >40 000 U/l[11]. ACTD was given intravenously at a dose of 1.25 mg/m^2 every 14 days. The response rate using the same GOG criteria was 94%. The two patients who failed to respond to pulse therapy were changed to five-day ACTD, one patient responded, and the other was switched to MTX followed by hysterectomy. The specimen contained a focus of choriocarcinoma, and the patient received combination chemotherapy.

12.6 LOW-RISK METASTATIC TROPHOBLASTIC DISEASE

Virtually all patients with non-metastatic and low-risk metastatic disease can be cured using single-agent MTX or ACTD. Review of the clinical course of 48 patients with low-risk metastatic GTT treated with primary single-agent chemotherapy revealed that although all patients achieved sustained remission, 25 (51%) required a second single-agent regimen, and seven (14%) needed combination chemotherapy[31]. An average of 3.4 courses of chemotherapy was necessary to achieve remission, and six patients (12%) underwent resection of resistant tumor foci. Primary single-agent chemotherapy is a reasonable treatment option in patients with low-risk metastatic disease, although a higher first-line failure rate should be anticipated.

In patients with vaginal metastases, the prognosis depends mainly on the extent of the disease[32]. A favorable response to chemotherapy was observed in low risk patients with vaginal metastases.

12.7 SUMMARY

The GOG clinical trials indicate that intramuscular weekly MTX and single-dose ACTD in NMGTD patients are effective, safe, inexpensive and convenient. Traditional therapy consists of ACTD administered intravenously at 10–12 μg/kg per day for five days or MTX administered intramuscularly or intravenously at 0.4 μg/kg per day for five days. The cycle is repeated after a rest of seven days. A mean of three courses, or approximately six weeks, is required to reach a normal hCG level with either single-dose or five-day ACTD. Eighty-one per cent of patients treated with single-dose ACTD experienced toxicity, although <10% had severe symptoms of nausea and vomiting which were the most common adverse effects.

High-dose MTX–CVF rescue, which usually consists of 1 mg/kg MTX every day for four doses alternating with CVF rescue, has a remission rate of >90% and lack of significant toxicity[4]. However, a later study had an MTX–CVF failure rate of 28%[33]. There is some question about the pharmacological effect of CVF rescue on MTX since low drug levels were noted prior to the CVF dose; the decrease in toxicity may be an effect of the schedule rather than the CVF rescue[34].

A comparison in cost between pulse ACTD, five day ACTD, intramuscular MTX, five-day MTX and eight-day MTX–CVF indicates that single-dose ACTD or intramuscular MTX greatly reduces cost[8,10]. Single-dose ACTD is comparable to conventional alternatives. Because of the efficacy and toxicity profile, pulsed ACTD appears superior to current standard therapy in terms of convenience and cost effectiveness. Weekly MTX may be superior to pulsed ACTD because of less gastrointestinal toxicity.

Others have used single-agent intravenous 5-fluorouracil infusion and oral etoposide, which have similar complete response rates to those of MTX regimens[35,36]. Five-day MTX has a high incidence toxicity (21%)[16]. Intramuscular MTX has minimal hematological (grades 1 and 2) and gastrointestinal toxicity (grades 1 and 2). Five-day fluorouracil infusion has the most severe toxicity. Oral etoposide is associated with alopecia and amenorrhea along with significant hematological and gastrointestinal toxicity.

Although survival is excellent when MTX and folinic acid are used, in one large report 20% of low-risk patients had to change treatment because of the development of drug resistance, and 6% needed to change treatment because of drug-induced toxicity[37]. At another institution, patients were treated with either weekly MTX or MTX and folinic acid[38]. Weekly MTX was equally effective and less toxic than the eight-day MTX–folinic acid regimen. Efforts should continue to identify new chemotherapy protocols that maximize remission rates and minimize toxicity and hospitalization.

Alternating five-day chemotherapy with MTX and ACTD as primary treatment for non-metastatic gestational disease was studied in nine patients with a 100% complete response[39]. Stomatitis was universal and mild to moderate. Thirty-seven patients with NMGTD were treated with one or more cycles of oral MTX following intramuscular MTX as part of induction therapy, with remission in 31 patients (84%), indicating that this is safe, easily administered and effective[40].

None of the regimens may approach the ideal, yet, single-agent therapy has much to offer when appropriately given to the patient with low-risk trophoblastic disease.

REFERENCES

1. Soper, J.T. (1993) Management of gestational trophoblastic disease. *Oncolocy*, **7**, 68–74.
2. Hammond, C.B., Hertz, R., Ross, G.T. *et al.* (1967) Primary chemotherapy for non-metastatic gestional trophoblastic neoplasms. *Am. J. Obstet. Gynecol.*, **98**, 71–8.
3. Wong, L.C., Choo, Y.C. and Ma, H.K. (1985) Methotrexate with citrovorum factor rescue in gestational trophoblastic disease. *Am. J. Obstet. Gynecol.* **152**, 59–62.
4. Berkowitz, R.S. and Goldstein, D.P. (1979) Methotrexate with citrovorum factor rescue for nonmetastatic gestational trophoblastic neoplasms. *Obstet. Gynecol.*, **54**, 725–8.
5. Berkowitz, R.S., Goldstein, D.P., Jones, M.A. *et al.* (1980) Methotrexate with citrovorum factor rescue: reduced chemotherapy toxicity in the management of gestational trophoblastic neoplasms. *Cancer*, **45**, 423–6.
6. Khoo, S.K. and Jones, I.S.C. (1980) Medium-dose methotrexate/folinic acid regimen in the chemotherapy of gestational trophoblastic disease. *Med. J. Aust.*, **1**, 317–20.
7. Goldstein, D.P., Saracco, P., Osanthanondth, H.F.T. (1978) Methotrexate with citrovorum factor rescue with gestational trophoblastic neoplasms. *Obstet. Gynecol.*, **51**, 93–6.
8. Homesley, H.D., Blessing, J.A., Rettenmaier, M. *et al.* (1988) Weekly intramuscular methotrexate for nonmetastatic gestational trophoblastic disease. *Obstet. Gynecol.*, **72**, 413–8.
9. Homesley, H.D., Blessing, J.A., Schlaerth, J. *et al.* (1990) Rapid escalation of weekly intramuscular methotrexate for nonmetastatic gestational trophoblastic disease: a Gynecologic Oncology Group study. *Gynecol. Oncol.*, **39**, 305–8.
10. Twiggs, L. (1983) Pulse actinomycin D trophoblastic scheduling in non-metastatic gestational neoplasia: cost-effective chemotherapy. *Gynecol. Oncol.*, **16**, 190–5.
11. Petrilli, E.S., Twiggs, L.B., Blessing, J.A. *et al.* (1987) Single-dose actinomycin-D treatment for nonmetastatic gestational trophoblastic disease: a prospective Phase II trial of the Gynecologic Oncology Group. *Cancer*, **60**, 2173–6.
12. Koonings, P.P. and Schlaerth, J.B. (1993) CA-125: a marker for persistent gestational trophoblastic disease? *Gynecol. Oncol.*, **49**, 240–2.
13. Vasilev, S.A., Schlaerth, J.B., Ahn, C. and Sauer, M.V. (1994) Serum progesterone monitoring in post-molar surveillance. *Gynecol. Oncol.*, **54**, 288–91.
14. Homesley, H.D. (1994) Development of single-agent chemotherapy regimens for gestational trophoblastic disease. *J. Reprod. Med.*, **39**, 185–92.
15. Yedema, K.A., Verheijen, R.H., Kenemans, P. *et al.* (1993) Identification of patients with persistent trophoblastic disease by means of a normal human chorionic gonadotropin regression curve. *Am. J. Obstet. Gynecol.*, **168**, 787–92.
16. Soper, J.T., Clarke-Pearson, D.L., Berchuck, A. *et al.* (1994) 5-day methotrexate for women with metastatic gestational trophoblastic disease. *Gynecol. Oncol.*, **54**, 76–9.
17. Soper, J.T., Evans, A.C., Conaway, M.R. *et al.* (1994) Evaluation of prognostic factors and staging in gestational trophoblastic tumor. *Obstet. Gynecol.*, **84**, 969–73.
18. Smith, D.B., Holden, L., Newlands, E.S. and

Bagshawe, K.D. (1993) Correlation between clinical staging (FIGO) and prognostic groups with gestational trophoblastic disease. *Br. J. Obstet. Gynaecol.*, **100**, 157–60.

19. Kim, D.S., Moon, H., Kim, K.T. *et al.* (1986) Effects of prophylactic chemotherapy for persistent trophoblastic disease in patients with complete hydatidiform mole. *Obstet. Gynecol.*, **67**, 690–4.
20. Womack, C. and Elston, C.W. (1985) Hydatidiform mole in Nottingham: a 12 year retrospective epidemiological and morphological study. *Placenta*, **6**, 93.
21. Mangili, G., Spagnolo, D., Valsecchi, L. and Maggi, R. (1993) Transvaginal ultrasonography in persistent trophoblastic tumor. *Am. J. Obstet. Gynecol.*, **169**, 1218–23.
22. Carter, J., Fowler, J., Carlson, J. *et al.* (1993) Transvaginal color flow Doppler sonography in the assessment of gestational trophoblastic disease. *J. Ultrasound Med.*, **12**, 595–9.
23. Jaffe, R. (1993) Investigation of abnormal first-trimester gestations by color Doppler imaging. *J. Clin. Ultrasound*, **21**, 521–6.
24. Hsieh, F.J., Wu, C.C., Lee, C.N. *et al.* (1994) Vascular patterns of gestational trophoblastic tumors by color Doppler ultrasound. *Cancer*, **74**, 2361–5.
25. Tepper, R., Shulman, A., Altaras, M. *et al.* (1994) The role of color Doppler flow in the management of nonmetastatic gestational trophoblastic disease. *Gynecol. Obstet. Invest.*, **38**, 14–17.
26. Park, Y.W., Kim, K.D., Cho, J.S. *et al.* (1994) The utilization of Doppler ultrasonography with color flow mapping in the diagnosis and evaluation of malignant trophoblastic tumors. *Yonsei Med. J.*, **35**, 329–35.
27. Hsieh, F.J., Wu, C.C., Chen, C.A. *et al.* (1994) Correlation of uterine hemodynamics with chemotherapy response in gestational trophoblastic tumors. *Obstet. Gynecol.*, **83**, 1021–5.
28. Lurain, J.R. (1990) Gestational trophoblastic tumors. *Semin. Surg. Oncol.*, **6**, 347–53.
29. Berkowitz, R.S., Goldstein, D.P. and Bernstein, M.R. (1986) Ten years' experience with methotrexate and folinic acid as primary therapy for gestational trophoblastic disease. *J. Gynecol. Oncol.*, **23**, 111–18.
30. Elit, L., Covens, A., Osborne, R. *et al.* (1994) High-dose methotrexate for gestational trophoblastic disease. *Gynecol. Oncol.*, **54**, 282–7.
31. DuBushter, B., Berkowitz, R.S., Goldstein, D.P. and Bernstein, M.R. (1991) Management of low-risk metastatic gestational trophoblastic tumors. *J. Reprod. Med.*, **36**, 36–9.
32. Wong, L.C., Ngan, H.Y., Collins, R.J. and Ma, H.K. (1990) Vaginal metastases in gestational trophoblastic disease. *Asia Oceania J. Obstet. Gynecol.*, **16**, 123–6.
33. Smith, E.B., Weed, J.D., Tyrey, L. *et al.* (1982) Treatment of nonmetastatic gestational trophoblastic disease: results of methotrexate alone versus methotrexate–folinic acid. *Am. J. Obstet. Gynecol.*, **144**, 88–92.
34. Rotmensch, J., Rosenshein, N., Donehower, R. *et al.* (1984) Plasma methotrexate levels in patients with gestational trophoblastic regimens. *Am. J. Obstet. Gynecol.*, **148**, 730–4.
35. Sung, H.C., Wu, P.C. and Yang, H.Y. (1984) Re-evaluation of 5-fluorouracil as a single therapeutic agent for gestational trophoblastic neoplasms. *Am. J. Obstet. Gynecol.*, **150**, 69–75.
36. Wong, L.C., Choo, Y.C. and Ma, H.K. (1986) Primary oral etoposide therapy in gestational trophoblastic disease. *Cancer*, **58**, 14–17.
37. Bagshawe, K.D., Dent, J., Newlands, E.S. *et al.* (1989) The role of low-dose methotrexate and folinic acid in gestational trophoblastic tumours (GTT). *Br. J. Obstet. Gynaecol.*, **96**, 795–802.
38. Gleeson, N.C., Finan, MA., Fiorica, J.V. *et al.* (1993) Nonmetastatic gestational trophoblastic disease: weekly methotrexate compared with 8-day methotrexate–folinic acid. *Eur. J. Gynaecol. Oncol.*, **14**, 461–5.
39. Rose, P.G. and Piver, M.S. (1989) Alternating methotrexate and dactinomycin in nonmetastatic gestational trophoblastic disease. *J. Surg. Oncol.*, **41**, 148–52.
40. Barter, J.F., Soong, S.J., Hatch, K.D. *et al.* (1989) Treatment of nonmetastatic gestational trophoblastic disease with sequential intramuscular and oral methotrexate. *Gynecol. Oncol.*, **33**, 82–4.
41. *Society of Gynecologic Oncologists Staging Handbook*, 1st edn, 1994.

TREATMENT OF METASTATIC GESTATIONAL TROPHOBLASTIC TUMORS

13

John R. Lurain

In the late 1950s and early 1960s, Hertz and colleagues at the US National Cancer Institute (NCI) first demonstrated the efficacy of chemotherapy in the treatment of metastatic gestational trophoblastic disease (GTD)[1,2]. They obtained complete remissions in 47% of patients with methotrexate alone[1] and in 74% of patients treated with both methotrexate and actinomycin D sequentially[2]. These investigators also recognized that successful outcome of therapy was dependent to a large extent on duration of disease, height of the pretreatment human chorionic gonadotropin (hCG) level, presence or absence of brain or liver metastases, and expertise in the use of the chemotherapy drugs. Over 95% of patients who were diagnosed early and treated vigorously were cured, whereas patients in whom there was a delay in diagnosis and consequently more extensive disease had only a 36% remission rate.

This observation led to the recognition of certain prognostic factors which placed patients with trophoblastic tumors at higher risk of treatment failure: (1) longer than four months from the antecedent pregnancy event to diagnosis; (2) pretreatment hCG level >100 000 U/24 h urine or >40 000 U/l serum; (3) metastases to sites other than the lung and vagina; (4) an antecedent term gestation; and (5) previous failed therapy. Most major US trophoblastic disease centers have used a clinical classification system based on these prognostic factors, originally described by the NCI investigators, to determine treatment and report results. In this system, patients are divided into three disease groups: non-metastatic; low-risk metastatic; and high-risk metastatic. High-risk refers to patients whose disease is not likely to be cured by single-agent chemotherapy and who are at the highest risk of treatment failure. In 1983, the World Health Organization (WHO) adopted a prognostic scoring system proposed by Bagshawe based on the patients' age, parity and type of antecedent pregnancy, interval between antecedent pregnancy and trophoblastic tumor event, hCG level, paternal and maternal blood type, number and site of metastases, largest tumor mass and previous chemotherapy. Factors affecting prognosis are assigned numerical values that, when added together, are used to divide patients into low-risk (≤4), middle-risk (5–7), and high-risk (≥8) groups[3].

Patients with low-risk metastatic GTD can still be treated with single-agent chemotherapy, while patients with high-risk metastatic disease, based on the presence of one or more of these prognostic factors and/or a WHO score ≥8, are now generally

Gestational Trophoblastic Disease.
Edited by B.W. Hancock, E.S. Newlands and R.S. Berkowitz.
ISBN 0 412 63100 8

treated more aggressively with initial combination chemotherapy with or without adjuvant radiotherapy or surgery. The benefit of this approach was first noted at the John I. Brewer Trophoblastic Disease Center in 1968. Patients with high-risk disease who were initially treated with the triple chemotherapy regimen of methotrexate, actinomycin D and cyclophosphamide or chlorambucil (MAC) had a survival rate of 65%, whereas the rate for similar patients who were treated initially with a single agent followed by MAC as secondary therapy was 39%[4]. In 1973, Hammond *et al.*[5] reported the results of therapy in 91 patients with metastatic GTD. Seventy-one 'good-prognosis' patients were treated initially with single-agent chemotherapy with a 98.6% survival. Of 17 'poor prognosis' patients, seven received initial single-agent chemotherapy followed by MAC combination chemotherapy if resistance developed, and 10 were treated initially with MAC. Only one of seven patients (14%) treated with single-agent chemotherapy followed by MAC survived as compared to seven of 10 patients (70%) treated initially with MAC.

Others have subsequently confirmed the value of initial combination chemotherapy in treating patients with high-risk metastatic GTD[6–9]. The added toxicity of such combination chemotherapy, however, does not appear to warrant its use in patients with less extensive metastatic disease, in which survival can be anticipated to approach 100% with the use of single-agent chemotherapy. It is imperative, therefore, that patients with metastatic trophoblastic tumors be chosen for treatment with single-agent or multi-agent chemotherapy based on careful attention to selection criteria in order to ensure the best outcome with the least morbidity.

13.1 LOW-RISK METASTATIC DISEASE

Patients categorized into the low-risk metastatic disease group should be treated with single-agent chemotherapy with methotrexate or actinomycin D, according to one of the protocols described in Table 13.1.

Table 13.1 Chemotherapy for low-risk metastatic gestational trophoblastic tumors

Methotrexate 0.4 mg/kg i.v. or i.m. q.d. × 5 d; repeat every 12–14 d (7–9-day window)
Actinomycin D 10–13 μg/kg i.v. q.d. × 5 d; repeat every 12–14 d (7–9-day window)
Methotrexate 1 mg/kg i.m. days 1, 3, 5, 7; folinic acid 0.1 m/kg i.m. days 2, 4, 6, 8; repeat every 15–18 d (7–10-day window)

The weekly methotrexate or biweekly single-dose actinomycin D protocols currently in use for non-metastatic post-molar gestational trophoblastic tumors should not be employed for treatment of metastatic disease. Methotrexate should be avoided if there is an abnormality in hepatic or renal function, or if effusions or large theca lutein cysts are present. At the Brewer Trophoblastic Disease Center, we prefer to begin treatment with a five-day methotrexate regimen unless contraindicated and to administer the drugs sequentially; that is, when resistance to the first drug occurs, the second drug is begun. Patients who develop resistance to sequential single-agent chemotherapy are then treated with combination chemotherapy, as for high-risk disease.

Several studies have demonstrated the high curability of low-risk metastatic GTD when appropriate therapy is administered (Table 13.2). Ross and co-workers were the first investigators to identify the highly favorable prognosis in this group of patients, curing 20 of 21 patients (95%) with relatively non-toxic sequential methotrexate and actinomycin D chemotherapy[2]. Subsequent reports from Brewer *et al.*[4], Hammond *et al.*[5,11], Goldstein and co-workers,[10,12,14], Bagshawe[6], Jones and Lewis[8,13] and Lurain *et al.*[9] documented virtually 100% cures with low-risk metas-

Table 13.2 Treatment of low-risk metastatic gestational trophoblastic tumors with single-agent chemotherapy

Reference	*No. of patients*	*Remission*	
		No.	*%*
Ross *et al.*[2]	21	20	95
Goldstein[10]	29	29	100
Hammond *et al.*[5]	71	70	99
Jones and Lewis[8]	6	6	100
Hammond *et al.*[11]	55	55	100
Goldstein and Berkowitz[12]	95	95	100
Lurain *et al.*[9]	69	69	100
DuBeshter *et al.*[15]	48	48	100
Soper *et al.*[16]	52	52	100

tatic disease using initial single-agent chemotherapy.

DuBeshter *et al.*[15] at the New England Trophoblastic Disease Center treated 48 patients with low-risk metastatic gestational trophoblastic tumors with single-agent methotrexate or actinomycin-D between 1965 and 1990. All patients achieved sustained remission, although 51% required a second single-agent regimen, 14% needed combination chemotherapy, and 12% underwent resection of resistant tumor foci. Combination chemotherapy was more often required following the use of methotrexate–folinic acid protocols (30%) than single-agent methotrexate or actinomycin D (4%).

More recently, Soper *et al.*[16] at the Southeastern Regional Trophoblastic Disease Center retrospectively analyzed 52 patients with low-risk metastatic GTD treated with five-day cycles of intramuscular methotrexate repeated every 12–14 days. Sixty per cent achieved primary remission with a median of three cycles of methotrexate. Therapy was changed because of drug resistance in 19% and toxicity in 21%. Only two patients (4%) required multi-agent therapy, one of whom also underwent hysterectomy. Pre-therapy hCG >10 000 U/l was associated with the development of drug resistance. Sustained remission was achieved in all patients.

At the Brewer Center we treated 92 low-risk metastatic disease patients with initial single-agent chemotherapy between 1962 and 1992. All patients were cured; 72 (78.3%) required only one drug with or without hysterectomy, 19 (20.4%) received two drugs sequentially, and one (1.1%) needed multi-agent chemotherapy. Of the 70 patients treated only with chemotherapy, 21 (30%) required a change in chemotherapy because of drug resistance (24.6%) or toxicity (9.8%)[16a].

It is apparent from these reports that 30–50% of patients will develop resistance to the first chemotherapeutic agent and require alternate treatment. It is, therefore, very important to carefully monitor patients undergoing treatment for evidence of drug resistance (plateau or rise in hCG level and/or development of new metastases) so that a change to a second agent can be made at the earliest possible time. Approximately 10–15% of patients treated for low-risk metastatic disease with sequential single-agent chemotherapy will require combination chemotherapy with or without surgery to achieve complete remission. Surgery may be

Table 13.3 Treatment of high-risk metastatic gestational trophoblastic tumors with MAC

Reference	*No. of patients*	*Remission*	
		No.	*%*
Hammond *et al.*[5]	63	42	67
Jones and Lewis[8]	15	12	80
Berkowitz *et al.*[17]	14	10	71
Gordon *et al.*[19]	32	20	63
Lurain and Brewer[18]	46	29	63

From Lurain, J. R. (1994) High-risk metastatic gestational trophoblastic tumors: current management. *J. Reprod. Med.*, **39**, 217–22.

necessary to eradicate persistent disease in the uterus, if all evidence of metastatic disease has disappeared and if the hCG remains elevated despite repeated courses of chemotherapy, or rarely to excise isolated pulmonary metastases[11,16]. Hysterectomy may also be incorporated into the initial management of the patient with low-risk metastatic disease resulting in a higher likelihood of single-agent chemotherapy success, fewer courses of chemotherapy, and a shorter duration of treatment[11].

13.2 HIGH-RISK METASTATIC DISEASE

Patients categorized as having high-risk metastatic gestational trophoblastic tumors, based on the aforementioned prognostic factors, should be treated with combination chemotherapy. Until the mid-1980s, the primary multi-drug regimen used as initial therapy in these patients was MAC: methotrexate, 15 mg intravenously or intramuscularly; actinomycin D, 0.5 mg intravenously; and cyclophosphamide, 3 mg/kg intravenously, or chlorambucil, 10 mg by mouth, with each drug given for five days per course. Berkowitz *et al.* modified this triple therapy to include slightly higher doses of methotrexate, 1.0 mg/kg intramuscularly on days 1,3,5 and 7, with folinic acid, 0.1 mg/kg intramuscularly on days 2, 4, 6 and 8[17]. The interval between courses was 9–14 days. After three to four courses of such therapy, treatment often needed to be changed to single-agent chemotherapy because of the cumulative toxicity and inability to treat the patient as often as desired.

With the use of initial MAC chemotherapy in the treatment of high-risk patients, reported cure rates ranged from 63% to 80% (Table 3.13). Hammond and colleagues originally reported curing 42 (67%) of 63 high-risk patients treated from 1966 to 1979[11]. Jones and Lewis obtained an 80% remission rate in 15 high-risk patients treated with MAC[8]. All three deaths in their series occurred in patients with brain and/or liver metastases, and all patients who were at high risk because of high hCG levels or prolonged duration of disease only were cured. In 1985 we reported on the treatment of 73 high-risk patients with MAC; 63% of 46 treated primarily were cured. Factors that were determined to influence response to treatment were clinicopathological diagnosis of choriocarcinoma, metastases to sites other than the lung and/or vagina, antecedent term gestation and presence of three or more high-risk factors[18]. Berkowitz and associates[17] and Gordon *et al.*[19] reported similar results.

Table 13.4 EMA-CO regimen for high-risk metastatic gestational trophoblastic tumors

Day	*Drug*	*Dose*
1	Etoposide	100 mg/m^2 i.v. infusion over 30 min
	Actinomycin D	0.5 mg i.v. push
	Methotrexate	100 mg/m^2 i.v. push
		200 mg/m^2 i.v. infusion in 1000 ml 5% dextrose in water over 12 h
2	Etoposide	100 mg/m^2 i.v. infusion over 30 min
	Actinomycin D	0.5 mg i.v. push
	Folinic acid	15 mg i.m. or by mouth every 12 h for 4 doses beginning 24 h after start of methotrexate
8	Cyclophosphamide	600 mg/m^2 i.v.
	Vincristine	1.0 mg/m^2 i.v. push

Repeat cycle on days 15, 16 and 22 (every 2 weeks).
i.v., intravenous; i.m., intramuscular.

In the mid-1970s, Bagshawe introduced the seven-drug, nine-day CHAMOCA protocol, employing hydroxyurea, actinomycin D, methotrexate with folinic acid rescue, cyclophosphamide, vincristine and doxorubicin for the treatment of high-risk patients. Using the CHAMOCA regimen primarily in treating 72 patients over a five-year period, Begent and Bagshawe reported an 82% remission rate[20]. The causes of death in 13 patients were initial extent of disease (6), drug resistance (5), infection (1) and leukemia (1). Wong *et al.* confirmed the effectiveness of this regimen, also achieving an 82% complete remission rate in 50 high-risk patients[21].

In a randomized clinical trial comparing MAC and CHAMOCA for primary treatment of high-risk patients, the Gynecologic Oncology Group (GOG) found that the cure rate was higher in patients who were treated initially with the MAC regimen (95%) as compared with the CHAMOCA regimen (70%)[22]. The primary remission rates for the two protocols were similar, 73% (16/22) for MAC and 65% (13/20) for CHAMOCA; however, five of six patients failing MAC were cured subsequently by additional chemotherapy and surgery versus only one of seven patients failing CHAMOCA. Life-threatening toxicity occurred in 45% of patients receiving CHAMOCA as compared to 9% of patients on the MAC regimen. This study was criticized because the two treatment groups were not stratified for risk factors, resulting in patients with the highest prognostic scores being in the CHAMOCA treatment group. Nevertheless, the study demonstrated that MAC was as effective as CHAMOCA in treating high-risk patients and that it was certainly less toxic.

After the discovery that etoposide was a very effective chemotherapeutic agent for gestational trophoblastic tumors, Newlands *et al.* formulated the EMA-CO regimen employing etoposide, high-dose methotrexate with folinic acid rescue, actinomycin D, cyclophosphamide and vincristine (Table 13.4). They originally reported survival in 83% of 36 patients treated primarily with the EMA-CO regimen[23]. A more recent report from Charing Cross Hospital, London, updating their experience with this regimen demonstrated an 80% complete clinical response rate and 82% survival with minimal

Table 13.5 Treatment of high-risk metastatic gestational trophoblastic tumors with EMA-CO

	Primary therapy				*Secondary therapy*			
	Complete response		*Survival*		*Complete response*		*Survival*	
Reference	*No.*	%	*No.*	%	*No.*	%	*No.*	%
Newlands *et al.*[24]	53/66[a]	80	62/72	82	57/72	82	64/72	89
Bolis *et al.*[25]	16/17	94	15/17	88	10/14	71	9/14	64
Schink *et al.*[26]	10/12	83	12/12	100				
Soper *et al.*[39]	4/6	67			13/16	81	15/22[b]	68[b]

[a]Ten patients who died of the initial disease before a response to EMA-CO could be assessed were excluded from the response analysis.
[b]All patients, primary and secondary chemotherapy.
Modified from Lurain, J.R. (1994) *Journal of Reproductive Medicine*, **38**, 217–22.

toxicity in 76 high-risk patients who had received no prior chemotherapy (Table 13.5)[24]. Bolis *et al.* reported an initial complete response rate of 94% and survival in 88% of 17 patients with high-risk disease treated primarily with EMA-CO. Only one patient failed to achieve an initial complete response, and three patients (19%) relapsed from remission. Significant toxicity, mainly myelosuppression, was observed in 39% of patients[25].

We recently reported the results of a prospective study evaluating the efficacy and toxicity of EMA-CO for initial treatment of patients with high-risk metastatic gestational trophoblastic tumors at the Brewer Trophoblastic Disease Center between 1986 and 1991[26]. Ten of 12 patients (83%) had complete responses to EMA-CO. Two patients had partial responses, and one patient with an initial complete response relapsed four months after completing therapy; all three were salvaged with cisplatin/etoposide with or without bleomycin chemotherapy. Overall survival was 100%, with all 12 patients remaining disease free at a median follow-up of 28 months.

A total of 64 treatment cycles were administered to the 12 patients, and toxicity was not life threatening. In eight of 64 treatment cycles neutropenia occurred, necessitating a one-week treatment delay. Anemia was common, but a transfusion was required in only two chemotherapy cycles. Peripheral neuropathy occurred in two patients. Stomatitis, associated with 18% of treatment cycles, was generally mild. All patients developed alopecia. Reproductive function was preserved in nine patients, all of whom had normal menstrual cycles. Four subsequent pregnancies in three patients resulted in two uncomplicated term deliveries, one preterm delivery and 1 hydatidiform mole complicated by postmolar trophoblastic tumor.

Soper and colleagues[27] treated 22 high-risk patients with EMA-CO. Four (67%) of six patients receiving primary therapy and 13 (81%) of 16 patients receiving secondary therapy had complete responses. Six (35%) of the 17 complete responders developed recurrences within six months of therapy. Overall, 15 (68%) patients have remained without evidence of disease after completing therapy. Grade 4 hematological toxicity was associated with 11% of 126 treatment cycles in 23% of patients; non-hematologic toxicity was uncommon.

Quinn *et al.*[28] from Australia treated 35 patients with metastatic trophoblastic disease with EMA-CO. Most of the patients had high-risk features and all had WHO scores >4. The survival rate was 89%. All four deaths occurred in patients who had hepatic and/or central nervous system metastases, one of whom had a placental site tumor. Treatment was generally well tolerated and toxicity was mild. Treatment delays were necessary on only 52 occasions and grade 4 neutropenia was associated with only five of the 359 treatment cycles.

Other chemotherapeutic agents with proven activity in trophoblastic tumors are cisplatin, bleomycin and ifosfamide. These drugs have been used in combination with vinblastine or etoposide to produce cures in some high-risk patients who have failed initial multi-agent chemotherapy[20,24,29–33]. When these agents are used as components of primary therapy, however, significant cumulative toxicity often occurs before a complete response is accomplished. As demonstrated in the GOG trial comparing MAC with CHAMOCA and also in the EMA-CO reports, the ultimate cure rate often depends on the success of salvage chemotherapy. If the initial chemotherapy regimen results in problematic cumulative toxicity as seen with the MAC, CHAMOCA, cisplatin/bleomycin, and ifosfamide-containing regimens, then the ability to deliver adequate salvage therapy is severely compromised. The EMA-CO regimen is very well tolerated, requiring only one night in the hospital every two weeks, with minimal acute and cumulative toxicity. Chemotherapy is continued until three consecutive normal hCG levels are reached and two to four courses have been given after the first normal hCG level.

When central nervous system (CNS) metastases are present, whole brain irradiation (3000 cGy in 200 cGy fractions) is usually given simultaneously with the initiation of chemotherapy[9,34,35]. Brain irradiation has the dual purpose of being both tumoricidal and hemostatic. Yordan *et al*. reported that death due to CNS involvement occurred in 11 of 25 patients (44%) treated with chemotherapy alone, but in none of 18 patients treated with brain irradiation and chemotherapy[34]. During radiotherapy, the methotrexate infusion dose in the EMA-CO protocol is increased to 1 g/m^2, and 30 mg of folinic acid is given every 12 h for three days, starting 32 h after the infusion begins. As an alternative to brain irradiation, the Charing Cross Hospital group has recommended intrathecal as well as high-dose intravenous methotrexate[23,24,36]. Eighty-six per cent of their patients with brain lesions achieved complete remission with this intensive chemotherapy regimen[37]. Overall, 50–80% of patients with brain metastases can be cured by using these treatment plans.

Liver metastases from choriocarcinoma are particularly ominous since the reported survival of patients with hepatic lesions ranges from 0 to 40%[7,9,38,39]. Most patients with liver metastases have extensive disease when they present for treatment, and this is the primary reason for treatment failure. These patients are at significant risk from serious hepatic bleeding, especially during the first course of chemotherapy. Some authors have recommended whole-liver irradiation to 2000 cGy over two weeks combined with systemic chemotherapy if metastases are present in order to reduce morbidity and mortality from hemorrhage[5, 7,8]. This concept cannot be supported by the literature, and we do not use liver irradiation at the Brewer Center. The technique of selective hepatic artery occlusion has been shown to be effective in controlling hemorrhage from hepatic metastases from choriocarcinoma[40]. Some authors have recommended hepatic artery infusion chemotherapy, but no results of the technique have been reported[41].

Adjuvant surgical procedures, especially hysterectomy and thoracotomy, may be of use in removing known foci of chemotherapy-resistant disease[11,42]. Mutch *et al*. reported that 17 of 28 patients with recurrent gestational trophoblastic tumors had surgery as part of their therapy. Twelve of 14 who underwent hysterectomy had histological evidence of uterine disease, and 10 (71%) survived. Four of nine patients (44%) who underwent thoracotomy with pulmonary wedge resection of resistant choriocarcinoma survived[43]. Surgery may also play a role in therapy for high-risk disease as a means of controlling tumor hemorrhage, relieving bowel or urinary obstruction, treating infection or dealing with other life-threatening complications. Selective angiographic embolization of the uterine arteries may also be employed to control uterine or pelvic tumor bleeding in lieu of surgical intervention[44].

13.3 SUMMARY

Single-agent chemotherapy utilizing standard doses of methotrexate or actinomycin D has resulted in cure of essentially all patients with low-risk metastatic gestational trophoblastic tumors. Approximately 30–50% of patients in this category will develop resistance to the first chemotherapeutic agent, including as many as 10–15% who will require multi-agent chemotherapy with or without surgery to achieve complete remission.

Intensive, multimodality therapy with

appropriate combination chemotherapy (EMA-CO or some variation of it) and adjuvant radiotherapy and surgery, when indicated, has resulted in cure rates of 80–90% in patients with high-risk metastatic gestational trophoblastic tumors. It is clear, however, that approximately 20% of high-risk patients will fail first-line combination chemotherapy. Most of these patients will have a clinicopathological diagnosis of choriocarcinoma, metastases to sites other than the lung and vagina, more than eight metastases and/or failed previous chemotherapy, resulting in high WHO scores (⩾8)[38,39]. They initially respond well to treatment, only to have their hCG levels plateau before achieving complete remission or to relapse after initial remission. In order to cure these patients, we must first use an aggressive regimen of weekly chemotherapy and avoid treatment interruption until hCG levels have normalized. For selected patients who develop drug-resistant choriocarcinoma, surgical resection of sites of resistant disease, usually in the uterus or lungs, remains an important component of the treatment plan. Thereafter, continued salvage chemotherapy with cisplatin/etoposide in combination with bleomycin or ifosfamide will result in a cure for most patients. New technology, such as the use of colony-stimulating factors to prevent treatment delays or dose reductions[45], or high-dose chemotherapy with or without autologous bone marrow transplantation or peripheral stem cell support[46,47], may play an important role in the future management of patients who develop drug resistance.

REFERENCES

1. Hertz, R., Lewis, J., Jr and Lipsett, M.D. (1961) Five years experience with chemotherapy of metastatic choriocarcinoma and related tumors in women. *Am. J. Obstet. Gynecol.*, **82**, 631–40.
2. Ross, G.T., Goldstein, D.P., Hertz, R. *et al.* (1965) Sequential use of methotrexate and actinomycin D in the treatment of metastatic choriocarcinoma and related trophoblastic diseases in women. *Am. J. Obstet. Gynecol.*, **93**, 223–9.
3. World Health Organization Scientific Group on Gestational Trophoblastic Diseases (1983) Gestational Trophoblastic Diseases *WHO Tech. Rep. Ser. 692*.
4. Brewer, J.I., Eckman, T.R., Dolkart, R.E. *et al.* (1971) Gestational trophoblastic disease: a comparative study of the results of therapy in patients with invasive mole and with choriocarcinoma. *Am. J. Obstet. Gynecol.*, **109**, 335–40.
5. Hammond, C.B., Borchert, L.G., Tyrey, L. *et al.* (1973) Treatment of metastatic trophoblastic disease: good and poor prognosis. *Am. J. Obstet. Gynecol.*, **115**, 451–7.
6. Bagshawe, K.D. (1976) Risk and prognostic factors in trophoblastic neoplasia. *Cancer*, **38**, 1373–85.
7. Surwit, E.A. and Hammond, C.B. (1980) Treatment of metastatic trophoblastic disease with poor prognosis. *Obstet. Gynecol.*, **55**, 565–70.
8. Jones, W.B. and Lewis, J.L., Jr (1974) Treatment of gestational trophoblastic disease. *Am. J. Obstet. Gynecol.*, **120**, 14–20.
9. Lurain, J.R., Brewer, J.I., Torok, E.E. *et al.* (1982) Gestational trophoblastic disease: treatment results at the Brewer Trophoblastic Disease Center. *Obstet. Gynecol.*, **60**, 354–60.
10. Goldstein, D.P. (1972) The chemotherapy of gestational trophoblastic disease: principles of clinical management. *JAMA*, **220**, 209–13.
11. Hammond, C.B., Weed, J.C., Jr and Currie, J.L. (1980) The role of operation in the current therapy of gestational trophoblastic disease. *Am. J. Obstet. Gynecol.*, **136**, 844–56.
12. Goldstein, D.P. and Berkowitz, R.S. (1982) Nonmetastatic and low-risk metastatic gestational trophoblastic neoplasms. *Semin. Oncol.*, **9**, 191–7.
13. Jones, W.B. (1981) Management of low-risk metastatic gestational trophoblastic disease. *J. Reprod. Med.*, **26**, 213–17.
14. Berkowitz, R.S., Goldstein, D.P. and Bernstein, M.R. (1986) Ten years' experience with methotrexate and folinic acid as primary therapy for gestational trophoblastic disease.

Gynecol. Oncol., **23**, 111–18.

15. DuBeshter, B., Berkowitz, R.S., Goldstein, D.P. *et al.* (1991) Management of low-risk metastatic gestational trophoblastic tumors. *J. Reprod. Med.*, **36**, 36–9.

16a. Roberts, J.P. and Lurain, J.R. (1996) Treatment of low-risk metastatic gestational trophoblastic tumour with single-agent chemotherapy. *Am. J. Obstet. Gynecol.*, **174**, 1917–24.

16. Soper, J.T., Clarke-Pearson, D.L., Berchuck, A. *et al.* (1994) Five-day methotrexate for women with metastatic gestational trophoblastic disease. *Gynecol. Oncol.*, **54**, 76–9.

17. Berkowitz, R.S., Goldstein, D.P. and Bernstein, M.R. (1984) Modified triple chemotherapy in the management of high-risk metastatic gestational trophoblastic tumors. *Gynecol. Oncol.*, **19**, 173–81.

18. Lurain, J.R. and Brewer, J.I. (1985) Treatment of high-risk gestational trophoblastic disease with methotrexate, actinomycin D and cyclophosphamide chemotherapy. *Obstet. Gynecol.*, **65**, 830–6.

19. Gordon, A.N., Gershenson, D.M., Copeland, L.J. *et al.* (1985) High-risk metastatic gestational trophoblastic disease. *Obstet. Gynecol.*, **65**, 550–6.

20. Begent, R.H.J. and Bagshawe, K.D. (1982) The management of high-risk choriocarcinoma. *Semin. Oncol.*, **9**, 198–203.

21. Wong, L.C., Choo, Y.C. and Ma, H.K. (1986) Modified Bagshawe's regimen in high-risk gestational trophoblastic disease. *Gynecol. Oncol.*, **23**, 87–93.

22. Curry, S.L., Blessing, J.A., DiSaia, P.J. *et al.* (1989) A prospective randomized comparison of methotrexate, actinomycin D and chlorambucil (MAC) versus modified Bagshawe regimen in 'poor-prognosis' gestational trophoblastic disease. *Obstet. Gynecol.*, **73**, 357–62.

23. Bagshawe, K.D. (1984) Treatment of high-risk choriocarcinoma. *J. Reprod. Med.*, **29**, 813–20.

24. Newlands, E.S., Bagshawe, K.D., Begent, R.H.J. *et al.* (1991) Results with EMA/CO (etoposide, methotrexate, actinomycin D, cyclophosphamide, vincristine) regimen in high risk gestational trophoblastic tumors, 1979–1989. *Br. J. Obstet. Gynecol.*, **98**, 550–7.

25. Bolis, G., Bonazzi, C., Landoni, F. *et al.* (1988) EMA/CO regimen in high-risk gestational trophoblastic tumor. *Gynecol. Oncol.*, **31**, 439–44.

26. Schink, J.C., Singh, D.K., Rademaker, A.W. *et al.* (1992) Etoposide, methotrexate, actinomycin D, cyclophosphamide, and vincristine for the treatment of metastatic, high-risk gestational trophoblastic disease. *Obstet. Gynecol.*, **80**, 817–20.

27. Soper, J.T., Evans, A.C., Clarke-Pearson, D.L. *et al.* (1994) Alternating weekly chemotherapy with etoposide–methotrexate–dactinomycin / cyclophosphamide–vincristine for high-risk gestational trophoblastic disease. *Obstet. Gynecol.*, **83**, 113–17.

28. Quinn, M., Murray, J., Friedlander, M. *et al.* (1994) EMACO in high-risk gestational trophoblastic disease; the Australian experience. *Aust. NZ J. Obstet. Gynaecol.*, **34**, 90–2.

29. Gordon, A.N., Kavanagh, J.J., Gershenson, D.M. *et al.* (1986) Cisplatin, vinblastine, and bleomycin combination therapy in resistant gestational trophoblastic disease. *Cancer*, **58**, 1407–10.

30. DuBeshter, B., Berkowitz, R.S., Goldstein, D.P. (1989) Vinblastine, cisplatin and bleomycin as savage therapy for refractory high-risk metastatic gestational trophoblastic disease. *J. Reprod. Med.*, **34**, 189–92.

31. Theodore, C., Azab, M., Droz, J.-P. *et al.* (1989) Treatment of high-risk gestational trophoblastic disease with chemotherapy combinations containing cisplatin and etoposide. *Cancer*, **64**, 1824–8.

32. Azab, M., Droz, J.-P., Theodore, C. *et al.* (1989) Cisplatin, vinblastine, and bleomycin combination in the treatment of resistant high-risk gestational trophoblastic tumors. *Cancer*, **64**, 1829–32.

33. Sutton, G.P., Soper, J.T., Blessin, J.A. *et al.* (1992) Ifosfamide alone and in combination in the treatment of refractory malignant gestational trophoblastic disease. *Am. J. Obstet. Gynecol.*, **167**, 489–95.

34. Yordan, E.L., Schlaerth, J., Gaddis, O. and Morrow, C.P. (1987) Radiation therapy in the management of gestational choriocarcinoma metastatic to the central nervous system. *Obstet. Gynecol.*, **69**, 627–30.

35. Weed, J.C., Jr, Woodward, K.T. and Hammond, C.B. (1982) Choriocarcinoma metastatic

to the brain: therapy and prognosis. *Semin. Oncol.*, **9**, 208–12.

36. Athanassion, A., Begent, R.H.J., Newlands, E.S. *et al.* (1983) Central nervous system metastases of choriocarcinoma: 23 years' experience at Charing Cross Hospital. *Cancer*, **52**, 1728–35.
37. Rustin, G.J., Newlands, E.S., Begent, R.H. *et al.* (1989) Weekly alternating etoposide, methotrexate and actinomycin D/vincristine and cyclophosphamide chemotherapy for the treatment of CNS metastases of choriocarcinoma. *J. Clin. Oncol.*, **7**, 900–4.
38. Lurain, J.R., Casanova, L.A., Miller, D.S. *et al.* (1991) Prognostic factors in gestational trophoblastic tumors: a proposed new scoring system based on multivariate analysis. *Am. J. Obstet. Gynecol.*, **164**, 611–16.
39. Soper J.T., Evans, A.C., Conaway, M.R. *et al.* (1994) Evaluating prognostic factors and staging in gestational trophoblastic tumor. *Obstet. Gynecol.*, **84**, 969–73.
40. Crumbine, F.C., Rosenshein, N.B., Brereton, H.D. and Kaufman, S.L. (1980) Management of liver metastases from gestational trophoblastic neoplasia. *Am. J. Obstet. Gynecol.*, **137**, 959–61.
41. Song, H., Zia, Z., Wu, B. and Wang, Y. (1979) 20 years' experience in chemotherapy of choriocarcinoma and malignant mole. *Chin. Med. J.*, **92**, 677–87.
42. Soper, J.T. (1994) Surgical therapy for gestational trophoblastic disease. *J. Reprod. Med.*, **39**, 168–74.
43. Mutch, D.G., Soper, J.T., Babcock, C.J. (1990) Recurrent gestational trophoblastic disease. *Cancer*, **66**, 978–82.
44. Vogelzang, R.L., Nemcek, A.A., Skrtic, Z. *et al.* (1991) Uterine arteriovenous malformations: primary treatment with therapeutic embolization. *J. Vasc. Intervent. Radiol.*, **2**, 517–22.
45. Hartenbach, E.M., Saltzman, A.K., Carter, J.R. *et al.* (1995) A novel strategy using G-CSF to support EMA/CO for high-risk gestational trophoblastic disease. *Gynecol. Oncol.*, **56**, 105–8.
46. Collins, R.H., Jr, White, C.S., Stringer, C.A. and Fay, J.W. (1991) Successful treatment of refractory gestational trophoblastic neoplasm with high-dose etoposide and cyclophosphamide. *Gynecol. Oncol.*, **43**, 317–19.
47. Lotz, J.P., Andre, T., Donsimoni, R. *et al.* (1995) High-dose chemotherapy with ifosfamide, carboplatin, and etoposide combined with autologous bone marrow transplantation for the treatment of poor-prognosis germ cell tumors and metastatic trophoblastic disease in adults. *Cancer*, **75**, 874–85.

DIFFERENCES IN MANAGEMENT AND TREATMENT: A CRITICAL APPRAISAL 14

Barry W. Hancock

Gestational trophoblastic disease (GTD) is such a rare condition, with acknowledged geographical and cultural differences in behavior, that it is not surprising that management and treatment philosophies should vary across the world. In developed health care systems:

1. accurate registration and follow-up data are usually available, and often reported on a formal basis;
2. clinical management (diagnosis, staging and treatment) is usually undertaken by health professionals skilled in the care of these specialized conditions according to agreed local (and sometimes national) protocols;
3. the disease is usually detected in 'early' stages and follow-up is not usually a problem.

In less developed countries, particularly in Asia, Africa, South America and the Indian subcontinent:

1. population-based incidence and outcome data are less easy to come by;
2. treatment is undertaken in hospitals by caring but not necessarily specialized staff, with suboptimal health care and drug resources;
3. patients often present late in their disease, and adequate follow-up is often impossible.

Differences in management between different treatment centers in the West (particularly between the USA and UK) are largely a reflection of the 'local' experience and expertise of the center, and of patient expectation and medicolegal consequences. For example, patients in the USA are far more likely at the present time to sue their clinician for not giving 'appropriate' treatment as soon as possible, particularly if the treatment when it has to be given is more complicated and problematic.

14.1 CLINICAL PRESENTATION

In contemporary gynecological practice there is now general awareness of the protean clinical manifestations of gestational GTD and the need to refer such cases to 'expert' centers. When such patients present to other clinicians, particularly with non-gynecological symptoms and signs (the classic examples being respiratory or central nervous system presentations), the diagnosis is often delayed, primarily because it comes a long way down the list of differential diagnoses.

However, in some countries, even where a formal or semi-formal registration exists,

Gestational Trophoblastic Disease.
Edited by B.W. Hancock, E.S. Newlands and R.S. Berkowitz.
ISBN 0 412 63100 8

referral to a center may not be made – either at the request of the patient or more likely a feeling on the part of the attending physician that he or she is competent to undertake the full clinical care of that patient! There is now, however, a growing body of evidence suggesting that patients with rare cancers are best treated in special centers[1].

In developing countries, patients frequently present with advanced local or metastatic disease and may never be referred to expert centers – either because of the difficulties on the part of the patient in actually traveling to that center or because of the non-existence of such a center.

The UK registration, screening and treatment facility is generally regarded as the ideal model for the management of GTD; the excellent results in those patients who eventually come to treatment are a testament to the success of this surveillance scheme. In other developed countries, particularly in the USA, large university hospital centers have been established for treatment; these are, however, few designated registration and screening systems and patients are referred from local practitioners (most often gynecologists) often at presentation but also when problems start to develop, for example with persistent GTD or less commonly gestational trophoblastic tumor (GTT) resistant to treatment. In the UK, such patients are rarely seen and then most often from overseas; this is a particular feature of the Charing Cross (London) center practice.

14.2 MANAGEMENT

If it is accepted that patterns of presentation vary then obviously management protocols will be adapted to take into account these local factors. There is no conclusive evidence to suggest that there are major variations in the natural history of GTD once detected, yet more patients will be treated for persistent GTD or GTT in the USA (approximately 20%) than in the UK (less than 10%).

The level of investigation undertaken depends on:

1. the availability and 'up-to-dateness' of those investigations available;
2. the requirements of the staging/prognostic scoring systems being used;
3. clinical research into new investigational methods being undertaken at the time.

The availability of sophisticated human chorionic gonadotropin (hCG) assay systems and high-technology scanning facilities has led (sometimes) in developed countries to a more intensive investigation of patients, but as yet this has not influenced clinical management protocols, most of which are based on traditional (and largely unchanged) staging/prognostic scoring systems relying broadly on clinical criteria, simple radiological tests and a satisfactory broad-spectrum βhCG assay. Whilst undoubtedly computed tomography or magnetic resonance imaging scans, immunoscintigraphy and sophisticated (e.g. color Doppler) ultrasonography give more information regarding individual patients[2–4], many authorities still recommend that the basic investigations should simply include clinical assessment, βhCG assay, chest radiology and abdominal ultrasonography, and will make their treatment decisions on the basis of these evaluations.

14.3 TREATMENT

Hysterectomy remains a reasonable option for fit, usually older, patients with family completed and to whom sterilization is acceptable – the risk of persistent GTD falls from 20% to below 10%[5].

Very few experts disagree on the management of locally advanced/bulky or grossly metastatic disease, proven choriocarcinoma or very high βhCGs. Once the diagnosis has been established (clinical evaluation, evacuation curettage, hCG levels) most authorities would institute chemotherapy without much delay.

For non-metastatic disease the situation is different. The criteria for starting chemotherapy vary from center to center. The place for prophylactic chemotherapy (i.e. at the time of molar evacuation) is still being debated. This would seem a valuable option for patients with high-risk complete moles in countries where clinical or technical resources are not available to monitor patients, or where patients may be non-compliant. The risk of persistent GTD and/or metastases is reduced from about 50% to 10%[6]. In centers where facilities for treatment and follow-up are optimal, the role for prophylactic chemotherapy can be disputed:

1. there is unnecessary exposure (albeit brief), to chemotherapy in over half of such patients;
2. protection against persistent GTD is incomplete;
3. a false sense of security (possibly with inadequate follow-up) might be engendered.

For this reason many centers rely on a close clinical and biochemical (βhCG) monitoring in all cases following adequate evacuation.

The indications for treating persistent GTD vary significantly, particularly between the USA and the UK (where a more conservative approach is adopted). In the USA a standard recommendation is that if hCG levels increase or plateau over a period of three or more consecutive weeks, immediate work-up and treatment for post-molar GTD are indicated[6]. At the other end of the spectrum UK clinicians advocate a more expectant policy, and in low-risk cases we are prepared to wait up to six months following these patients with serial hCG estimations, provided the hCG is falling. At the Sheffield center we treat only 5% of our registered patients[7,8], compared with 8% at Charing Cross and approximately 20% in the USA[9]. Patient selection may have some bearing on this – in Sheffield we rarely have patients referred with other than newly diagnosed disease; we do not have patients who have proved difficult management problems to other clinicians (e.g. chemotherapy resistance). In addition we have 'traditionally' requested a second dilatation and curettage in patients with persistent GTD derived from low-risk moles – we are currently re-evaluating this policy which to many colleagues is outmoded. However, we do not have an 'inferior' cure rate – 98% overall – from this ultra-conservative policy!

The risks of treating a greater proportion of patients are theoretically the same as those quoted for prophylactic chemotherapy – mainly exposure of twice as many patients to toxic therapy. In practice, however, chemotherapy though associated with short-term side effects has not led to major long-term sequelae – in particular on future pregnancy outcomes, and only a slight increase in second cancers[10].

The regimen of chemotherapy given varies in type, schedule and with clinical treatment criteria. Here, staging/prognostic groupings become highly relevant – there is clearly a need to distinguish low-risk from high-risk molar disease and particularly which factors relate to persistent GTD and to chemotherapy resistance. There are a large number of classification schemes for both scoring and staging GTD, none of which has gained universal acceptance, reflecting both 'personal preference' on the part of the proponents and users of the particular system and also that there are deficiencies in all of them[11]. The World Health Organization (WHO) (and the Charing Cross system from which it is derived) and the National Institutes of Health (NIH) systems are the oldest and still the most widely used. They are not true staging systems but define (with reasonable accuracy and equivalence) prognostic categories requiring 'high-risk' (multi-agent) or 'low-risk' (single-agent) chemotherapy. The revised International Federation of Gynecology and Obstetrics (FIGO) system now includes prognostic as well as anatomical criteria; its predictive value remains to be evaluated.

The Charing Cross group, using their own scoring system, select three groups for differing intensities of therapies; most centers, however, define two groups only. Single-agent low-dose methotrexate (with folinic acid rescue) remains the most popular therapy worldwide for truly low-risk GTD. However, actinomycin D given as a single treatment every 14 days has also been shown to be effective treatment[12] and there are no controlled data comparing these two agents. Methotrexate has its own particular problems and even ardent proponents of this therapy admit that toxicity curtails the use in over 5% of patients (the associated pleurisy can be particularly debilitating). Actinomycin D causes alopecia, myelosuppression and more nausea and vomiting. Despite the fact that this might seem to be a more cost-effective way of managing treatment (i.e. two-weekly intravenous day case injections rather than alternate-day intramuscular injections) patients often prefer the latter particularly if this can be done in the community. Also there are more data on methotrexate (than on actinomycin D) as to the lack of long-term carcinogenicity.

A proportion of patients will be resistant to single-agent chemotherapy but usually respond to multi-agent regimens.

For high-risk (Charing Cross intermediate- and high-risk) tumors multi-agent chemotherapy (MAC, CHAMOCA, EMACO) are given with good results; even when these patients are chemoresistant salvage regimens (incorporating agents such as cisplatin) are successful in the majority of patients.

Again, our more conservative (Sheffield) approach[13] does not lead to inferior treatment results in our patient population; 3196 cases were registered between 1 May 1986 and 30 April 1994 – approximately 400 per annum. During this time 166 patients have required chemotherapy for persistent GTD. Based on their Charing Cross risk score, patients were assigned to low (score 7 or less) or high (8 or more) risk categories receiving low-dose methotrexate or moderate-dose methotrexate, with actinomycin D/etoposide, treatment regimens respectively (Table 14.1). In the low-risk group 78% (113 of 145) of patients were cured with no further treatment; all methotrexate-resistant cases responded to actinomycin D/etoposide. In the high-risk groups 76% (16 of 21) were cured with first-line intensive treatment therapy; two of the five not responding were successfully salvaged with a cisplatin/etoposide/cyclophosphamide regimen in association with surgical resection of metastases. Three patients have died (all from tumor-related problems); all were atypical in histopathological type.

Table 14.1 Current treatment regimens (Sheffield, UK)

'Low risk' group (maximum score 7)
Low-dose methotrexate (MTX): 50 mg i.m. alternating days × 4 doses
Folinic acid: 7.5 mg p.o. 24 h after each MTX
7-day interval *et seq.*

MTX resistance
Actinomycin D: 500 μg i.v. daily × 3
Etoposide: 100 mg/m^2 i.v. daily × 3
7-day interval *et seq.*

'High risk' group (score 8 or more)
MTX: 300 mg/m^2 i.v. in 12 h
Folinic acid: 15 mg six-hourly × 8 doses commencing 24 h after start of MTX

7-day interval then:
Actinomycin D: 500 μg i.v. daily × 3
Etoposide: 100 mg/m^2 i.v. daily × 3
7-day interval *et seq.*

14.4 CONCLUSIONS

For the optimal management of GTD (allowing for geographical and cultural variations), it is possible to recommend the following.

1. Patients diagnosed with GTD should be formally registered and monitored through a purpose-designated screening center.
2. Clinical management should be by expert specialist multidisciplinary health professionals.
3. All staging/scoring systems have deficiencies but are appropriate guides to clinical management when used by clinicians familiar and expert in interpretation of the particular system.
4. An assay that detects all forms of hCG, such as a βhCG radioimmunoassay, is to be preferred.
5. Standard (i.e. non-research) investigations should be appropriate to that information required for the staging/scoring system being used.
6. Prophylactic chemotherapy is acceptable for those patients with high-risk molar disease where monitoring facilities are suboptimal.
7. Hysterectomy is an option for older patients with low-risk molar disease not requiring to maintain fertility.
8. Low- and high-risk categories can be defined, though some overlap is inevitable.
9. For low-risk GTD single-agent chemotherapy with methotrexate or actinomycin D is appropriate; methotrexate is generally considered the less toxic in the short and long term.
10. For high-risk GTD multi-agent chemotherapy (usually incorporating methotrexate, actinomycin D and etoposide) is recommended.
11. Relapse after first-line chemotherapy for high-risk disease can generally be salvaged by alternative chemotherapy regimens (plus surgical resection when needed).
12. In the optimal situation almost 100% success can be achieved in the treatment of GTD.

REFERENCES

1. Spiller, C.A. (1994) Centralised treatment, entry to trials and survival. *British Journal of Cancer*, **70**, 352–62.
2. DeBaz, D.P. and Lewis, T.J. (1995) Imaging of gestational trophoblastic disease. *Seminars in Oncology*, **22**, 130–41.
3. Tang, K.S., Nakielny, R.A. and Hancock, B.W. (1993) Computerised tomographic (CT) scanning of the abdomen in the investigation of persistent trophoblastic disease: How necessary is it? *Journal of Cancer Care*, **2**, 222–4.
4. Lorigan, P.C., O'Sullivan, M.P., Peck, R.J. *et al*. (1994) Imaging techniques for persistent gestational trophoblastic disease. *British Journal of Cancer*, **70**, (22), 16.
5. Bahar, A.M., El-Ashnehi, N.S. and Senthilselvan, A. (1989) Hydatidiform mole in the elderly: hysterectomy or evacuation. *International Journal of Obstetrics and Gynaecology*, **29**, 233–8.
6. Goldstein, D.P. and Berkowitz, R.S. (1995) Prophylactic chemotherapy of complete molar pregnancy. *Seminars in Oncology*, **22**, 157–60.
7. Doreen, M.S. (1993) Gestational trophoblastic diseases: a review of their presentation and management. *Clinical Oncology*, **5**, 46–56.
8. Sheridan, E., Hancock, B.W., Smith, S.C. *et al*. (1993) Gestational trophoblastic disease: experience of the Sheffield (United Kingdom) supraregional screening and treatment service. *International Journal of Oncology*, **3**, 149–55.
9. Kennedy, A.W. (1995) Persistent non-metastatic gestational trophoblastic disease. *Seminars in Oncology*, **22**, 161–5.
10. Newlands, E.S., Rustin, G.J.S., Lutz, J.M. *et al*. (1995) Chemotherapy for gestational trophoblastic tumours may increase the incidence of second tumours and may cause a premature menopause. *Proceedings of American Society of Clinical Oncology*, **14**, 269.

11. Greenfield, A.W. (1995) Gestational trophoblastic disease: prognostic variables and staging. *Seminars in Oncology*, **2**, 142–8.
12. Schlaerth, J.B., Morrow, C.P., Nalick, R.H. *et al*. (1984) Single-dose Actinomycin-D in the treatment of post molar trophoblastic disease. *Gynecologic Oncology*, **19**, 53–6.
13. Loryan, P.C., Nevin, J., Radstone, C. *et al*. (1995) Etoposide and actinomycin D (EA) for methotrexate (MTX) resistant, low-risk persistent gestational trophoblastic disease (GTD) and EA with MTX (MEA) for high-risk GTD. *European Journal of Cancer*, **31A**, S244.

ROLE OF SURGERY 15

David R. Millar

Chemotherapy has established itself as the cornerstone of treatment in gestational trophoblastic disease (GTD), with cure rates of over 95% to be expected even in metastatic carcinoma.

Before the days of chemotherapy the best that surgery had to offer was 40% five-year survival when the disease was thought to be confined to the uterus and only 20% in the presence of metastases[1].

One corollary of modern management is that the study of autopsy material and the histological examination of the excised uterus play an ever decreasing role in diagnosis, so that many cases of GTD are cured without establishing whether the case was one of invasive mole (IM) or choriocarcinoma (CC).

Surgery still has an important place in the management of hydatidiform mole and a subsidiary role in the treatment of persistent GTD and this will be covered under the headings listed below:

- Evacuation of hydatidiform mole
- Diagnosis of persistent GTD
- Place of hysterectomy in treatment
- Conservative uterine surgery
- Surgery for metastatic disease
- Special techniques to control hemorrhage
- Placental site trophoblastic tumor
- Non-gestational choriocarcinoma
- Pre- and postoperative care.

15.1 EVACUATION OF HYDATIDIFORM MOLE

The widespread use of ultrasonic scanning in early pregnancy has led to the frequent diagnosis of molar pregnancy before spontaneous, or even threatened abortion intervenes. Because the risks of vaginal hemorrhage, and of other serious complications such as hyperemesis and pregnancy hypertension, increase with gestational age evacuation of the mole is recommended as soon as possible after the diagnosis is made. The only rare exception to this rule is when an apparently normal fetus accompanies the mole[2]. Usually this means a partial mole with a triploid fetus which will result in missed abortion or in fetal death soon after miscarriage, but a fetus with a normal appearance on ultrasound may be a twin accompanying the mole and capable of survival. Under these circumstances a spell of conservative management to a stage of fetal viability may be tried, although spontaneous mid-trimester abortion, or the need to intervene because of other molar complications, are the more common end results.

Gestational Trophoblastic Disease.
Edited by B.W. Hancock, E.S. Newlands and R.S. Berkowitz.
ISBN 0 412 63100 8

15.1.1 SUCTION CURETTAGE AND OXYTOCICS

The method of choice for the evacuation of a mole is cervical dilatation and the use of a suction catheter under general anesthesia but epidural, spinal or paracervical blocks may be used in selected cases.

Oxytocic agents play an important complementary role in reducing hemorrhage. Prostaglandins, mifepristone[3] and oxytocin can be used singly or in combination to induce abortion medically, but curettage is seldom avoided as the mole is usually expelled incompletely. Moreover, medical abortion has been accepted as leading to a higher incidence of post-molar disease[4].

More recent evidence has suggested that the prognosis relates to gestational age and not to the use of oxytocics, which have been selectively employed in more advanced pregnancies[5,6].

In contrast to induced abortion when a fetus is present, there is no gestational age at which the evacuation of a mole by the suction method is contraindicated. When the pregnancy has progressed beyond the first trimester an infusion of oxytocin (30–40 U/l) is advised during the evacuation and the cross-matching of blood is a reasonable precaution. As a mixture of blood and molar tissue enters the suction bottle it is difficult to assess the true blood loss and pulmonary edema due to excessive transfusion is a hazard[2]. Therefore, especially after 16 weeks of gestational age, central venous pressure monitoring may be a wise precaution during the operation.

When the evacuation of the uterus is complete an injection of ergometrine (0.25 mg intravenously or 0.5 mg intramuscularly) is indicated. Anesthetists may be reluctant to use this long-established oxytocic because it can cause hypertension and vomiting, but there is no better agent for controlling hemorrhage from the placental site by causing a sustained uterine contraction. It is contraindicated only in the presence of severe hypertension. Suction curettage is so efficient that hysterotomy for mole is only considered in the rare situation that a viable fetus is present.

The tissue obtained from the uterus should be sent for pathological examination, but Elston was not able to show that even expert histology could predict which cases would require treatment for persistent disease[7,8].

Because rhesus iso-immunization can occur with a true classical mole and the coexistence of a fetus (partial mole) is difficult to exclude, it is recommended that anti-D γ-globulin be given to non-immunized rhesus-negative mothers after the evacuation.

15.1.2 HYSTERECTOMY

Primary hysterectomy, especially for the older parous woman with hydatidiform mole (HM), was advocated in Singapore based on the increased risk of post-molar disease with age[9]. This radical treatment reduced the number of deaths from CC in the days before chemotherapy but did not prevent invasive disease and may even promote the vascular dissemination of trophoblast[4,10].

Although a woman over 35 years of age is much more likely to have a molar pregnancy and its malignant sequelae, in our experience, and in the published work of others[10], she does not have a worse prognosis, in terms of response to treatment, if persistent GTD ensues. So we reserve primary hysterectomy for mole for a few older women who request sterilization, and for the patient who presents with a rare but serious complication such as uterine sepsis or perforation.

The removal of the uterus does not prevent the need for registration of the mole and for careful follow-up for malignant sequelae.

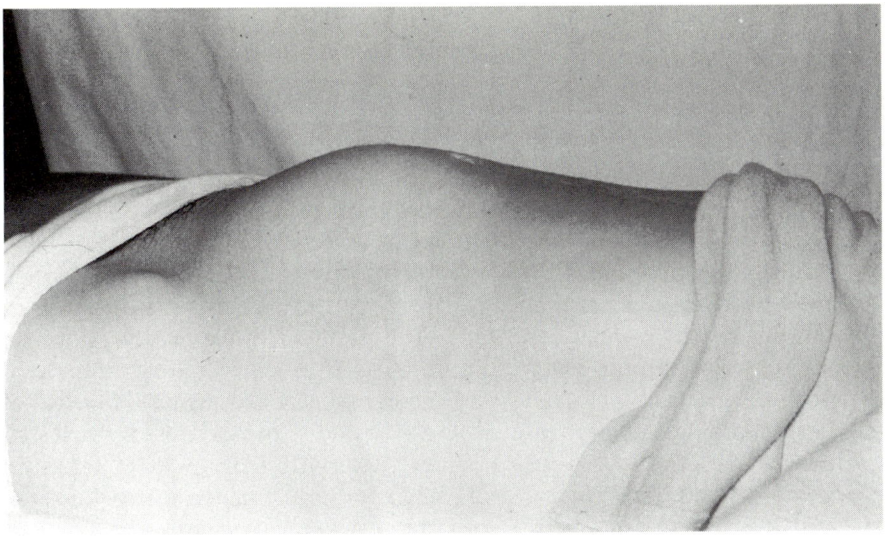

Figure 15.1 Lower abdominal swelling due to large theca lutein cysts.

15.1.3 OVARIAN CYSTS

Occasionally a laparotomy may be required for complications arising from the presence of theca lutein cysts in association with a mole. Torsion or hemorrhage may demand an oophorectomy, but in general these cysts should be left alone as they resolve completely when the human chorionic gonadotropin (hCG) levels return to normal (Figure 15.1).

15.1.4 PROPHYLACTIC CHEMOTHERAPY

We do not recommend that methotrexate or other anticancer agents be given to cover the evacuation of HM. Thus, some 95% of our patients avoid having cytotoxic chemotherapy which can cause serious complications even in small doses. The 5% of post-molar patients who require chemotherapy in the north of England start their treatment with no previous exposure to the drugs and this may reduce the problem of drug resistance[11]. A randomized controlled trial of prophylactic chemotherapy in molar pregnancy is at present in progress to establish whether the above policy is correct.

15.1.5 MOLAR ECTOPIC PREGNANCY

Although there are fewer than 100 reported cases there is no reason why the incidence of HM in ectopic pregnancy should be any different from that in uterine pregnancy. Usually the diagnosis is made only after salpingectomy but there have been some reports of the correct diagnosis having been made by ultrasound[12].

The trend of dealing with ectopic pregnancy laparoscopically leads to a greater risk of disseminating trophoblast within the peritoneal cavity. A review of American laparoscopists suggested that this risk might merit follow-up by hCG assays after all salpingectomies[13]. Certainly, ectopic moles need the usual period of monitoring and if there are malignant sequelae chemotherapy is equally effective.

15.2 DIAGNOSIS OF PERSISTENT TROPHOBLASTIC DISEASE

15.2.1 REPEAT CURETTAGE

The use of a sharp curette was not mentioned in the section on evacuation of a mole because it increases the risk of uterine perforation, may cause synechiae and Asherman's syndrome (where the uterine cavity is obliterated by adhesions) and may encourage trophoblastic emboli by opening up tissue planes deep to the decidua.

Instead, many gynecologists advocate an exploration with a sharp curette one or two weeks after molar evacuation, when the uterus is firm and involuted. This routine is unnecessary if hCG levels are falling satisfactorily and if there is no significant vaginal blood loss[14].

It is not uncommon for patients with persistent disease to arrive at the treatment center only after the referring doctor has carried out multiple fruitless curettage procedures for continued vaginal bleeding. The invasive trophoblast in these cases is deep within the myometrium and is inaccessible to the curette. An ultrasonic scan looking for tissue within the endometrial cavity is most valuable in detecting those cases where exploration is worthwhile. When an experienced gynecologist has repeated the evacuation once without relieving the bleeding any patient whose hCG levels remain elevated should be referred for chemotherapy.

15.2.2 ENDOSCOPY

Laparoscopy has been used to detect invasive disease in the uterus and intra-abdominal metastases but its use in diagnosis has been replaced almost completely by the accuracy of modern ultrasound scanning. Therapeutic laparoscopy may be of benefit in aspirating fluid from thecalutein cysts which are causing symptoms. Hysteroscopy, like curettage, is of limited value because invasive disease is not visible in the endometrial cavity.

15.2.3 HYSTERECTOMY

Those women who develop CC soon after a normal pregnancy usually present with postpartum hemorrhage and, when the bleeding is severe, it is not uncommon for the correct diagnosis to be made only after emergency hysterectomy. When secondary postpartum bleeding is persistent or recurrent an hCG assay should always be requested before considering hysterectomy or internal iliac artery ligation. Prompt chemotherapy may control the bleeding and preserve the uterus.

15.3 THE PLACE OF HYSTERECTOMY IN TREATMENT

In modern management two main indications for hysterectomy are well established, namely to control severe uterine hemorrhage and to eliminate disease which is confined to the uterus and which has proved to be resistant to chemotherapy[15].

Vaginal bleeding is a problem most commonly in the early days of treatment and it is always worth instituting or persisting with a chemotherapeutic regimen for several days despite heavy bleeding because the drugs do reduce the vascularity of the trophoblastic tumor. However, if the patient's condition continues to deteriorate despite transfusion hysterectomy becomes an option, along with selective embolization of the pelvic vessels which will be discussed later.

There is a wide variation in the reported incidence of hysterectomy. In 1980 the team at Duke University, North Carolina, published a series of 257 cases of GTD in which the uterus was removed in more than a quarter overall and in 32% of patients with metastases. Evidence was presented that early hysterectomy reduced the duration of treatment and surgery was favored particularly in those who had completed their families[16].

A recent Polish review included 178 patients with GTD, all treated by chemotherapy, of whom 29% had hysterectomy (10% before treatment started and 19% during treatment)[17]. On the other hand, the Singapore group selected those cases of CC which did not respond to chemotherapy and their hysterectomy rate was only 1.5%[18].

In a review of high-risk cases from Charing Cross Hospital, London[19], 8.8% of 148 patients were subjected to hysterectomy as a salvage procedure, but in only two of the 13 patients was the operation deemed to be of major benefit, largely because in nine cases the pathologist could not find active residual disease in the uterus. This was probably because the surgery was done as a last resort after prolonged chemotherapy.

The special principles of surgery in these cases, in order to minimize the risk of causing trophoblastic emboli, are that the vessels draining the uterus should be ligated at an early stage and the uterine tissues should be handled as gently as possible.

15.3.1 SHEFFIELD EXPERIENCE

In the 20 years between the start of molar registration in 1973 and 1992 the North of England Trophoblastic Tumour Centre treated 333 women with chemotherapy (5.7% of all registered patients, but less than 5% of post-molar cases as one-eighth of the total were postpartum and post-abortal cases of proven CC).

Twenty (6%) of all the treated patients had already had a hysterectomy, usually for hemorrhage, in the referring center (Table 15.1). Five of these were done for uncontrollable postpartum hemorrhage due to CC.

Among the post-molar cases, those women who bled heavily vaginally usually proved to have CC whereas, when the operation was done for severe intraperitoneal bleeding from disease penetrating the uterus, this proved more often to be IM.

The remaining three cases of hysterectomy in this group were patients with atypical histology: two with placental site trophoblastic tumor and one with a dimorphic tumor with elements of endometrial carcinoma as well as CC. Two of these eventually died of their disease.

Hysterectomy was undertaken on 24 occasions during chemotherapy in Sheffield (7.2%) and 15 of these were for drug resistance (Table 15.2). It has been our practice to operate when second-line chemotherapy (usually a combination of methotrexate, ac-

Table 15.1 Gestational trophoblastic disease: hysterectomy prior to chemotherapy

Postpartum hemorrhage (CC)	5
Post-molar hemorrhage	
Vaginal (CC)	4
(IM)	1
Peritoneal (CC)	2
(IM)	5
Atypical disease (2 died)	3
	20 (6%)

Table 15.2 Gestational trophoblastic disease: hysterectomy during chemotherapy

Choriocarcinoma	
Residual uterine disease	
No further chemotherapy	6
Cured after further chemotherapy	6
Died of metastases	1
Vaginal hemorrhage	4
Patient's request	3
Invasive mole	
Resistant to chemotherapy	2
Peritoneal hemorrhage	2
	24 (7.2%)

tinomycin D and etoposide) fails to lower the hCG levels and when we are sure that there is no more than minimal disease outside the uterus. We cover the operation with either methotrexate or etoposide and have never experienced problems with wound healing in the convalescent period.

Eight of these 15 patients (six with CC and two with IM) required no further chemotherapy. The cases of IM had massive well differentiated disease which seemed to be particularly resistant to chemotherapy.

Only one patient in this high-risk group was not cured and she was one of the first to be treated in Sheffield in 1974. In retrospect this was a fruitless operation as she proved later to have brain metastases.

An interesting histopathological observation in this group of resistant tumors is that there is not, as one might expect, a necrotic layer of growth surrounding the active disease. Typically there is a peripheral shell of active tumor round a necrotic core, so the resistance to chemotherapeutic attack is not due to the inability of the drug to reach the malignant cells. (Figures 15.2 and 15.3).

Three patients were reluctant to continue with their chemotherapy for psychological or social reasons. We agreed to their request for hysterectomy and they all did well. The last six women required emergency hysterectomy for severe bleeding despite chemotherapy and again the observation was made that the vaginal hemorrhages were from true CC while those that bled into the abdomen had IM. Figure 15.4 shows a typical example of a uterus with penetrating IM. This was a young unmarried girl of 19 who fortunately later married and was able to adopt children, but this case prompted our interest in reviewing the place of conservative uterine surgery for such patients.

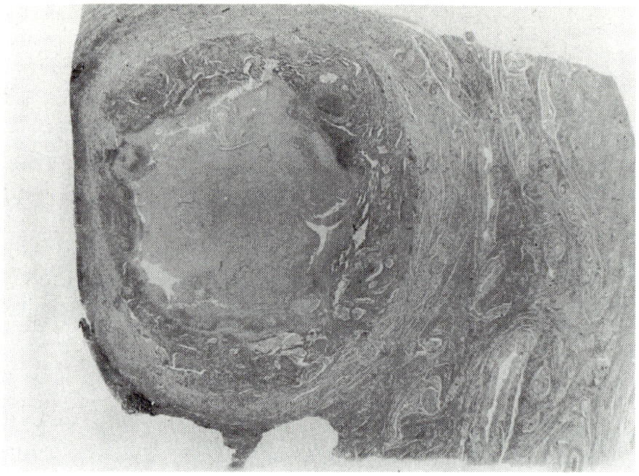

Figure 15.3 Histological section of similar lesion.

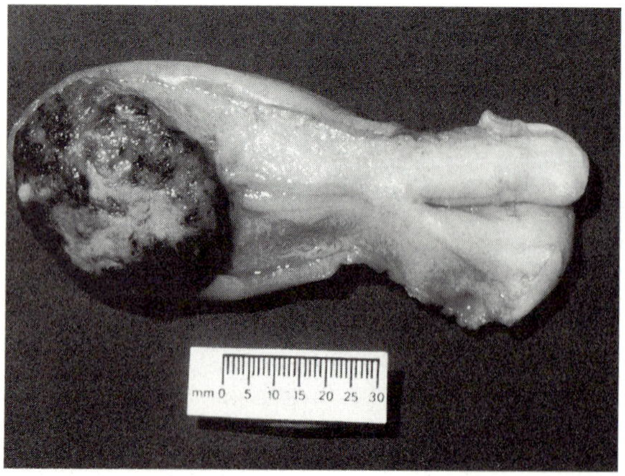

Figure 15.2 Uterus showing large deposit of resistant CC.

15.4 CONSERVATIVE UTERINE SURGERY

In 1965 there was a report from the Mayo Clinic describing five patients whose invasive molar tissue was removed by local excision from the uterus[20]. None had chemotherapy and none developed malignant sequelae. The progression from a villous to an avillous tumor is rare.

Two further papers from Japan describe cases where foci of invasive mole were excised, many of the patients subsequently delivering healthy babies[21,22].

More recently a Chinese group has reported on 25 cases where they removed

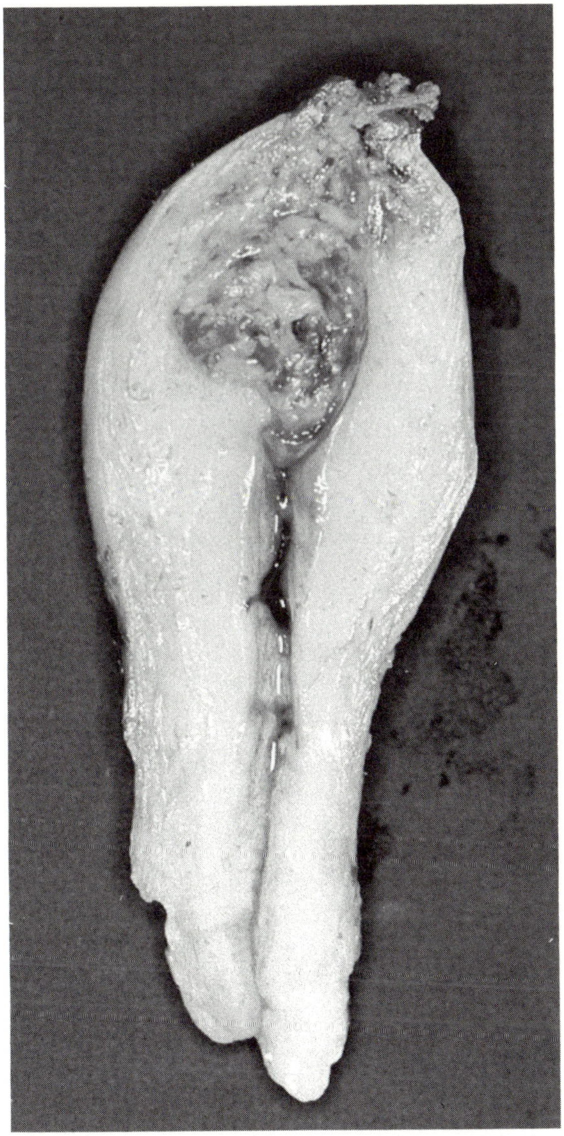

Figure 15.4 Uterus showing a penetrative invasive mole which caused severe intraperitoneal hemorrhage.

nodules of 'malignant trophoblastic tumor' from the uterus by hysterotomy to preserve the fertility of nulliparous women[23].

In Sheffield we have treated six patients after the referring surgeons, operating for intraperitoneal hemorrhage, had merely sutured the uterine perforation or had excised the invasive disease and repaired the uterus. Four were clear cases of IM, but one showed areas of villous tumor suggesting transition to CC, and the last was frank postpartum CC. All these patients did well after chemotherapy and one has since conceived. The conclusion is that, when one is dealing with a malignant disease as responsive to chemotherapy as GTD, then the normal rules of cancer surgery may not apply. In young nulliparous women it may be quite reasonable to carry out a local excision of a bleeding invasive trophoblastic tumor from the uterus and buy time to cure the disease medically, thus preserving their fertility. In our experience most of these tumors will prove not to be CC, but even if they are the results of removing isolated metastases from lung and brain (see below) suggest that local excision combined with chemotherapy can be successful.

15.5 SURGERY FOR METASTASES

This is a growing point in the overall treatment of GTD. It is a general principle of cancer surgery that the presence of metastases tends to make the disease inoperable. The early triumphs of chemotherapy in the 1960s and 1970s relegated surgery to a subsidiary role. Bagshawe, in particular, conducted a successful campaign to discourage gynecologists from removing the uterus[24].

As the cure rate in GTD approached 95% attempts were made to salvage the remaining cases by removing residual resistant disease at first by hysterectomy and pulmonary metastectomy, but later from the brain and other sites. The success of these interventions has encouraged a trend towards earlier surgery when falls in the levels of hCG in response to chemotherapy do not suggest early remission. Surgical 'debulking' can reduce the duration and increase the success of chemotherapy.

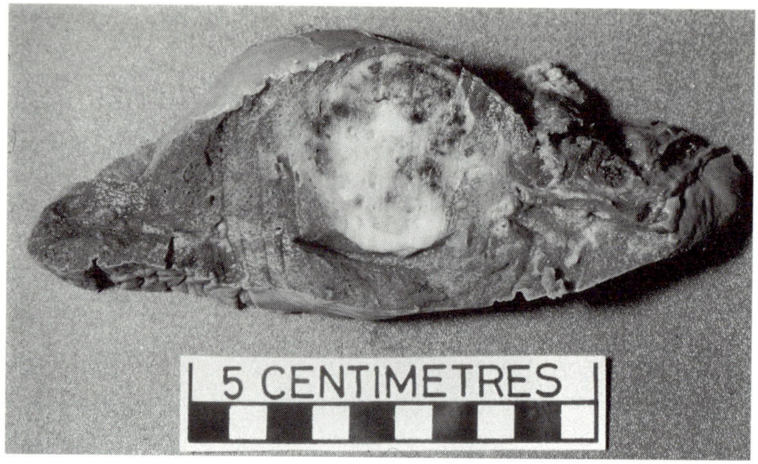

Figure 15.5 Section of lung containing metastatic CC.

15.5.1 THORACOTOMY (Figure 15.5)

The lead in chest surgery for metastatic GTD has come from the Far East. The Hong Kong group were not encouraged by their early results[25] but in the 1980s the Chinese achieved 50% remission in a review of 43 drug-resistant cases[26]. Later, there were 11 survivals out of 13 thoracotomies in Singapore (85%), but their enthusiasm was tempered by being unable to confirm the presence of viable tumor histologically in six specimens[27].

A review of 27 years experience from Japan suggested that when they operated on as many as 40% of their cases with pulmonary metastases their survival rates increased to 80%[28]. Remission of 100% was achieved when four criteria were satisfied: a persistent hCG level below 100 U/l, a 'good-risk' patient and metastases confined to the lung which could be removed at one operation.

The latest in a succession of reviews comes from the Memorial Sloan Kettering Center in New York[28], where intervention was restricted to highly selected cases of resistance to chemotherapy. Six out of their nine cases (66.7%) achieved remission and histological changes were reported which were considered to be characteristic of drug-resistant metastases. If possible the pulmonary veins should be clamped as early as possible in the procedure to prevent trophoblastic embolism.

Clearly, there is an important place for thoracotomy in GTD and it may be that the more conservative centers should intervene somewhat earlier in cases showing a poor response to chemotherapy before the tumor becomes totally resistant.

15.5.2 CRANIOTOMY (Figure 15.6)

The majority of autopsies for CC show brain metastases, so the prevention and treatment of these lesions play a major part in improving the results. Chemotherapeutic agents have a variable penetration through the blood–brain barrier and intrathecal methotrexate is an important addition to the drug regimen.

In 1983, Charing Cross Hospital, London, reported their experience monitoring in the pre-computed tomography (CT) scan era and they had achieved remission in only 17 of their 69 cases with brain metastases, but there were five remissions among

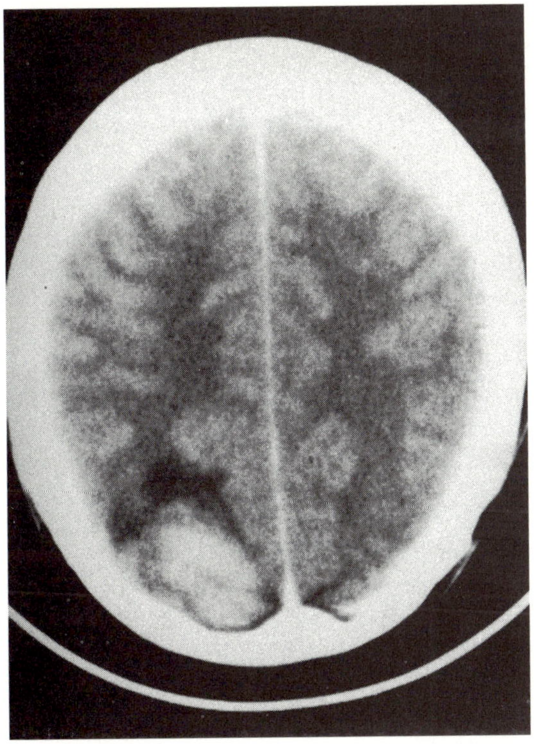

Figure 15.6 CT scan showing brain metastasis of CC later removed surgically.

the seven patients who were selected for craniotomy[30]. Emergency craniotomy may occasionally be indicated for cerebral hemorrhage or increasing intracranial pressure.

Postmortem studies have shown that more than half of isolated brain metastases are resectable neurosurgically, so, as with lung disease, there is an increasing tendency to consider surgery[28]. For single accessible metastases CT-directed craniotomy may make the surgery very precise. Indeed, it is now UK policy to resect accessible deposits before starting chemotherapy because of the risk of precipitating hemorrhage.

Radiotherapy to the brain has played an important part in the salvage of cases of CC, especially when metastases are multiple or inaccessible, and recent advances in stereotactic radiotherapy using multiple radioactive sources may result in this becoming the method of choice for these cases.

15.5.3 GASTROINTESTINAL METASTASES

Bowel involvement in CC is usually a late phenomenon and when it occurs the lesions are often multiple and so are not amenable to surgical removal. Obstruction and perforation of the bowel may require a traditional emergency laparotomy.

15.5.4 LIVER METASTASES

The question of surgery only arises in advanced and neglected cases where there may be massive bleeding into the liver. The best chance of controlling the bleeding, without the serious risk to the patient involved in hepatic surgery is to pass a catheter into feeding vessels under radiographic control and attempt embolization (see below). However, arterial occlusion in the liver is hampered by anatomical variations in the hepatic artery and because the rich collateral blood supply limits its effect[31,32].

15.5.5 VAGINAL METASTASES

Deposits of CC in the vagina are often the first clinical sign of metastatic disease. They are notoriously vascular but fortunately are usually very sensitive to chemotherapy (Figures 15.7 and 15.8). Biopsy should be avoided even when the true pathology is in doubt, and heavy bleeding is best controlled by packing the vagina for a few hours.

15.6 SPECIAL TECHNIQUES TO CONTROL HEMORRHAGE

Two situations arise when patients with GTD, or its aftermath, may suffer from severe hemorrhage.

Firstly, the bleeding may be a manifestation of untreated or poorly controlled dis-

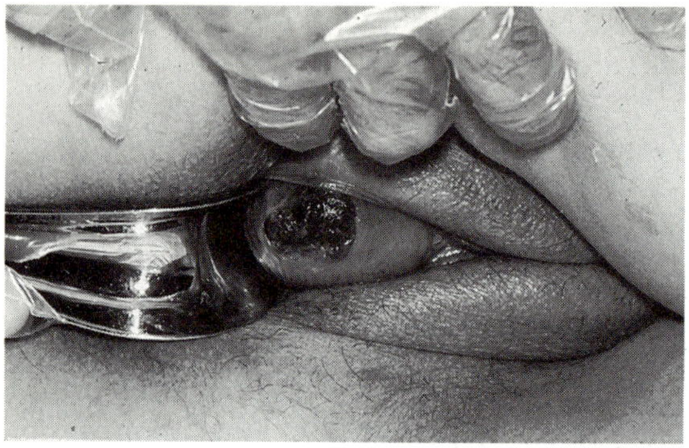

Figure 15.7 Vaginal metastasis before single-dose MXT.

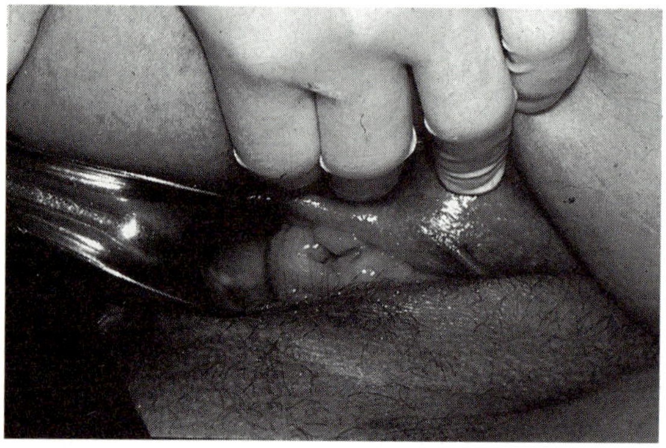

Figure 15.8 Vaginal metastasis after single-dose MXT.

ease. Angiography in molar pregnancy, and when its malignant sequelae have appeared, reveals gross arteriovenous malformations within the tumors and it is not surprising that such abnormal vessels bleed heavily when they are breached.

Secondly, even after cure of GTD the vascular spaces previously filled by tumor, especially within the myometrium, may persist as arteriovenous fistulae or aneurysms[33]. In the past uterine hemorrhage in both these clinical situations usually has led to hysterectomy. A better understanding of the pathology and new diagnostic and therapeutic techniques now allow bleeding to be controlled without removing the uterus.

15.6.1 SELECTIVE EMBOLIZATION

There are few parts of the body that cannot be reached by modern interventional radiologists. Having passed a flexible catheter into the vessels feeding a tumor or vascular malformation, the injection of steel coils, Gelfoam pellets, polyvinyl alcohol particles or liquid polymers have all been used to control bleeding by embolization. These techniques may be used in GTD, especially for vaginal hemorrhage from pelvic tumors and also for hepatic bleeding[34].

Severe menorrhagia from post-molar arteriovenous malformations has also been successfully controlled and at least two reports describe patients who went on to have successful pregnancies[35,36].

15.6.2 VESSEL LIGATION

Before selective embolization was introduced gynecologists who wished to avoid hysterectomy in cases of severe uterine hemorrhage usually tried ligating one or both internal iliac arteries. Pelvic anastomoses are so good that even the bilateral operation rarely caused dangerous ischemia within the pelvic organs, most worrying being the bladder. This operation may still be used where a skilled interventional radiologist is not available but after the ligation of iliac vessels pelvic angiography may not be possible.

Vaginal bleeding from uterine vascular malformations may also be controlled by ligation of the feeding vessels. The author was associated with the successful ligation of a post-molar uterine aneurysm which was deemed by the radiologists to be too extensive for embolization (Figures 15.9 and 15.10). This patient was later delivered of her first child by Cesarean section[37]. Some of the surgical details of this operation, which has not to our knowledge been described

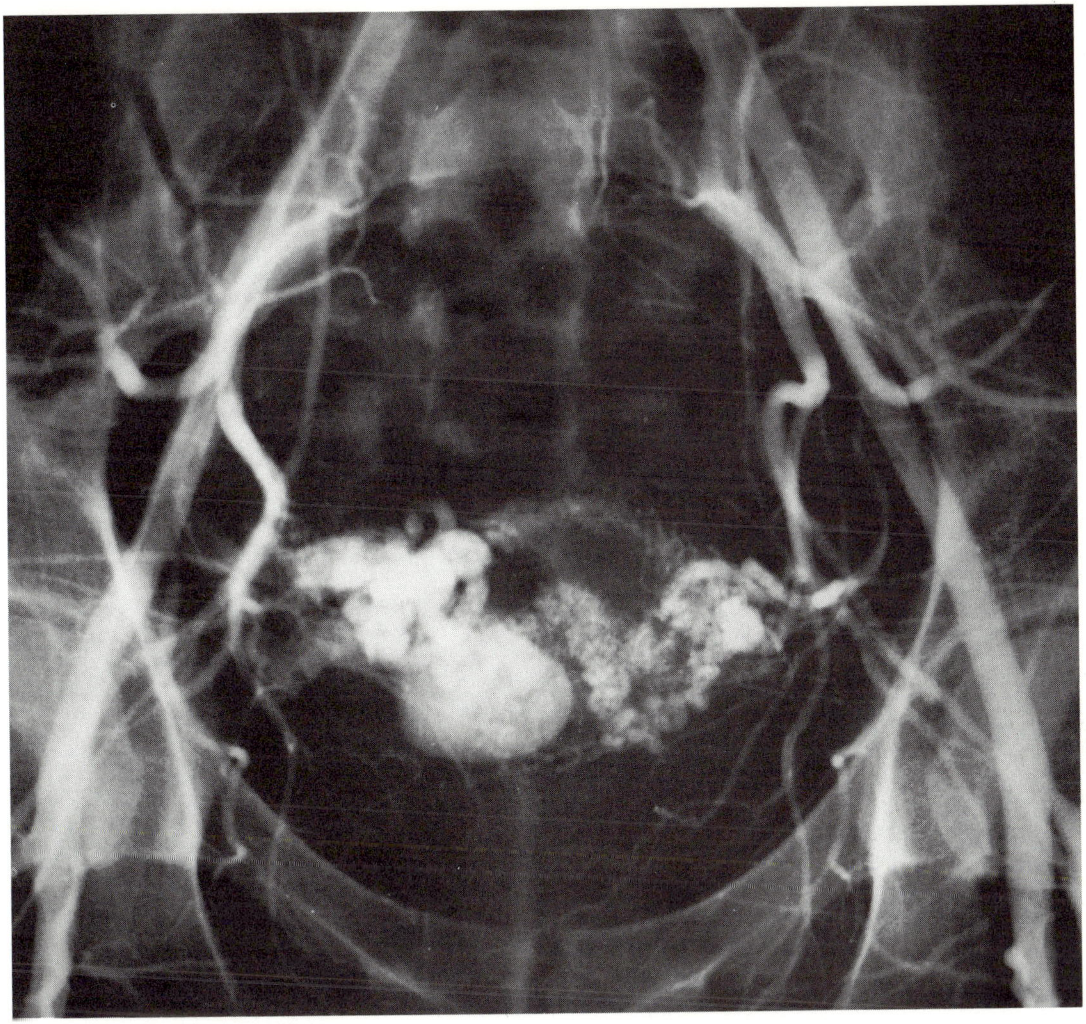

Figure 15.9 Angiogram showing aneurysm of uterine wall before ligation.

previously, are given here.

Having exposed the uterus myomectomy techniques were used to control uterine bleeding. A soft rubber catheter was used as a tourniquet round the uterine isthmus, passed through windows in the broad ligaments and clamped with a large artery forceps. Also light intestinal clamps were placed on the infundibulopelvic ligaments. The roof of the aneurysm was then opened and the vessels entering it were serially tied off with polyglycolic acid ligatures. The aneurysmal cavity was then obliterated with deep sutures and control of the bleeding confirmed by releasing the haemostats.

15.7 PLACENTAL SITE TROPHOBLASTIC TUMOR

First described in 1976 when it was called a 'trophoblastic pseudotumor'[38] this rare form of GTD, lacking the dimorphic picture

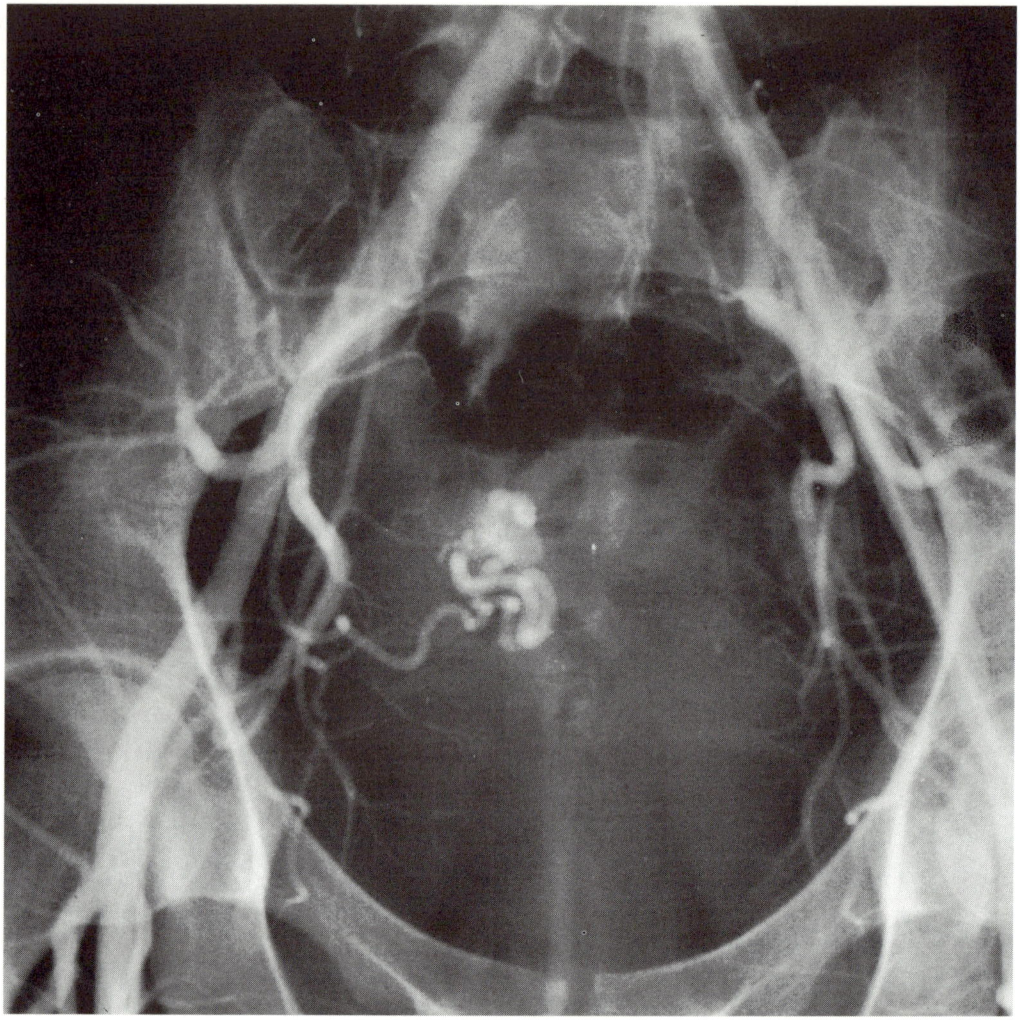

Figure 15.10 Angiogram showing aneurysm of uterine wall after ligation.

of cyto- and syncytio-trophoblast characteristic of CC, is very unpredictable in its malignant potential. Most are cured by timely hysterectomy alone but others spread to the pelvic lymph glands and farther afield, running a more aggressive course, sometimes lasting many years[39].

Cases have been recognized only after patients with persistent GTD have failed to respond to conventional chemotherapy and characteristically the levels of hCG secreted by the tumor are low. The diagnosis may be confirmed, in cases where the histology is unavailable or in doubt, by finding raised levels of placental lactogen (hPL).

The standard treatment is by total hysterectomy, conserving the ovaries which are seldom involved[40]. Some surgeons have reported regional lymph node dissection[41] but this is unnecessary in most cases. If the tumor is outside the uterus, or if it recurs, then a response to standard chemotherapy may be seen and radiotherapy also may have a place.

15.8 NON-GESTATIONAL CHORIOCARCINOMA

Sporadic case reports keep appearing of primary CC in extragenital sites and sometimes there is not even a history of an antecedent pregnancy. However, these cases are likely either to be metastatic tumors where the uterine primary has regressed without recognition or they may represent the malignant transformation with trophoblastic differentiation in tumors arising at other sites, e.g. carcinoma of the bronchus. Primary ovarian CC, on the other hand, does exist and is part of a germ cell tumor (teratoma or dysgerminoma).

The ovary has usually been removed before the diagnosis is made, but if malignant tissue persists it will secrete hCG and sequential assays are invaluable during follow-up. These tumors also respond well to chemotherapy.

15.9 PRE- AND POSTOPERATIVE CARE

Those women who come to surgery with GTD suffer from a number of complications which need attention prior to anesthesia.

15.9.1 HEMATOLOGICAL

Vaginal bleeding frequently leads to anemia and a bleeding tendency in trophoblastic disease may be aggravated by coagulation failure[42]. Those patients who have been receiving chemotherapy may be short of leucocytes and platelets. Therefore, a full blood count and clotting screen along with the grouping and cross-matching of blood for pre- or intraoperative transfusion are essential.

15.9.2 RESPIRATORY

Some women present with respiratory difficulties due to multiple trophoblastic tumor emboli from the pelvic veins. These patients may need respiratory support on a ventilator[43]. Others may have pulmonary edema due to the over-transfusion of blood or electrolytes or from cardiac failure associated with pregnancy hypertension, and diuretics may be indicated.

15.9.3 METABOLIC

Renal and liver function tests are necessary, especially after prolonged chemotherapy.

15.9.4 ENDOCRINE

High levels of hCG (usually $>10^6$U/l) may be associated with high levels of thyrotropic hormone. A small number of these patients show frank hyperthyroidism and to avoid a thyroid crisis they require treatment with potassium iodide and β-blocker drugs[44].

15.9.5 INFECTIVE

A few patients may have uterine sepsis especially after repeated curettage. If there is an offensive discharge bacteriological swabs should be taken from the vagina and where there is a significant pyrexia blood cultures are indicated.

Appropriate antibiotic therapy should be given, preferably before surgery, but in cases of emergency intervention antibacterial cover with metronidazole or another agent which covers anaerobic organisms is the treatment of choice.

15.9.6 POSTOPERATIVE CARE

All the above problems may be carried over into the convalescent period if not fully controlled before surgery. In addition there may have been operative blood loss which needs continued transfusion. An accurate fluid balance chart is essential at least for a few days and the anesthetist may advise care in a high dependency unit until the patient's condition is stable. After major pelvic surgery an indwelling catheter is advisable to check on urinary output and avoid the inconvenience of a bed-pan for one or two days at least.

15.10 SUMMARY

Hydatidiform mole should be evacuated as soon as possible after diagnosis using suction curettage supplemented by oxytocic agents. Curettage is seldom required thereafter. Chemotherapy has transformed the prognosis for women with CC but surgery plays a vital role in the control of hemorrhage and should be regarded as more than just 'salvage' treatment when cases of persistent GTD are not responding well to drugs. In order to make an optimal decision when to intervene surgically it is invaluable for a gynecologist to be a member of the team in each trophoblastic tumor center.

REFERENCES

1. Brewer, J.I., Smith, R.T. and Pratt, G.B. (1963) Choriocarcinoma: absolute 5-year survival rates of 122 patients treated by hysterectomy. *American Journal of Obstetrics and Gynecology*, **85**, 841–3.
2. Schlaerth, J.B. (1984) Methodology of molar termination, in *Clinical Obstetrics and Gynecology*, Vol. 27(i) (ed. C.P. Morrow), Harper & Row, Philadelphia, pp. 192–198.
3. Bates, A., Pinto, A. and Evans, J. (1994) Termination of molar pregnancy using mifepristone and gemeprost. *British Journal of Obstetrics and Gynaecology*, **101**, 637–8.
4. Stone, M. and Bagshawe, K.D. (1979) An analysis of the influence of maternal age, gestational age, contraceptive method and the primary mode of treatment of patients with hydatidiform mole on the incidence of subsequent chemotherapy. *British Journal of Obstetrics and Gynaecology*, **86**, 782–92.
5. Flam, F., Lundstrom, V. and Pettersson, F. (1991) Medical induction prior to surgical evacuation of hydatidiform mole: is there a greater risk of persistent trophoblastic disease? *European Journal of Obstetrics, Gynaecology and Reproductive Biology*, **42**, 57-60.
6. Ratnam, S.S. and Prasad, R.N.V. (1990) Medical management of abnormal pregnancy, in *Clinical Obstetrics and Gynaecology*, Vol. 4. Baillière Tindall, London pp. 361–74.
7. Elston, C.W. (1978) Trophoblastic tumours of the placenta, in *Pathology of the Placenta* (ed. H. Fox), Saunders, London, pp. 368–425.
8. Elston, C.W. (1984) The pathology of trophoblastic disease: current status, in *Clinics in Obstetrics and Gynaecology* (ed. H. Fox), Saunders, London, pp. 135–52.
9. Tow, W.S.H. (1966) The influence of primary treatment of hydatidiform mole on its subsequent course. *Journal of Obstetrics and Gynaecology of the British Commonwealth*, **73**, 544–52.
10. Curry, S.L., Hammond, C.B., Tyrey, L. *et al.* (1975) Hydatidiform mole, diagnosis, management and long-term follow up. *Obstetrics and Gynecology*, **45**, 1–8.
11. Bagshawe, K.D. (1976) Risk and prognostic factors in trophoblastic neoplasia. *Cancer*, **38**, 1373–85.
12. Asseryanis, E., Schurz, B., Eppel, W. *et al.* (1993) Late complication of tubal pregnancy visualised with color Doppler ultrasound: case report (in German), *Ultraschall in der Medizin*, **14**(4), 180-1.
13. Cartwright, P.S. (1991) Peritoneal trophoblastic implants after surgical management of tubal pregnancy. *Journal of Reproductive Medicine*, **36**, 523-4.
14. Schlaerth, J.B., Morrow, C.P. and Rodriguez, R.N. (1990) Diagnostic and therapeutic curettage in gestational trophoblastic disease. *American Journal of Obstetrics and Gynecology*, **162**, 1465–71.
15. Lewis, J.L., Jr, Ketcham, A.J. and Hertz, R. (1966) Surgical intervention during chemotherapy of gestational trophoblastic neoplasms. *Cancer*, **19**, 1517–22.
16. Hammond, C.B., Weed, J.C. and Currie, J.L. (1980) The role of operation in the current therapy of gestational trophoblastic disease. *American Journal of Obstetrics and Gynecology*, **136**, 844–58.
17. Sablinska, B., Kietlinska, Z. and Zielinski, J. (1993) Chemotherapy combined with surgery

in the treatment of gestational trophoblastic disease. *European Journal of Gynaecological Oncology*, **14** (Suppl.), 146–51.

18. Ratnam, S.S. and Ilancheran, A. (1982) Disease of the trophoblast, in *Clinics in Obstetrics and Gynaecology*, Vol. 9 (ed. R.H. Philpott), Saunders, London, pp. 539–64.
19. Newlands, E.S., Bagshawe, K.D., Begent, R.H.J. *et al.* (1991) Results with the EMA/CO regimen in high risk GTD, 1979 to 1989. *British Journal of Obstetrics and Gynaecology*, **98**, 550–7.
20. Wilson, R.B., Beecham, C.T. and Symmonds, R.E. (1965) Conservative surgical management of chorioadenoma destruens. *Obstetrics and Gynecology*, **28**, 814–20.
21. Mitani, Y., Jimi, S., Takao, N. and Sashikata, T. (1967) Partial resection of the uterus for chorio-adenoma destruens, in *Proceedings of the Vth World Congress of Gynaecology and Obstetrics* (eds C. Wood and W.A.W. Walters), Butterworth, Sydney, p. 416.
22. Takeuchi, S. (1982) Nature of invasive mole and its rational management. *Seminars in Oncology*, **9**, 181.
23. Shi, Y.F. and Fang, Q. (1993) Hysterotomy and focal ectomy of malignant trophoblastic tumor (in Chinese). *Chung-Hua Fu Chan Ko Tsa Chih*, **28**, 613–5, 636.
24. Bagshawe, K.D. (1967) Correspondence in *British Medical Journal*, 15 April, p. 178 and 29 July, p. 309.
25. Wong, L.C. and Ma, H.K. (1963) Persistent chest opacity in trophoblastic disease: is thoractomy justified? *Australian and New Zealand Journal of Obstetrics and Gynaecology*, **23**, 101–7.
26. Xu, L.-T., Sun, C.-F., Wang, Y.-E. and Song, H.-Z. (1985) Resection of pulmonary metastatic choriocarcinoma in 43 drug resistant patients. *Annals of Thoracic Surgery*, **39**, 257–9.
27. Kumar, J., Ilancheran, A. and Ratnam, S.S. (1988) Pulmonary metastases in gestational trophoblastic disease: review of 97 cases. *British Journal of Obstetrics and Gynaecology*, **95**, 70–4.
28. Ishizuka, N. and Tomoda, Y. (1990) Surgical treatment of metastasis, in *Gestational Trophoblastic Disease*, University of Nagoya Press, Nagoya, pp. 108–17.
29. Jones, W.B., Romain, K., Erlandson, R.A. *et al.* (1993) Thoracotomy in the management of gestational choriocarcinoma. *Cancer*, **72**, 2175–81.
30. Athanassiou, A., Begent, R.H.J., Newlands, E.S. *et al.* (1983) Central nervous system metastases of choriocarcinoma: 23 years experience at Charing Cross Hospital. *Cancer*, **52**, 1728–35.
31. Barnard, D.E., Woodard, K.T., Yancy, S.G. *et al.* (1986) Hepatic metastases in choriocarcinoma: report of 15 cases. *Gynecologic Oncology*, **25**, 73–83.
32. Grumbine, F.C., Rosenhein, N.B., Brereton, H.D. and Kaufman, S.L. (1980) Management of liver metastasis from gestational trophoblastic neoplasia. *American Journal of Obstetrics and Gynecology*, **137**, 959–61.
33. Cockshott, W.P. and deV. Hendrickse, J.P. (1967) Persistent arteriovenous fistulae following chemotherapy of malignant trophoblastic disease. *Radiology*, **88**, 329–33.
34. Green-Thompson, R.W. (1987) Surgery in the management of gestational trophoblastic disease. *Baillieres Clinical Obstetrics and Gynaecology*, **1**(2) 293–317.
35. Chapman, D.R. and Lutz, M.H. (1985) Report of a successful delivery after nonsurgical management of a choriocarcinoma-related pelvic arteriovenous fistula. *American Journal of Obstetrics and Gynaecology*, **153**, 155–7
36. Tacchi, D. and Loose, H.W. (1988) Successful pregnancy after selective embolisation of a post-molar vascular malformation. *British Journal of Obstetrics and Gynaecology*, **95**, 814–17.
37. Belli, A.-M., Hemingway, A.P., Neal, F.E. and Millar, D.R. (1989) Arteriovenous malformation of the uterus related to trophoblastic disease: a case for surgery or embolisation? *Journal of Interventional Radiology*, **4**, 118–21.
38. Kurman, R.J., Scully, R.E. and Norris, H.J. (1976) Trophoblastic pseudotumor of the uterus: 12 cases. *Cancer*, **38**, 1214–26.
39. Finkler, N.J. (1991) Placental site trophoblastic tumor: diagnosis, clinical behavior and treatment. *Journal of Reproductive Medicine*, **36**, 27–30.
40. Hoffman, J.S., Silverman, A.D., Gelber, J. and Cartun, R. (1993) Placental site trophoblastic tumor: a report of radiologic, surgical and pathologic methods of evaluating the extent

of the disease. *Gynecologic Oncology*, **50**, 110–14.

41. Berkowitz, B.J., Jones, J.G., Merkatz, I.R. and Runowicz, C.D. (1990) Ovarian conservation in placental site trophoblastic tumor. *Gynecologic Oncology*, **37**, 239–43.
42. Tsakok, F.H.M., Koh, S. and Ratnam, S.S. (1976) Coagulation and fibrinolysis in intact hydatidiform molar pregnancy. *British Medical Journal*, **ii**, 1481–4.
43. Twiggs, L.B., Morrow, C.P. and Schlaerth, J.B. (1979) Acute pulmonary complications of molar pregnancy. *American Journal of Obstetrics and Gynecology*, **135**, 189–94.
44. Norman, R.J., Green-Thompson, R.W., Jailal, I. *et al*. (1981) Hyperthyroidism in gestational trophoblastic neoplasia. *Clinical Endocrinology*, **15**, 395–401.

GENERAL REFERENCES

Ma, H.-K., Wong, L.C. and Ngan, H.Y.S. (1990) The modern management of trophoblastic disease, in *Recent Advances in Obstetrics and Gynaecology*, Vol. 16 (ed. J. Bonnar), Churchill Livingstone, Edinburgh, pp. 3–23.

Soper, J.T. (1994) Surgical therapy for gestational trophoblastic disease. *Journal of Reproductive Medicine*, **39**, 168–74.

Soper, J.T., Mutch, D.G. and Hammond, C.B. (1987) The role of surgery, in *Gestational Trophoblastic Disease* (eds A.E. Szulman and H.J. Buchsbaum), Springer-Verlag, Berlin, pp. 159–69.

World Health Organization (1983) Gestational trophoblastic diseases. *WHO Technical Report No. 692*.

PSYCHOSOCIAL CONSEQUENCES OF GESTATIONAL TROPHOBLASTIC DISEASE

16

Lari B. Wenzel

Gestational trophoblastic disease (GTD) comprises a spectrum of interrelated diseases including partial and complete molar pregnancy and choriocarcinoma with varying propensity for invastion and metastasisf[1–4]. Despite the presence of widespread metastases, persistent gestational trophoblastic tumors (GTT) are highly curable with chemotherapy[2–6]. However, psychological shock is anticipated and understandable when the woman and her partner discover that their pregnancy is considered potentially cancerous and life threatening. It is within this context that we begin to address issues central to psychological, social and sexual adaptation during an assumed period of heightened anxiety.

Although a cure is generally anticipated, inherent psychosocial stressors exist for the patient and her partner. These stressors include loss of a pregnancy, a potentially life threatening diagnosis, surgical treatment and/or chemotherapy, and delay of future pregnancy. This diagnosis consequently poses a challenge to the woman and her partner since both are required to rapidly shift their sense of hopefulness and joy related to the pregnancy to a necessary challenge to manage a potentially life threatening condition.

This unique set of circumstances has led to investigation of the psychosocial impact of GTD. This chapter outlines several issues considered germane to a comprehensive understanding of the psychosocial issues and implications. First, a brief discussion of interpretations of childbearing is reviewed to provide a foundation to understand the distress which may occur if a pregnancy is threatened and abruptly halted, as is the case with GTD. Second, related psychosocial issues of female malignancy are addressed to underscore the potential sense of threat involving this diagnosis. Third, specific studies relevant to psychosocial aspects of GTD are critically discussed concerning the patient's response, as well as her partner's response to illness and its ramifications. Finally, a clinical model for assessment and intervention is provided with future recommendations.

16.1 ASPECTS OF FEMALE IDENTITY AND CHILDBEARING

All cultures have considered the ability to conceive and bear children as important to women. Historically, reproductive capacity for women has usually been closely tied to concepts of 'femininity' and gender identity. It has been stated that once having been pregnant, there is no return to a pre pregnant psychology[7].

Gestational Trophoblastic Disease.
Edited by B.W. Hancock, E.S. Newlands and R.S. Berkowitz.
ISBN 0 412 63100 8

Consequently, when considering a diagnosis of GTD and its inherent abnormality, the initial psychological concomitants of GTD could be compared to high-risk pregnancies, where either maternal or fetal factors will adversely affect the outcome of pregnancy. For example, it has been noted that since the concept of motherhood carries so many social expectations and feelings, a woman's self-esteem may be affected by the knowledge that her pregnancy is 'imperfect'[8]. The concept of 'imperfection' can be extended with GTD to feeling 'flawed', or lacking in femininity.

16.2 PSYCHOSOCIAL ISSUES OF FEMALE MALIGNANCY

The past decade has provided rich data relating to psychosocial and psychosexual concerns arising from pelvic malignancy diagnoses. Generally, these studies suggest that women with early-stage potentially curable disease do well over time, with 'islands of disruption' in areas of sexual functioning and body image[9]. In fact, despite the emotional trauma of a cancer diagnosis, those who remain disease free cope well and resume their life patterns.

It is important to recognize, however, those women who would be considered at high risk for more prolonged psychological disturbance. Generally, women with pelvic malignancies at high risk for psychological distress are generally younger (age <50 years), with self-perceived inadequate social support, a lower socioeconomic status, a premorbid psychiatric history (particularly depression), and more advanced disease with protracted treatment. These factors provide a parallel pertinent to the GTD population.

Obvious disruption in the reproductive cycle with a potentially life threatening disease creates a number of psychological and physical challenges to young women. Although GTD is presumably physically less permanent and debilitating than other pelvic malignancies, one might anticipate 'islands of disruption' in sexuality and self-image, and subtle changes in marital relationships at least during the time of active treatment and follow-up.

16.3 PSYCHOLOGICAL, SOCIAL AND SEXUAL ADAPTATION FOR WOMEN WITH GESTATIONAL TROPHOBLASTIC DISEASE

It is recognized that women diagnosed with GTD have undergone a unique series of stressors in a brief period of time: suffering the loss of a pregnancy, receiving a diagnosis of a potentially life threatening illness, undergoing a surgical procedure, possibly undergoing chemotherapy, and delay of future pregnancy for at least one year. With these concomitant stressors, one might hypothesize that women may suffer deleterious effects psychologically, socially, maritally and perhaps sexually.

Several retrospective studies have described psychosocial variables which appear altered as a result of the GTD diagnosis and treatment. It is likely that results of these studies are dependent on the cultural perspective regarding such concepts as society's view of women, childbearing, and the type and amount of medical information preferentially communicated to women with an illness. Chinese researchers have considered the cultural perspective of their community in defining a woman's role and meaning within that society[10]. They recognized that when a woman is unable to bear children she may label herself inadequate, particularly since the capability of a couple to have children is very much regarded as the responsibility of the woman.

To better understand these assumptions, as well as the psychosocial aspects of GTD, they consecutively selected 105 Chinese residents of Hong Kong to study their emotional responses to GTD and its effects on family life. GTD was categorized as either molar pregnancy ($n = 53$), or persistent gestational trophoblastic disease ($n = 53$). The majority of patients (71%) thought the disease occurred by chance, while 25% considered themselves responsible for the disease.

Fear was a predominant emotional response, either because they knew 'something was wrong' or, in the case of patients with persistent disease, it was directed more toward malignancy and its possible association with death. Fear of future pregnancy, congenital abnormality and/or infertility persisted, despite reassurance from physicians. In addition 34% of the molar pregnancy patients reported an emotional impact of the loss of the pregnancy.

Not surprisingly, the persistent disease patients appeared to have a significantly greater sense of pessimism, depression and insecurity related to their future as compared to the molar disease group. In total, however, only a relatively small proportion of combined groups admitted that their outlook on life had changed as a result of the disease.

The Chinese researchers also examined the important aspect of the patients' questioning of role change and feelings of adequacy or worth as a woman, when confronted with a disease that challenges the traditional female role. Indeed, a small percentage of both molar and persistent disease groups felt inadequate as a wife, and as a woman, due to the pregnancy loss.

Issues of self-worth and worthiness as a woman were again addressed with a similar population of women in Boston, who had achieved complete remission[11]. Although patients were assured that full recovery was anticipated, they acknowledged experiencing shifts in self-esteem, marital relationships, and attitudes toward future pregnancies. Similar to the Chinese population, those treated with chemotherapy expressed feelings of defectiveness, sadness and loss.

More recently, 76 women from the New England Trophoblastic Disease Center who had been diagnosed with GTD were retrospectively assessed to determine their current mood status, marital satisfaction, sexual functioning, response to illness, and report of the most stressful event occurring within the past year[12]. Data were analyzed according to disease type to include partial mole, complete mole and non-metastatic persistent GTD or metastatic disease.

Although the Chinese study found only moderate differences retrospectively between molar versus persistent disease patients, we observed that the metastatic disease group displayed significantly greater mood disturbance, actually elevated into the clinically significant range of distress. Patients with metastatic disease also had significantly greater levels of distress in response to the illness.

Specifically, the women with metastatic disease were more likely to state that more than one year from diagnosis was needed before life seemed back to normal, and were more likely to desire emotional support from a mental health care professional after completing the study questionnaires. The heightened response profile of this disease category requires that proactive attention be provided through an initial comprehensive psychosocial evaluation for all patients with metastatic disease, and follow-up counseling available for patient and partner at regular intervals.

Other subcategories of women were identified through this study as potentially at higher risk for distress. For example, women with active disease reported significantly greater levels of distress in response to the illness than those in gonadotropin remission. Women with active disease appear more likely to suffer negative feelings toward self which they attribute to the disease, they feel less attractive and less of a woman, and are consequently more likely to report negative sexual thoughts or experiences. They also appear understandably more preoccupied with the disease.

Although these retrospective psychosocial studies carry methodological flaws, results overall suggest that GTD challenges the patient's psychological set as she adjusts to certain elements of uncertainty, actual or feared, related to the disease. In fact, across disease types, GTD patients report experiencing clinically significant levels of anxiety, anger, fatigue, confusion and sexual problems.

One very important and unique psychosocial variable surrounds the issue of pregnancy. Cross-culturally and secondary to their GTD experience, women are significantly impacted by pregnancy concerns for protracted periods of time. These issues appear to take a great toll on the woman's overall adjustment, regardless of specific disease category. Correlated to this specific issue, it appears that women without children display a greater fear that the disease has made them less attractive to their mate, as well as suffering a more negative impact on their sense of self and well-being[13]. The emotional issue of pregnancy clearly deserves clinical attention as a unique stressor for this population of women, particularly during the active follow-up phase of care.

16.4 EFFECTS OF GESTATIONAL TROPHOBLASTIC DISEASE ON THE RELATIONSHIP WITH PARTNERS

Although there is burgeoning discussion on the psychosocial impact of malignancies on women, there has been a conspicuous absence of information related to the effects of the disease on partners of the affected woman. This has left us historically with only one window in which to assess the impact of diagnosis and treatment over time. Yet, given the interplay of issues of a disease occurring as a reproductive anomaly, it seems clear that at least some psychosocial or sexual aspects of the disease may impact on the partner.

A parallel discussion has ensued regarding partners of high-risk pregnancy patients, in which it has been noted that partners experience anxiety and concern about the health of fetus and mother, yet feel unable to voice worries for fear of adding to the woman's burdens. In addition, they may experience resentment towards her illness, or guilt for creating the problem[14]. Similar concepts can and should be addressed for couples affected by GTD, despite the fact that little attention has been paid to partners' responses.

It is assumed that both the patient and her partner face stressors secondary to the diagnosis and treatment of GTD. One obvious factor warranting assessment and attention is the marital relationship. Upon query of a partner's willingness to complete companion questionnaires assessing psychosocial status, stressors accompanying the diagnosis did not appear to affect overall marital satisfaction[10,15]. In fact, females and males rated their marriages overall as highly satisfactory regardless of the type of GTD or its treatment.

Differences were, however, observed between males and females concerning sexual functioning. Generally, women were significantly more likely to report a sexual desire problem, and attribute desire difficulties to ill health, stress or, not uncommonly, the diagnosis of GTD. Interestingly, although men and women were equally likely to attribute sexual dysfunction to the disease during the active phase of treatment, women were significantly more likely to continue to pursue this attribution as a prolonged, hidden stressor of sexual disturbance, even after disease remission.

GTD does appear to affect the quality of the woman's sexual functioning, with a proportion of women suffering long-term consequences which they attribute to the disease. The primary dysfunction was described as a loss of sexual desire. In the absence of prospective data, however, one might validly question whether the desire problem possibly pre-dated the GTD, particularly given the frequency of sexual desire problems in the general non-clinical population of women[16].

Nevertheless, to the extent that women may be attributing sexual dysfunction to GTD, it is necessary to consider that on a fundamental level it was sexual activity with their partner, and consequences of that activity (i.e. pregnancy), that led to the disease. It follows then that fear, self-blame, spousal blame, guilt or anger could be an inherent area for exploration in the sexual dysfunction. However, given the high level of marital satisfaction reported by both patient and partner, the most likely way for the negative feelings to manifest would be sexually. Sexual dysfunction would then remove any disapproving feeling that might otherwise be directed toward the 'supportive' spouse.

Although changes in sexual activity may be predictable, reasons for this change may vary culturally. As previously discussed, American women reported sexual desire problems. Interestingly, the Chinese sample also reported a form of sexual dysfunction[10]. However, they either decreased or abstained from activity out of fear of future pregnancy.

An additional point addressing relationship issues bears mention. It appears that regardless of disease type, if GTD has been diagnosed within a year, both patient and partner are likely to label this diagnosis as the most stressful event occurring in both of their lives. Although the impact of the disease on the patient has been assumed, this piece of data highlights the significant impact the disease has on her partner as well, and underscores the importance of including the partner clinically.

16.5 MEETING THE NEEDS OF PATIENTS AND PARTNERS

In contrast to Western medicine, Chinese counterparts suggest that the physician should sensitively judge what information, and how much, should be imparted to a particular patient. Regardless of philosophical choice, it is clear that a certain level of understanding is required of the patient in order to enhance prolonged compliance, which is vital to a full recovery. Consequently, a minimum standard of care should involve education related to the disease, treatment and treatment side effects, reassurance related to a generally favorable prognosis, and reassurance that no deleterious effects will occur on subsequent pregnancies after cure from GTD has been attained. This minimum standard would help to enhance compliance and hopefully allay fears.

It is hoped, however, that most practitioners would exceed minimum standards to address some additionally salient psychological, social and sexual issues related to this disease, and when possible to encourage the patient and partner to attend clinical meetings with the physician and staff. This approach would help to enhance support within the relationship, and is likely to foster a more open discussion of concerns. Within this context, sexual problems may be addressed.

We do recognize that not all people desire a complete education regarding their disease. This may be either culturally driven or a result of the individual's predetermined manner of coping with stress. Similarly, not all patients or couples may desire counseling to reduce personal turmoil. A couple may prefer leaving uncomfortable issues untouched.

Consequently, one may reserve complete psychosocial assessment and interventions to those targeted at 'high-risk' for distress. We can begin to anticipate the women, and couples, who appear to be at risk for psychological and behavioral morbidity. This assessment would optimally occur at the time of diagnosis, or early in the treatment process, with follow-up during the recovery/'one year' post-treatment period.

At the time of diagnosis, it is recommended that one assess for psychiatric comorbidity, particularly depression, which increases risk for emotional adjustment difficulties, comorbidity with other chronic illnesses, robustness of social support within the partnership, as well as the social support network and socioeconomic status. These factors provide important early information on risk for morbidity[9].

Additional GTD-specific 'high-risk' factors have been identified. For women with either active disease, a diagnosis within the past year, no children, or metastatic disease, proactive attention should be provided through an initial comprehensive psychosocial evaluation and follow-up contact with staff to provide education, reassurance and counseling as indicated. This approach should assist in decreasing the severity of emotional reactions, and provide the patient and her partner with the needed support to sustain them in this 'crisis' until remission is achieved. When indicated, this is likely to reduce the magnitude of mood disturbances experienced by women with metastatic disease, provide coping skills for dealing with the challenges of the disease and treatment, and enhance communication between the patient and her partner.

16.6 RECOMMENDATIONS FOR FUTURE INVESTIGATIONS

Prospective cohort or clinical trial studies which include a quality of life component have recently become a valued undertaking, as the field of obstetrics and gynecology recognizes the importance of examining the emotional, social and physical functioning issues which accompany procedures to treat benign[17] or malignant gynecological disease[18]. Such studies assist in elucidating the efficacy of particular gynecological procedures through the perspective of the patient, underscoring aspects of life which she values. Whether in the clinical or research setting, one should always ask what specific dimensions of quality of life are likely to be affected by the disease and treatment[19].

A similar approach could be advanced to address the quality of life needs of the patient with GTD. To date, no prospective analyses have addressed psychological, social or sexual issues which accompany the disease trajectory. Consequently, the logical next step would involve prospective assessment of quality of life issues known and suspected to affect women with GTD.

It is recommended that health-related quality of life should be assessed by the patient, and should reflect the evaluation of a number of dimensions affecting her life at that moment[19]. Generally, most experts in this field perceive quality of life as a multidimensional construct that includes several key dimensions. These include physical functioning, disease and treatment-related symptoms, psychological functioning and social functioning. Additional considerations in the evaluation of quality of life may include spiritual or existential concerns, sexual functioning and body image, and satisfaction with health care. Pertinent issues for the GTD patient would include her fear of future pregnancy, as well as indirect effects of the disease on the partnership (i.e. self-blame, guilt).

GTD quality of life assessment measures and data could be incorporated into clinical practices. Thus, clinicians can learn to monitor the effects of treatment by periodic assessment of quality of life in addition to the objective assessment of clinical response. These assessments would also serve to identify problems that can be addressed by the clinicians or other members of the health care team.

Such standardized assessments may provide assistance in treatment decision-making and outcome evaluation. Over time, development of a reliable and valid measurement practice would assist international trophoblastic centers to collaborate in objective quantification of quality of life issues so vital to this population of women. Ultimately, inclusion of the partner's response to disease variables would serve as an additional window of opportunity to examine and appropriately intervene in quality of life issues impacting the woman with GTD.

REFERENCES

1. Curry, S.L., Hammond, C.B., Tyrey, L. *et al.* (1975) Hydatidiform moles: diagnosis, management, and long-term follow-up of 347 patients. *Obstetrics and Gynecology*, **45**, 1–8.
2. Lurain, J.R. and Brewer, J.I. (1985) Treatment of high-risk gestational trophoblastic disease with methotrexate, actinomycin D and cyclophosphamide chemotherapy. *Obstetrics and Gynecology*, **65**, 830–6.
3. Goldstein, D.P. and Berkowitz, R.S. (1982) *Gestational Trophoblastic Neoplasms: Clinical Prinicples of Diagnosis and Management*, Saunders, Philadelphia, pp. 1–301.
4. Jones, W.B., Lewis, J.L., Jr and Lehr, M. (1975) Monitor of chemotherapy in the gestational trophoblastic neoplasm by the radioimmunoassay of the beta-subunit of human chorionic gonadotropin, *American Journal of Obstetrics and Gynecology*, **121**, 669–773.
5. Gordon, A.N., Gershenson, D.M., Copeland, L.J. *et al.* (1989) High-risk metastatic gestational trophoblastic disease: further stratification into two clinical entities, *Gynecologic Oncology*, **34**, 54–6.
6. Bagshawe, K.D. (1976) Risk and prognostic factors in trophoblastic neoplasia, *Cancer*, **38**, 1373–83.
7. Bibring, G., Dwyer, T., Huntington, D. *et al.* (1961) A study of the psychological processes in pregnancy and the earliest mother–child relationship. *Psychoanalytic Study of Child*, **16**, 9–72.
8. Jones, M.B. (1986) The high-risk pregnancy, in *Nursing Assessment and Strategies for the Family at Risk*, 2nd edn (ed. S.H. Johnson), Lippincott, Philadelphia, pp. 111–28.
9. Andersen, B.L. (1994) Surviving cancer. *Cancer*, **74**, 1484–95.
10. Ngan, H.Y.S. and Tang, G.W.K. (1986) Psychosocial aspects of gestational trophoblastic disease in Chinese residents of Hong Kong. *Journal of Reproductive Medicine*, **31**, 173.
11. Berkowitz, R.S., Marean, A.R., Hamilton, N. *et al.* (1980) Psychological and social impact of gestational trophoblastic neoplasia. *Journal of Reproductive Medicine*, **25**, 14–16.
12. Wenzel, L.B., Berkowitz, R.S., Robinson, S.E. *et al.* (1992) The psychological, social, and sexual consequences of gestational trophoblastic disease. *Gynecologic Oncology*, **46**, 74–81.
13. Wenzel, L.B., Berkowitz, R.S., Robinson, S.E. *et al.* (1990) *Psychological, Social and Sexual Consequences of Gestational Trophoblastic Disease: A Retrospective Analysis*. Fifth World Congress on Gestational Trophoblastic Diseases, London.
14. Rogers, M.P. (1989) Psychological aspects of pregnancy in patients with rheumatic disease, in *Rheumatic Disease Clinics of North America*, (ed. R.B. Zuriev), Vol. 15(2), Saunders, Philadelphia, pp. 361–74.
15. Wenzel, L.B., Berkowitz, R.S., Robinson, S.E. *et al.* (1994) Psychological, social and sexual effects of gestational trophoblastic disease on patients and their partners. *Journal of Reproductive Medicine*, **39**(3), 163–7.
16. Leiblum, S.R. and Rosen, R.C. (1988) Changing perspectives on sexual desire, in *Sexual Desire Disorders*, 2nd edn (eds S.R. Leiblum and R.C. Rosen), Guilford Press, New York, pp. 9–10.
17. Carlson, K.M., Miller, B.A. and Fowler, F.J. (1994) The Maine women's health study: II. Outcomes of nonsurgical management of leiomyomas, abnormal bleeding, and chronic pelvic pain. *Obstetrics and Gynecology*, **83**, 566–72.
18. Monk, B., Wenzel, L.B. and Cella, D.F. (1985) Quality of Life component of the Gynecologic Oncology Group Protocol #152: A phase III randomized study of cisplatin and taxol with interval secondary cytoreduction versus cisplatin and paclitaxel in patients with suboptimal Stage III & IV epithelial ovarian cancer. Presentation to Gynecologic Oncology Group, San Francisco, February 1995.
19. Cella, D.F. and Cherin, E.A. (1988) Quality of life during and after cancer treatment. *Comprehensive Therapy*, **14**, 69–75.

LATE TOXICITY AFTER THERAPY OF GESTATIONAL TROPHOBLASTIC TUMORS

17

Gordon J.S. Rustin

17.1 INTRODUCTION

A higher proportion of patients with gestational trophoblastic tumors (GTT) is at risk of long-term toxicity than patients with almost any other tumor because of the very high cure rate. It is essential that we frequently audit our results so that the occurrence of late side effects is discovered. It may then be possible to modify the therapy to minimize risks. This chapter investigates several well-known late side effects of chemotherapy such as infertility and induction of second tumors as well as the psychological sequelae of both losing a pregnancy and having to receive therapy for cancer.

17.2 SECOND TUMORS

There is often suspicion when a patient develops a second tumor that it is related to the initial therapy. It must be realized, however, that Moertel *et al*.[1] found that 2.8% of patients with a primary cancer treated before the era of chemotherapy developed another primary of different tissue of origin. For certain cancer types there have been reports suggesting an increased risk. This could be due to an underlying genetic defect in patients with many solid tumors[2] or to the associated immunodeficiency in patients who have leukemia or lymphoma. Unlike other cancers there is no known somatic genetic defect or immunosuppression associated with GTT.

Most anticancer agents act by causing chromosomal damage to neoplastic cells but also cause damage particularly to rapidly proliferating normal tissue. It is therefore not surprising that this damage may be carcinogenic and teratogenic. Continuous collation and analysis of clinical and laboratory data on cytotoxic drugs currently in use suggest that alkylating agents, antitumor antibiotics, cisplatin, procarbazine and etoposide are either identified as carcinogens or under strong suspicion, whilst the antimetabolites emerge as relatively safe[3–5]. Many reports of second tumors associated with cytotoxic chemotherapy have described high total doses of alkylating agents given over a long period, in many cases continuously. It is not yet clear whether the second tumors seen after high-dose therapy and marrow grafting are related to the high-dose therapy or the large total amount of chemotherapy that these poor-risk patients had received.

Most patients who require chemotherapy for GTT fit into the low-risk prognostic group and over 75% of these low-risk patients are cured by treatment with just

Gestational Trophoblastic Disease.
Edited by B.W. Hancock, E.S. Newlands and R.S. Berkowitz.
ISBN 0 412 63100 8

methotrexate and folinic acid. Methotrexate has been shown to be a cocarcinogen in mice also receiving methylcholanthrene possibly through its immunosuppressive effect[6]. Methotrexate has not been found to be carcinogenic alone in mice, rats or hamsters but can induce chromosomal damage in human bone marrow cells[7]. Although there have been case reports of neoplasia occurring after its use in treating psoriasis, no increased risk of internal tumors was found in a study of 205 patients receiving intermittent oral methotrexate, compared to a matched control group[8].

The first case-control study of second tumor incidence after therapy of GTT investigated 457 long-term survivors treated between 1958 and 1978[9]. Methotrexate was given to all but two patients, and 261 (57%) also received other drugs. After a mean period of 7.8 years since the beginning of treatment and a total of 3522 patient-years of risk, second tumors had developed in two women but would have been expected in 3.5. One case of acute myelomonocytic leukemia developed 11 months after intensive chemotherapy over 13 months with eight different drugs, including etoposide and cyclophosphamide. The other second tumor was breast cancer developing 11 years after receiving methotrexate and folinic acid. The conclusion of that study was that methotrexate is not carcinogenic in the medium term.

During the years since that study was completed we were notified of other patients developing secondary leukemia. In 1987 Ratain *et al.*[10] suggested that etoposide had leukemogenic potential. He found that four of 24 patients who survived more than one year after being treated with it for non-small cell lung cancer developed leukemia. There have since been reports of an increased incidence of leukemias after either etoposide or tenoposide given to patients with acute lymphoblastic leukemia, germ cell tumors, small cell lung cancer, neuroblastoma and non-Hodgkin's lymphoma[11–14]. The risk of secondary acute myeloid leukemia (AML) has been shown to be related to increasing dose and more frequent schedule of administration of podophyllotoxins. A cumulative risk at six years of 12% was found in children receiving therapy twice weekly or weekly, whilst it was 1.6% or less in those receiving less frequent tenoposide or etoposide[11]. Among 1990 patients who received etoposide, usually three-weekly for germ cell tumors, 16 (0.8%) developed leukemia[14].

17.2.1 SECOND TUMORS AMONG PATIENTS TREATED AT CHARING CROSS HOSPITAL 1958–1990

In view of all the factors mentioned above and the increasing use of etoposide in the management of GTT, we reinvestigated the second tumor incidence among patients treated at the Charing Cross Hospital[15]. Between 1958 and 1990 1394 women were treated with chemotherapy for GTT. Questionnaires were sent to long-term survivors living in the UK. They were completed and returned by 93.1%. The remainder were flagged for death or developing further cancers by the Office of Population Census and Surveys. After 15 279 person years at risk, 37 second cancers were observed. In an aged-matched population 24.45 cancers would have been expected, giving a standardized incidence ratio of 1.51 (95% confidence interval (CI) 1.06–2.08, $p < 0.011$). There were significant increased ratios of myeloid leukemia (16.61, CI 5.40–38.9, $p < 0.000$), colon cancer (4.59, CI 1.48–10.7, $p < 0.005$), melanoma (3.41, CI 0.03–8.75, $p < 0.031$) and breast cancer, but only in those followed more than 25 years (5.79, CI 1.19–16.86, $p < 0.016$).

All but two patients received methotrexate but leukemias only developed in those receiving etoposide plus other cytotoxic drugs. The mean dose of etoposide received by 335 long-term survivors was 1852 mg/m^2. The dose given to those developing leukemia was between 1500 and 3000 mg/m^2. A short latency between initial chemotherapy and secondary leukemia is classically seen in etoposide-induced leukemia. In three cases the latency was less than 16 months and in another there was a 8 : 21 translocation and durable response to antileukemic therapy. This suggests that at least four of the leukemias were induced by etoposide.

This study confirmed the safety of methotrexate when given alone or with folinic acid. However, the late increased development of breast cancers in women who received methotrexate with other cytotoxic drugs has serious implications. If confirmed in another study it would add urgency to studies aimed at selecting those most likely to benefit from adjuvant therapy.

The observation that 1.5% of those women who received etoposide developed leukemia demonstrates the danger of giving this drug as initial therapy to women with GTT who are in the low-risk prognostic group. Approximately 80% of these women are cured by methotrexate and folinic acid alone[16]. The remaining 20% require additional cytotoxic drugs because of toxicity or resistance to methotrexate but will still be cured. Because of the risk of etoposide-induced leukemia we try and induce remission with actinomycin D if the reason for changing from methotrexate is toxicity or the human chorionic gonadotropin (hCG) levels plateau at a value less than 1000 U/l.

Those patients who have a prognostic score in the middle-risk group but are treated with methotrexate have a 69+% chance of having to change therapy because of drug resistance[16,17]. Prior to the introduction of etoposide two of 75 (2.7%) middle-risk patients died from their disease. This compares with a 1.5% risk of leukemia if they receive etoposide. As we have had no deaths from drug resistance in the middle-risk group since the introduction of etoposide, our policy is to offer these patients an informed choice. They can either receive initial methotrexate/folinic acid with a high expectation of having to change therapy or receive the etoposide-containing EMA-CO schedule from the outset, which will lead to a more certain and speedier remission but at the cost of total alopecia and 1.5% chance of later developing leukemia[18]. The balance of risk in the high-risk group definitely favors the initial use of the EMA-CO schedule as these patients have a risk of approximately 15% of dying from their disease.

17.3 EFFECT OF THERAPY ON GONADAL FUNCTION

17.3.1 FERTILITY

Women treated for GTT are almost all in the reproductive age group and many desire to bear children after recovering from therapy. Cytotoxic drugs are well recognized as a potential cause of sterility. Permanent ovarian failure has been reported in over 50% of women treated for Hodgkin's disease[19,20]. The factors associated with the gonadotoxic effect of chemotherapy include age, and dose, type and duration of therapy. It is clear among women treated for Hodgkin's disease that many of those treated below the age of 30 maintain menses during and following treatment. Human ovaries acquire their quota of oocytes before birth, following which there is no further proliferation of germ cells. This might explain why the ovary appears more resistant to the effects of chemotherapy than the testis. It might also suggest that antimetabolite cytotoxic drugs that require proliferation to be effective may cause less sterility than drugs such as alkylating agents that damage DNA of resting cells. Once the ovary is damaged by chemotherapy with follicle destruction and ovarian fibrosis the hormonal effects are far greater than after cytotoxic damage to the male gonad. There is an elevation of serum follicle-stimulating hormone (FSH) and luteinizing hormone (LH), with a decrease in serum estradiol. This leads to temporary or permanent amenorrhea and symptoms associated with the menopause.

It has been known since the 1970s that pregnancies can occur after chemotherapy of trophoblastic neoplasms[21]. The largest study of women treated for GTT analyzed the obstetric records of 445 women treated at the Charing Cross Hospital between 1958 and 1978[22]. Of the 217 women who wished to conceive, 187 (86%) succeeded in having at least one live birth, 23 (11%) conceived but did not achieve a live birth, and seven (3%) who wished to conceive failed to do so. The average age on completion of treatment was 24.9 years for those who had a live birth, 24.4 years for those who conceived but had no live birth and 24.4 years for those who failed to conceive. There were 125 women aged over 30 at the completion of treatment. All 23 of these who wanted to conceive did so, and 83% had one or more live births. There were more older women who did not wish to conceive and having become menopausal may have contributed to this decision.

Those women who were given three or more drugs in combination were less likely to have a live birth or to conceive at all when compared with those women given methotrexate alone or in combination with only one other drug ($p<0.001$). Etoposide could not be adequately assessed in that paper but was shown by Choo *et al.*[23] to cause ovarian dysfunction when given as a single agent. When a lower total dose of etoposide is given as part of sequential or combination schedules it does not appear to cause permanent sterility. Adewole *et al.*[24] found that 77% of 74 women who received etoposide and wished to conceive succeeded in having at least one live birth. When correcting for two patients with a previous history of infertility he found only six (8.1%) of the patients had true post-chemotherapy infertility problems. Ovarian function after cisplatin-based therapy has been studied in women with ovarian germ cell tumors[25]. Menstruation restarted in 16 of 17 women who had a remaining ovary and uterus after therapy.

We advise women not to get pregnant for one year after the completion of chemotherapy. The main reason for this advice is that most relapses occur during that period. It is difficult initially to differentiate between a relapse and a new pregnancy as both lead to a rise in hCG levels. It is possible that a relapse with metastatic disease could become apparent during an early subsequent pregnancy, though we have not seen this. Most patients recover from the acute toxicity of chemotherapy within a few weeks though alopecia and neurotoxicity take longer to recover and ototoxicity and renal damage rarely recover. The terminal half-life of cytotoxic drugs used in treatment of GTT can be up to several days, with cisplatin having long-term tissue binding. Even low concentrations of these drugs pose serious risks to the early fetus. Despite our advice 45 women conceived within one year of completing treatment. These conceptions resulted in 31 live births, one anencephalic stillbirth, seven miscarriages and six terminations.

17.3.2 TERATOGENICITY

Cytotoxic drugs have been implicated as teratogenic when given during pregnancy but it appears that their effects on later conceptions are less than their mutagenic potential might suggest. Ross found no excess of malformations in 78 infants born to women treated for trophoblastic diseases[26]. Among 368 conceptions following chemotherapy for GTT at the Charing Cross Hospital, there were two anencephalic stillbirths, and single cases of spina bifida, tetralogy of Fallot, talipes equinovarus, collapsed lung and umbilical hernia discovered within seven days of birth[22]. These congenital malformations were not significantly in excess of expected numbers in England and Wales. Children born to mothers who had received chemotherapy may be at increased risk of developing cancer though this has not become apparent from studying progeny of women treated for GTT. There were 455 women who answered the question in our questionnaire 'Has any of your children born since receiving chemotherapy had a serious illness?' Only 1% after low-risk, 0.9% after middle-risk and 0.6% after high-risk therapy answered yes and none reported any malignancies.

17.3.3 AGE OF MENOPAUSE

The menopause is considered to have occurred when menstrual cycles have ceased for more than one year, and there is no evidence of ovarian steroid hormone production. The age of menopause of women in developed countries is considered to be 52 years. Alkylating agents have been shown in mice to cause oocyte destruction, but for there to be a major effect on the reproductive lifespan over 80% of the oocytes need to be destroyed[27]. Mathematical models have been produced based on total follicle counts of ovaries obtained from women suddenly dying or removed at surgery[28]. They suggest a bi-exponential decline, with the faster decline occurring when numbers had fallen to 25 000 at the age of 37.5 years. The model predicts that a 50% reduction before age 30 years resulted in menopause being reached at 44 years and 0.6 year later for every subsequent year until age 37.5, after which it is reached at 48 years.

Many women develop ovarian failure during cytotoxic chemotherapy. Based on the comments above one could assume that provided over 20% of oocytes remain there would be recovery of ovarian function. However, despite recovery there is likely to be a reduction in the number of menstrual years. It has only recently become possible to confirm this as women successfully treated with chemotherapy in their twenties and thirties approach their expected age of menopause.

The questionnaires that were sent to women treated at the Charing Cross Hospital between 1958 and 1990 asking about second tumors also enquired about menstrual history since completing chemotherapy[15]. In case a prior molar pregnancy was associated with premature ovarian failure we also sent questionnaires to a 'control' group of women who had a molar pregnancy but who had not required chemotherapy and who had reached the age of 45. The mean age of menopause was recorded in questionnaires from 140 treated women and in 63 untreated controls. The mean age of menopause was 45.9 in treated women compared to 52.2 among untreated women ($p<0.000$). The greatest effect was seen in the women who had received high-risk chemotherapy but there was still a significant effect in women who only received low-risk therapy.

This finding, though expected, has several implications. Women who receive any form of chemotherapy should be told of the risk of an early menopause. This information could alter the age at which they intend to become pregnant. Becoming menopausal six years early will increase the risk of osteoporosis and cardiovascular disease in these women. They require advice regarding hormone replacement therapy to prevent these problems as well as to control symptoms associated with the menopause.

17.4 PSYCHOLOGICAL SEQUELAE

Emotional disturbance is commonly seen after pregnancy loss due to miscarriage. Interestingly Ngan and Tang found that among women who had a molar pregnancy those who required chemotherapy were less disturbed by the pregnancy loss than those who did not receive chemotherapy[29]. This may

Table 17.1 Anxiety or depression following chemotherapy for GTT

Ever sought or wanted help	280/974	29%
Due to treatment at Charing Cross	123/931	13%
Fear of cancer/recurrence	25/123	
Fear of treatment (not cancer)	20/123	
Isolation, need for counselling	34/123	
Adverse effect on marriage	10	
Fear of subsequent pregnancy	8	
Attempted suicide	1	
Contemplated suicide	1	

be due to those requiring chemotherapy being more preoccupied with their disease, chemotherapy and fear of death.

Many women are surprised that they become most depressed soon after completing chemotherapy. Their lives have been controlled by the need to get through chemotherapy and once finished they feel lost and have difficulty organizing their lives again. This is probably due to feeling physically weakened by the treatment, due to the disruption to their lives, delayed grief over their pregnancy loss and expectation of euphoria once treatment is finished. Warning patients that they may become depressed or not happy on completing chemotherapy often relieves the distress.

Table 17.1 gives the findings from our questionnaire that was sent to 1089 women after successful chemotherapy for GTT. Thirteen per cent who answered a question on anxiety and depression wrote that they had sought or wanted help for anxiety or depression secondary to treatment for GTT. Four per cent felt isolated and wanted but did not receive counselling. Patients treated for GTT at the Charing Cross Hospital are only followed by urine or serum hCG levels after completing chemotherapy and do not return to the clinic. Their local doctors need to be aware that a small proportion require counselling.

Berkowitz found that 80% of patients with gestational trophoblastic disease had a change in their outlook on life[30]. This was less commonly seen among Chinese women[29]. Decreased sexual activity has been noted often because of the fear of getting pregnant again and 44% of those who required chemotherapy reported more tense sexual relationships[30]. However, 87% of these American women felt that their marital relationships were either unchanged or closer as a result of their experiences with GTT, whilst marital problems were reported in only 1% of the Charing Cross patients.

REFERENCES

1. Moertel, C.G., Docherty, M.B. and Baggerstoss, A.H. (1961) Multiple primary malignant neoplasms: introduction and presentation of data. *Cancer*, **14**, 221–30.
2. Easton, D.F. (1994) The inherited component of cancer. *British Medical Bulletin*, **50**, 527–35.
3. Casciato, D.A. and Scott, J.L. (1979) Acute leukemia following prolonged cytotoxic agent therapy. *Medicine (Baltimore)*, **58**, 32–46.
4. Tucker, M.A. (1993) Secondary cancers, in *Cancer Principle and Practice of Oncology*, 4th edn (eds V. De Vita, S. Hellman and S.A. Rosenberg), Lippincott, Philadelphia, pp. 2407–16.
5. Halnan, K.E. and Rustin, G.J.S. (1990) Hazards of treatment, in *Treatment of Cancer*, 2nd edn (eds K. Sikora and K.E. Halnan), Chapman & Hall, London, pp. 853–72.
6. Barich, L.L., Schwartz, J. and Barich, D. (1962) Oral methotrexate in mice: a co-carcinogenic as well as an anti-tumour agent

to methylchlolanthrene-induced cutaneous tumours. *Journal of Investigative Dermatology*, **39**, 615–19.

7. Jenson, M.K. and Nyfors, A. (1979) Cytogenic effect of methotrexate on human cells *in vivo*: comparison between results obtained by chromosome studies on bone-marrow cells and blood lymphocytes and by the micronucleus test. *Mutation Research*, **64**, 339–43.
8. Bailin, P.L., Tindall, J.P., Roenigk, H.H., Jr *et al.* (1975) Is methotrexate therapy for psoriasis carcinogenic? A modified retrospective-prognosis analysis. *Journal of the American Medical Association*, **232**, 359–62.
9. Rustin, G.J.S., Rustin, F., Dent, J. *et al.* (1983) No increase in second tumors after cytotoxic chemotherapy for gestational trophoblastic tumors. *New England Journal of Medicine*, **308**, 473–6.
10. Ratain, M.J., Kamminer, L.S., Bitran, J.D. *et al.* (1987) Acute non lymphocytic leukemia following etoposide and cisplatin combination chemotherapy for advanced non-small carcinoma of the lung. *Blood*, **70**, 1412–17.
11. Pui, C.H., Ribeiro, R.C., Hancock, M.L. *et al.* (1991) Acute myeloid leukaemia in children treated with epipodophylotoxins for acute lymphoblastic leukaemia. *New England Journal of Medicine*, **325**, 1682–7.
12. Whitlock, J.A., Greger, J.P. and Lukens, J.N. (1991) Epipodophylotoxin-related leukaemia: identification of a new subset of secondary leukaemia. *Cancer*, **68**, 600–4.
13. Hawkins, M.M., Kinnier Wilson, L.M., Stovall, M.A. *et al.* (1992) Epipodophylotoxins, alkylating agents, and radiation and risk of secondary leukaemia after childhood cancer. *British Medical Journal*, **304**, 951–8.
14. Boshoff, C., Begent, R.H.J., Oliver, R.T.D. *et al.* (1995) Secondary tumours following etoposide containing therapy for germ cell cancer. *Annals of Oncology*, **6**, 35–40.
15. Newlands, E.S. Rustin, G.J.S., Lutz, J.-M. *et al.* (1995) Chemotherapy for gestational trophoblastic tumours (GTT) may increase the incidence of second tumours and may cause a premature menopause. *Proceedings of the American Society of Clinical Oncology*, **14**, 269 (Abstract 744).
16. Bagshawe, K.D. (1976) Risk and prognostic factors in trophoblastic neoplasia. *Cancer*, **38**, 1373–85.
17. Newlands, E.S., Bagshawe, K.D., Begent, R.H.J. *et al.* (1991) Results with the EMA/CO (etoposide, methotrexate, actinomycin D, cyclophosphamide, vincristine) regimen in hiqh risk gestational trophoblastic tumours, 1979 to 1989. *British Journal of Obstetrics and Gynaecology*, **98**, 550–7.
18. Newlands, E.S., Bagshawe, K.D., Begent, R.H.J. *et al.* (1986) Developments in chemotherapy for medium- and high-risk patients with gestational trophoblastic tumours (1979–1984). **93**, 63–9.
19. Clark, S.T., Radford, D., Crowther, R. *et al.* (1995) Gonadal function following chemotherapy for Hodgkin's disease: a comparative study of MVPP and a seven-drug hybrid regimen. *Journal of Clinical Oncology*, **13**, 134–9.
20. Schilsky, R.L. Lewis, B.J., Sherins, R.J. *et al.* (1980) Gonadal dysfunction in patients receiving chemotherapy for cancer. *Annals of Internal Medicine*, **93**, 109–14.
21. Van Thiel, D.H., Ross, G.T. and Lipsett, M.B. (1970) Pregnancies after chemotherapy of trophoblastic neoplasms. *Science*, **169**, 1326–7.
22. Rustin, G.J.S., Booth, M., Dent, J *et al.* (1984) Pregnancy after cytoxic chemotherapy for gestational trophoblastic tumours. *British Medical Journal*, **288**, 103–6.
23. Choo, Y.C., Chan, S.Y., Wong, L.C. *et al.* (1985) Ovarian dysfunction in patients with gestational trophoblastic neoplasia treated with short intensive courses of etoposide (VP-16-213). *Cancer*, **55**, 2348–52.
24. Adewole, I.F., Rustin, G.J.S., Newlands, E.S. *et al.* (1986) Fertility in patients with gestational trophoblastic tumors treated with etoposide. *European Journal of Clinical Oncology*, **22**, 1479–82.
25. Rustin, G.J.S., Pektasides, D., Bagshawe, K.D. *et al.* (1987) Fertility after chemotherapy for male and female germ cell tumours. *International Journal of Andrology*, **10**, 389–92.
26. Ross, G.T. (1976) Congenital anomalies among children born of mothers receiving chemotherapy for gestational trophoblastic neoplasms. *Cancer*, **37**, 1043–7.
27. Generoso, W.M., Stout, S.K. and Huff, S.W.

(1971) Effects of alkylating chemicals on reproductive capacity of adult female mice. *Mutation Research*, **13**, 171–89.
28. Faddy, M.J., Gosden, R.G., Gougeon, A. *et al.* (1992) Accelerated disappearance of ovarian follicles in mid-life: implications for forecasting menopause. *Human Reproduction*, **7**, 1342–6.
29. Ngan, H.Y.S. and Tang, G.W.K. (1986) Psychosocial aspects of gestational trophoblastic disease in Chinese residents of Hong Kong. *Journal of Reproductive Medicine*, **31**, 173–8.
30. Berkowitz, R.S., Marean, A.R. and Hamilton, N. (1980) Psychological and social impact of gestational trophoblastic neoplasia. *Journal of Reproductive Medicine*, **25**, 14–16.

FUTURE PROSPECTS 18

Edward S. Newlands, Ross S. Berkowitz and Barry W. Hancock

18.1 REFERRAL CENTERS FOR PATIENTS WITH GESTATIONAL TROPHOBLASTIC DISEASE

A major part of the success in the management of gestational trophoblastic disease (GTD) and gestational trophoblastic tumors (GTT) has been made possible by the development of regional or national centers for these patients' management. By focusing on the variations in clinical presentation, treatment, management and complications, the outlook for these patients has improved progressively over the past four decades. The success for any center managing GTD and GTT needs the following elements:

1. registration of patients with or at risk of GTD or GTT, comprising clinical background details and arranging for regular human chorionic gonadotropin (hCG) estimations on each patient;
2. a sensitive and reliable assay for hCG. This will be considered further below;
3. nursing and medical staff experienced in the management of the patients and their disease who can deal with the numerous queries both from their referring gynecologists and from the patients and their families;
4. the national or regional centers need to be in a position of good transport to enable patients to come for treatment and consultations;
5. a reliable postal service for sending the patients' samples to the center and for posting back the hCG results;
6. good patient compliance with sending hCG samples and attending for treatment.

The above requirements are met in the parts of the world where regional or national trophoblastic disease centers have developed. There are many countries where it would be possible to develop new regional or national centers along the lines of those already existing and where the basic requirements of a regional center could be put in place if there was appropriate co-operation between the gynecological community of that country and the health care providers. In countries where the above key elements for developing a regional center are lacking at present, clinicians dealing with this disease need to develop links with one of the existing regional centers in another country to discuss management policies and difficult cases. Dissemination of this expertise is one of the key purposes of this volume to describe the policies of some of the existing regional and national centers.

Gestational Trophoblastic Disease.
Edited by B.W. Hancock, E.S. Newlands and R.S. Berkowitz.
ISBN 0 412 63100 8

18.2 QUALITY CONTROL OF hCG ASSAYS

The key role of assays for hCG has been emphasized throughout this volume in the diagnosis, monitoring and clinical management of these patients. In Chapter 5, Professor Laurence Cole has brought together the key aspects of different hCG assays.

The range of biological functions of hCG which is produced throughout pregnancy remains unclear. On empirical grounds it would seem likely that hCG could perform both a growth-promoting and growth-modulating role in a normal pregnancy. It is possible that hCG and its fragments may also have a growth-promoting role for the abnormal trophoblastic cell in GTD and GTT. This could explain the clinically observed phenomenon that the abnormal trophoblast in GTD and GTT never grows clinically without producing detectable hCG.

Monoclonal antibodies have outstanding specificity but this may not be optimum in monitoring GTD and GTT since hCG exists in a number of forms: intact hCG, nicked hCG, free-intact and nicked β-subunits; β-subunit core fragments and free α-subunits. As Professor Cole has emphasized in Chapter 5, assays which are too specific for one form or other of hCG or its degradation products can underestimate or miss GTD and GTT. At present the recommendation for an hCG assay for screening, monitoring and following up patients with GTD and GTT is that the assay should detect all the main forms of hCG and its β-subunit fragments. There are differences in profile between a normal pregnancy, which produces a higher proportion of intact hCG, and GTD and GTT, which have a higher proportion of nicked and metabolic fragments of hCG. In the future it may be possible to subclassify different variants of GTD and GTT by the profile of the proportion of hCG and its metabolic degradation products that are produced.

A better understanding of the profile of hCG and its degradation products produced by different forms of GTD and GTT would help clarify some of the problems of monitoring patients whose serum or urine samples contain immunologically reactive substances that are detected in assays directed against the β-subunit of hCG. Many assays for hCG have allotted an upper limit of normal of 5 U/l. It is not all that rare for some patients to have values in the range of 5–20 U/l. With long-term follow-up, confidence increases in that whatever has been detected in the hCG assay does not appear to have biological significance or association with any other recognized disease. In monitoring GTD and GTT, it is more important that an assay has a small incidence of apparent false positivity, which can be clarified by follow-up over time, than have false negatives where the presence of GTD or GTT is missed.

18.3 MOLECULAR GENETICS

Our understanding of the molecular genetics of GTD and GTT has developed rapidly over the last two decades. However, at present we do not know whether there is a common genetic event which is the final cause of all the variants of GTD and GTT. In the future it will be important to identify what this mechanism or mechanisms are, both to understand the disease process better and to understand the process which makes gestational tumors so much more chemosensitive than the majority of the more common human cancers. At present we do not understand the maternal defect in the ovum which allows the abnormal fertilization to occur in complete and partial moles. There clearly is a maternal element in this process since there is an excess of complete moles in very young women and in women having pregnancies over the age of 40 and in particular over the age of 50. The role of the partner in the disease process remains very difficult to study.

Clearly, given the rapid developments in molecular genetics (Chapter 2), it is likely that we will continue to be able to subtype variants of GTD and GTT which will help clinical and management decisions. This is illustrated by the clinical heterogeneity of placental site trophoblastic tumors (PSTT) and the fact that these tumors can occur after both a normal biparental pregnancy and an androgenetic complete molar pregnancy.

Provided DNA is available from the tumor, patient and partner, the presence of paternal genes can now be usually confirmed, even from formalin-fixed blocks. The presence of paternal genes in the tumor is definitive proof of gestational origin. However, inability to detect paternal genes in a trophoblastic tumor cannot exclude gestational origin but can make it unlikely. Using multiple microsatellite polymorphisms, which fail to detect any paternal genes in the tumor, combined with an atypical clinical picture, can make it reasonably certain that the patient does not have a gestational tumor. Morphologically it is not always possible to distinguish gestational choriocarcinoma from tumors with extensive trophoblastic differentiation. This additional genetic information can alter clinical decision-making. If it seems very unlikely that the patient has a gestational tumor, then the management should be directed towards disease control and palliation since nearly all these patients will succumb from their disease. In contrast, patients with paternal genes in their tumor continue to have the good prognosis associated with gestational choriocarcinoma and most of these patients can be salvaged with appropriate treatment.

18.4 MOLECULAR BIOLOGY

While the precise molecular pathogenesis of hydatidiform mole and choriocarcinoma has not been determined, various oncogenes and growth factors have been studied in these tissues. Increased expression of p53 gene and c-fms has been reported in complete molar pregnancy[1,2]. Rearrangement of c-fms and amplification of c-myc has been shown in a study of five choriocarcinoma cell lines and increased c-myc and ras RNAs have been measured in choriocarcinoma[3,4]. However, it is important to emphasize that normal placentae have also been demonstrated to express high levels of several protooncogenes. Additional studies need to be pursued to further understand the potential relationship between alterations in the expression of various oncogenes and growth factors and the pathogenesis of GTD. Differential expression of oncogenes may also be of prognostic importance in identifying trophoblastic tumors with marked virulence.

Certain genes are only expressed on the maternal or paternal chromosomes (parental imprinting). Tumor formation has been associated with modification of parental imprinting and complete hydatidiform moles appear to have relaxation in parental imprinting. While the H19 gene is normally expressed in embryos only from the maternal allele, the H19 gene is expressed in complete molar trophoblast which does not contain maternal chromosomes[5]. Relaxation of parental imprinting may be important in the pathogenesis of trophoblastic neoplasia.

18.5 INTENSIVE CARE FOR PATIENTS PRESENTING WITH ADVANCED DISEASE

Patients with organ failure from GTD or GTT present a range of major medical problems. Some of these have been discussed in Chapter 11. These patients constitute one of the two subgroups of patients with GTT who die from their disease. Here the usual cause of death is organ failure from extensive disease before adequate chemotherapy can be given. The most common problem which needs intensive care support in these patients is respiratory failure from multiple pulmonary metastases. If the patient is breathless at rest before chemotherapy is started, it is likely that their respiratory function will deteriorate further when they start chemotherapy. This syndrome of presumed tumor lysis, inducing reduced pulmonary compliance and oxygen exchange, can present a major clinical dilemma. It is important not to ventilate the patient with high ventilation pressures which will disrupt the remaining compliant lung. Newer techniques of support are potentially available for these rare patients and include extracorporeal membrane oxygenation (ECMO). However, at present this technique continues to carry a significant mortality, particularly in patients with extensive hemorrhagic tumor since they need to be heparinized for this procedure.

Patients with single cerebral deposits from GTT which are superficial should usually have these removed at the initiation of therapy to minimize the chance of intracerebral hemorrhage. However, if there are multiple cerebral metastases, this is not possible and it is important to prevent cerebral edema developing at the initiation of therapy. The third major organ that can fail at the initiation of therapy in a patient with GTT is the liver. Extensive intrahepatic metastases which can hemorrhage can result in hepatic failure and major clotting problems. Provided the patient can be supported through the acute phase, recovery of liver function will occur as the tumor comes under control. However, it should be recognized that the presence of liver metastases in a patient with GTT continues to be a significant adverse prognostic factor.

18.6 HIGH-DOSE CHEMOTHERAPY WITH AUTOLOGOUS BONE MARROW TRANSPLANTATION

The techniques for performing high-dose chemotherapy with autologous bone marrow transplantation (ABMT) safely have improved rapidly over the last two decades. Advances have included peripheral blood stem cell harvest of the bone marrow which allows the collection of cell populations, allowing a more rapid engraftment and shorter hospital stays. From its initial experimental applications in the leukemias, this approach has been used increasingly widely in diseases such as the lymphomas, germ cell tumors and in patients with high risk forms of breast cancer. In the hematological malignancies and lymphomas, there is increasing evidence that this approach can salvage patients who would otherwise die from their disease with conventional dose chemotherapy[6]. There is evidence in the germ cell tumors that high-dose chemotherapy can salvage between 30% and 40% of patients with recurrent but still drug-sensitive disease[7].

It might be anticipated that this technique would be appropriate for patients with high-risk GTT. If this approach is going to be considered it is important that it is not reserved until the patient is moribund with drug-resistant tumor. No series has yet been reported in GTT using high-dose chemotherapy to indicate how successful this approach is going to be. Clearly this reflects the good outcome for the majority of patients with conventional treatment and the rarity of patients needing this salvage approach. From discussions about patients treated at other centers and from our own very limited experience, patients receiving high-dose chemotherapy with ABMT have not done well. While responses have been seen, these have not been maintained. Clearly this may reflect poor patient selection in that their disease had become highly drug resistant. In addition, at least some of the patients receiving high-dose chemotherapy with ABMT may not have had gestational tumors in the first place. In Figure 18.1 is a patient who had a widely metastatic tumor with an apparent primary in the uterus. Morphological choriocarcinoma was removed with the cranial metastasis but this

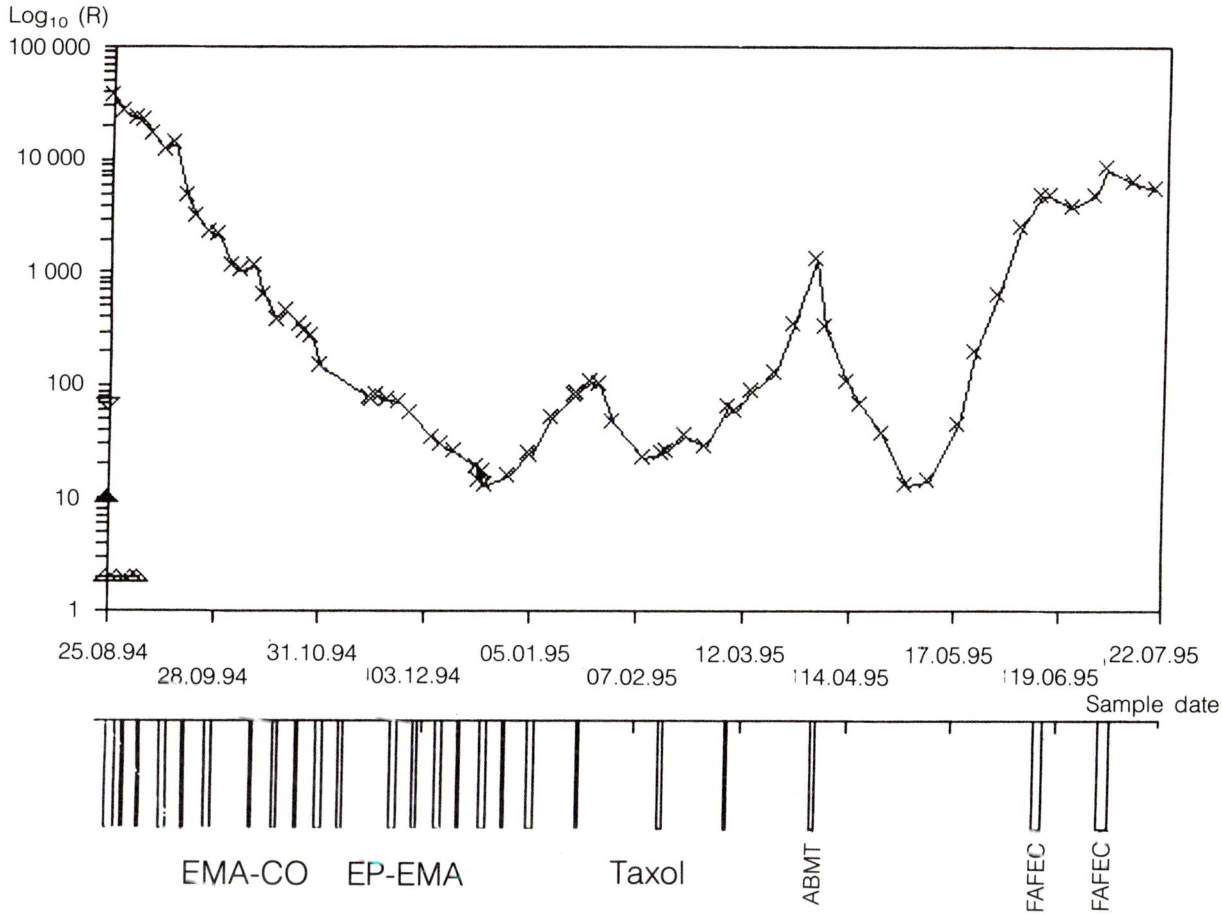

Figure 18.1 Patient presenting with widely metastatic disease involving the uterus, lungs and brain. Histology of necrotic tumor from the brain was compatible with choriocarcinoma but on molecular genetic analysis no paternal genes were detectable. After an initially good response to chemotherapy her disease became progressively more drug resistant to Taxol and had only a brief response to high-dose chemotherapy (etoposide, carboplatin and cyclophosphamide).

highly necrotic tumor did not contain detectable paternal genes. In this patient's case it is possible that she did not have a gestational tumor and the brevity of the response to high-dose chemotherapy is clearly very disappointing. It is clear that further experience needs to be obtained about using this approach in patients who have gestational rather than non-gestational trophoblastic tumors.

18.7 DEVELOPMENTS IN CHEMOTHERAPY FOR GTD AND GTT

At present we have a drug and treatment schedule with methotrexate and folinic acid that is clearly effective in patients with low-risk GTD and GTT, which has an acceptable toxicity profile both short and long term (Chapter 16). However, patients receiving combination chemotherapy do have to accept both the short-term side effects of more intensive chemotherapy such as reversible alopecia and myelosuppression, and the more worrying long-term safety profile of combination chemotherapy. As discussed in Chapter 16, these patients have to accept that there is a small long-term penalty in terms of second tumor induction. At present the balance of risks is clearly in favor of intensive chemotherapy since the risks of the patient's primary disease far outweigh the long-term risks of intensive chemotherapy. However, the increasing data on the incidence of acute myeloid leukemia in patients receiving etoposide[8] indicate that this drug should only be used in patients with disease that has become resistant to methotrexate or in high-risk patients from the outset. The incidence of second tumors following more intensive chemotherapy clearly confirms that we need to develop new chemotherapeutic agents that (1) hopefully have a better long-term safety profile and (2) have activity against GTD and GTT that have become resistant to currently established agents.

At present there is considerable excitement in medical oncology about the potential of a range of new anticancer agents that are coming through to the clinic. Some of these agents are shown in Table 18.1. The taxanes, paclitaxel and docetaxel, are a new class of anticancer agent with a new mechanism of action[9,10]. Both compounds are thought to act primarily by promoting the polymerization of tubulin. Both these compounds have shown activity in tumors that have become resistant to more standard agents and they have also shown activity in diseases which rarely respond to previously available chemotherapy. Paclitaxel has been most widely studied in ovarian adenocarcinoma and breast carcinoma and docetaxel is clearly active in small cell carcinoma of the lung. Paclitaxel has been shown to have activity against previously treated germ cell tumors and therefore is a candidate for evaluation of GTD and GTT[11].

Table 18.1 Anticancer compounds in development and of potential major clinical interest

Taxanes	Taxol (paclitaxel) Taxotere (docetaxel)
Camptothecins	Topotecan Irinatecan
Antimetabolites	Fludarabine 2-Chlorodexoyadenosine Gemcitabine Tomudex
Miscellaneous	Mixed amine platinum complexes Bryostatin Temozolomide

The camptothecins, topotecan and irinatecan, are also promising compounds with a new mechanism of action. In contrast to drugs such as etoposide, which inhibit topoisomerase II, the camptothecins inhibit topoisomerase I. Both these compounds have been shown to have significant antitumor activity against quite a wide range of cancers and, as they become available, need to be assessed in GTD and GTT[12,13].

A new generation of antimetabolites has been coming into the clinic and fludarabine and 2-chlorodeoxyadenosine have significant activity against hematological and lymphoid malignancies[14,15]. Gemcitabine has activity against some solid tumors[16,17], as does the thymidylate synthetase inhibitor, tomudex. Both gemcitabine and tomudex need to be evaluated in resistant GTD and GTT.

The mixed amine–platinum complexes have been developed to try and overcome the resistance to the established platinum complexes, cisplatin and carboplatin[18]. Experimentally, the data are good that these compounds can overcome resistance to the standard agents but at present clinical data are quite preliminary. Bryostatin is a novel antitumor agent which modulates the activity of protein kinase C[19]. This is an interesting compound but again the clinical development is in a very preliminary phase. Temozolomide is a new anticancer agent that has been in development since 1987[20]. It is orally bioavailable and is a well-tolerated agent which has shown significant activity against malignant melanoma and high-grade gliomas[21,22]. It is currently undergoing broader Phase II testing. It has been shown experimentally to be highly active against cell lines of germ cell tumors and therefore is again a potential candidate for assessment in patients with GTD and GTT.

Targeting cancer cells by exploiting specific antigens expressed on the tumor cell surface has been a long-term hope and aim for oncologists. One method of amplifying this therapeutic concept is antibody-directed enzyme prodrug therapy (ADEPT). If the active form of the prodrug has a very short half-life, then specific enzymatic activation of the prodrug on the tumor cell surface might increase the therapeutic index sharply. This approach is complex and continues in development but it has been shown to be active in choriocarcinoma xenografts experimentally[23,24].

The number of agents shown in Table 18.1 is far from exhaustive and it is likely that we will have other active compounds to assess in the gestational tumors in the coming decade. Clearly, however, the long-term safety profile of any new agent will not be available for many decades to come. It is therefore imperative that patients receiving novel and hopefully successful therapies are followed up for life so that any late side effects from their treatment can be evaluated. Only in this way will it be possible to reassure future generations of women receiving this treatment that there is a satisfactory balance of risk between their primary disease and the late side effects of the therapy that is being recommended.

18.8 COST EFFECTIVENESS OF CENTERS TREATING GTD AND GTT

Medical advances have improved the clinical management options available, but these together with demographic changes and the rise of expectations of a more health-conscious public are placing increasing demands on limited resources. Economic evaluation (value analysis) is therefore likely to assume increasing importance even with curable cancers such as GTD. In drawing up contracts purchasers (be they patients or their agents) are still uncertain as to what they should demand to achieve the best quality and most cost-effective care. The onus is on the expert provider to advise them of up-to-date practice in sensible terms. For example, it will be important to prove prospectively that specialist centers are essential to monitor and treat GTD. In less developed countries, where resources are scarce, the case for the provision of funds to care for these rare diseases will be difficult to justify unless cost effectiveness can be unequivocally demonstrated.

Whereas with palliative therapy there is an acknowledged lack of outcome measures, it is not difficult to establish the cost utility of treatment used in curing cancer. Health economists in the USA demonstrated that the successful treatment of teratoma in one year produced sufficient economic benefit to support all the drug development costs of the preceding 17 years of the National Cancer Institute's program[25]. Likewise, we have estimated[26] that the average cost of treating a patient with high-grade non-Hodgkin's lymphoma is no greater than £6000 (US $9000); the cost per life year saved on such patients is about £1000 (US $1500). In undertaking such calculations it is mandatory to include factors other than the cost of the chemotherapeutic agents; these will include time and other materials (including nursing/medical resources), and must take into account supporting investigations, out-

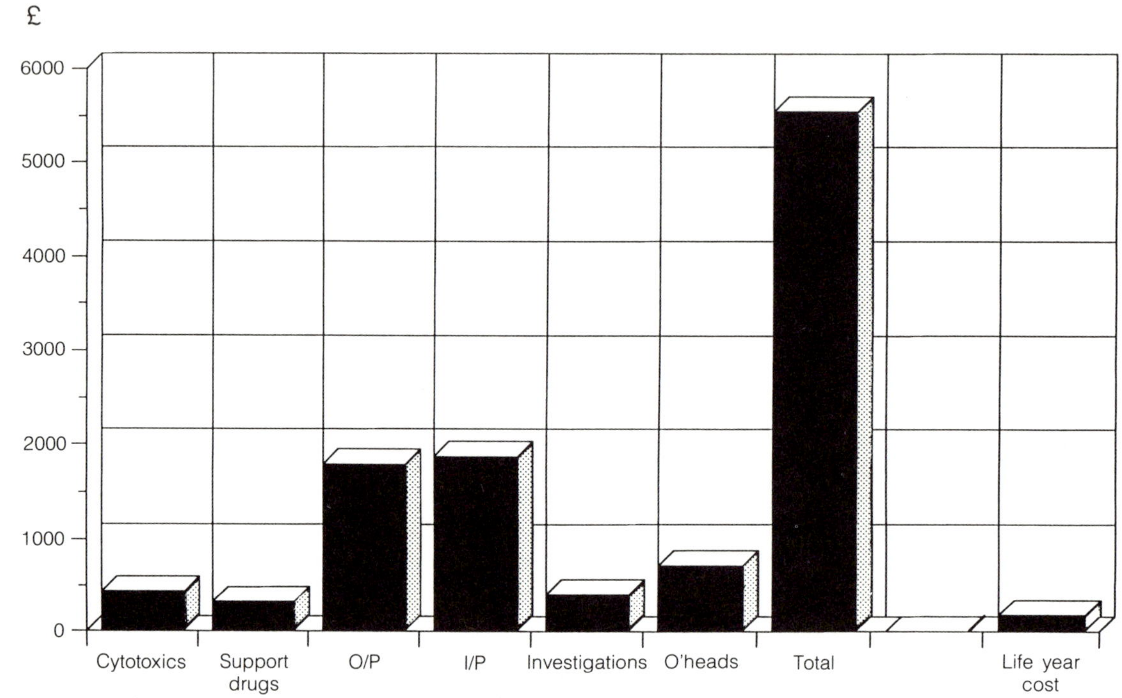

Figure 18.2 Approximate average costs of curative chemotherapy for gestational trophoblastic tumors: O/P, outpatient attendances; I/P, inpatient stays; Overheads, hospital overheads (15%).

patient and particularly in-patient care, as well as the 'hidden' costs such as hospital overheads, including an allowance for capital depreciation. In one model we have derived it is possible to break down the overall costs of treating particular cancers into individual treatment categories with recognized outcomes. It is then relatively easy to obtain real data on consumption of cytotoxic and supportive drugs by individual disease groups as well as the investigations undertaken, and to combine these with an agreed estimate of the costs of in-patient stay and out-patient visits. These can then be added together to gain an overall assessment of average costs of care. The value of a course of chemotherapy to a patient with cancer may be displayed best by calculating the number of months or years of benefit that the treatment will provide; with curable tumors treatment cost can then be justified in terms of extended life (survival costs), i.e. by cost per unit of survival time.

With GTT which are highly chemosensitive, good-quality normal life expectancy in excess of 95% for patients of childbearing age can be expected. The average cost for treating such a patient is approximately £5000 (US $7500), thus the cost per life year saved is less than £200 (US $300)[27] (Figure 18.2).

However, to offer comprehensive screening and monitoring facilities for GTD, as well as providing expert treatment, centers need more than just clinical staff and chemotherapeutic drugs. State-of-the-art information technology, expert computer technologists, a knowledgeable administrator with good secretarial back-up, and appropriate clinical chemistry (for accurate and well-interpreted hCG data) are all requirements that have to be built into the total cost to be charged for the service. In this ideal scenario costs are of course higher but in Sheffield, UK, even when total costs of the screening service are taken into account, the cost per life year saved is still less than £500 (US $750), which must make this one of the most cost-efficient of all specialist medical treatments available!

What are the changes for the future that are most likely to affect the balance of the cost–benefit equation?

Certainly there is likely to be a trend towards more out-patient or even domiciliary care – with better quality of life and less expense for patients, but with problems of effective supervision by the center.

New drugs and techniques are likely to make a significant impact on health care budgets. However, when evaluating the case for these it is important to assess the benefits in both clinical and monetary terms since decisions based solely on purchase costs may ignore advantages which in the long term may outweigh the initial price disadvantage. They must therefore be properly researched, with incorporation of economic evaluation as well as the standard clinical and quality measures.

With small numbers of patients being treated (even in specialist centers) the role of clinical trials is likely to increase. There should be more cross-center collaboration since it has been shown that multi-center controlled clinical trials, probably by standardization of treatment, often in collaboration with specialist centers, offer higher survival rates, particularly for less common cancers[28]. In addition, patients are generally willing to take part in such studies[29]. Funding of such clinical research must therefore remain a high priority.

Long-term management and sequelae must be taken into account in assessing global costs and benefits. The future is bright for patients with GTT; they can be cured by appropriate chemotherapy given under expert supervision. They are likely to lead productive lives, to remain fertile, and to be free of major long-term physical effects. However, both the short- and the long-term psychological trauma of having a potentially life-threatening illness requiring sometimes acutely toxic chemotherapy must not be underestimated; there may be a role for ongoing counselling or even personal rather than remote computerized follow-up.

REFERENCES

1. Cheung, A.N.Y., Srivastava, G., Chung, L.P. *et al.* (1994) Expression of the p53 gene in trophoblastic cells in hydatidiform moles and normal human placentas. *J. Reprod. Med.*, **39**, 223–7.
2. Cheung, A.N.Y., Srivastava, G., Pittulauga, S. *et al.* (1993) Expression of c-myc and c-fms oncogenes in hydatidiform mole and normal human placenta. *J. Clin. Pathol.*, **46**, 204–7.
3. Fujino, T. (1987) Analysis of c-onc genes in choriocarcinoma cells. *Hokkaido Igaku Zasshi*, **62**, 798.
4. Sarkar, S., Kacinski, B.M., Kohorn, E.I. *et al.* (1986) Demonstration of myc and ras oncogene expression by hybridization *in situ* in hydatidiform mole and in the Be Wo choriocarcinoma cell line. *Am. J. Obstet. Gynecol.*, **154**, 390–3.
5. Mutter, G., Stewart, C., Chaponot, M. *et al.* (1993) Oppositely imprinted genes H19 and insulin-like growth factor 2 are coexpressed in human androgenetic trophoblast. *Am. J. Hum. Genet.*, **33**, 1096–102.
6. Armitage, J.O. (1994) Bone marrow transplantation (Review article). *New Engl. J. Med.*, **330**, 827–38.
7. Lotz, J.-P., Andre, T., Donsimoni, R. *et al.* (1995) High dose chemotherapy with ifosfamide, carboplatin and etoposide combined with autologous bone marrow transplantation for the treatment of poor prognosis germ cell tumors and metastatic trophoblastic disease in adults. *Cancer*, **75**, 874–85.
8. Boshoff, C., Begent, R.H.J., Oliver, R.T.D. *et al.* (1995) Secondary tumours following etoposide containing therapy for germ cell cancer. *Ann. Oncol.*, **6**, 35–40.

9. Gelmon K. (1994) The taxoids: paclitaxel and docetaxel (Drug profile). *Lancet*, **344**, 1267–72.
10. Rowinsky, E.K. and Donehower, R.C. (1995) Paclitaxel (Taxol). (Review article). *New Engl. J. Med.*, **332**, 1004–14.
11. Motzer, R.J., Bajarin, D.F., Schwartz, L.H. *et al.* (1994) Phase II trial of paclitaxel shows antitumor activity in patients with previously treated germ cell tumors. *J. Clin. Oncol.*, **12**, 2227–83.
12. Slichenmyer, W.J., Rowinsky, E.K., Donehower, R.C. *et al.* (1993) The current status of camptothecin analogues as antitumor agents. *J. Natl. Cancer Inst.*, **85**, 271–91.
13. Potmesil, M. (1994) Camptothecins: from bench research to hospital wards. *Cancer Res.*, **54**, 1431–9.
14. Keating, M.J., O'Brien, S., Robertson, L.E. *et al.* (1994) The expanding role of fludarabine in hematologic malignancies. *Leuk. Lymphoma*, **14** (Suppl. 2), 11–16.
15. Hoffman, M,, Tallman, M.S., Hakimian, D. *et al.* (1994) 2-Chloro-deoxyadenosine is an active salvage therapy in advanced indolent non-Hodgkin's lymphoma. *J. Clin. Oncol.*, **12**, 788–92.
16. Lund, B., Hansen, O.P., Theilade, K. *et al.* (1994) Phase II study of Gemcitabine (2', 2'-difluorodeoxycyidine) in previously treated ovarian cancer patients. *J. Natl. Cancer Inst.*, **86**, 1530–3.
17. Anderson, H., Lund, B., Bach, F. *et al.* (1994) Single-agent activity of weekly Gemcitabine in advanced non-small-cell cancer: a Phase II study. *J. Clin. Oncol.*, **12**, 1821–6.
18. Harrap, K.R. (1995) Initiatives with platinum- and quinazoline-based antitumour molecules: fourteenth Bruce F Cain memorial Aware Lecture. *Cancer Res.*, **55**, 2761–6.
19. Jayson, G.C., Crowther, D., Prendiville, J. *et al.* (1995) A Phase I trial of Bryostatin 1 in patients with advanced malignancy using a 24 intravenous infusion. *Br. J. Cancer*, **72**, 461–8.
20. Newlands, E.S., Blackledge, G.R.P, Slack, J.A. *et al.* (1992) Phase I trial of Temozolomide (CCRG 81045; M&B 39831; NSC 362856). *Br. J. Cancer*, **65**, 287–91.
21. O'Reilly, S.M., Newlands, E.S., Glaser, M.G. *et al.* (1993) Temozolomide: A new oral cytotoxic chemotherapeutic agent with promising activity against primary brain tumours. *Eur. J. Cancer*, **29A**, 940–2.
22. Bleehen, N.M., Newlands, E.S, Lee, S.M. *et al.* (1995) Cancer Research Campaign Phase II trial of Temozolomide in metastatic melanoma. *J. Clin. Oncol.*, **13**, 910–13.
23. Springer, C.J., Bagshawe, K.D., Sharma, S.K. *et al.* (1991) Ablation of human choriocarcinoma xenografts in nude mice by antibody-directed enzyme pro-drug therapy (ADEPT) with three novel compounds. *Eur. J. Cancer*, **27**, 1361–6.
24. Bagshawe, K.D. (1993) Antibody-directed enzyme pro-drug therapy (ADEPT). *Adv. Pharmacol.*, **24**, 99–121.
25. Shibley, L., Brown, M., Schuttings, J. *et al.* (1990) Cisplatin-based combination chemotherapy in the treatment of advanced stage testicular teratoma: cost benefit analysis. *J. Natl. Cancer Inst.*, **82**, 186–92.
26. Hancock, B.W. and Baber, A. (1995) The cost effectiveness of cancer chemotherapy: a clinicians view. *Proc. R. Coll. Phys. Edinburgh*, **25**, 61–6.
27. Hancock, B.W. and Lorigan, P.C. (1994) *World Congress on Gestational Trophoblastic Diseases*, Hong Kong, Abstract 53.
28. Stiller, C.A. (1994) Centralised treatment, entry to trials and survival. *Br. J. Cancer*, **70**, 352–62.
29. Slevin, M., Mossman, J., Bowling, A. *et al.* (1995) Volunteers or victims: patients' views of randomised cancer clinical trials. *Br. J. Cancer*, **71**, 1270–4.

Index

Page numbers in **bold** refer to figures and page numbers in *italic* refer to tables. Abbreviations used in the index are: CC = choriocarcinoma; CHM = complete hydatidiform mole; CNS = central nervous system; GTD = gestational trophoblastic disease; GTT = gestational trophoblastic tumor; hCG = human chorionic gonadotropin; HM = hydatidiform mole; NETDC = New England Trophoblastic Disease Center; PHM = partial hydatidiform mole; PSTT = placental site trophoblastic tumor; PTD = persistent trophoblastic disease.